| Practical Approaches |

Laser and Light Treatment in Asian Skin

CCLMS Committee

KOONJA

Laser and Light Treatment in Asian Skin

By CCLMS Committee

1st Print : 2016-03-02
1st Publication : 2016-03-10

Publisher : Jooyeon Jang
Editor : Eunhee Cho
Text Designer : Seonmi Park
Cover Designer : Koonja Publishing
Illustrator : Lutronic & Koonja Publishing

Permissions may be sought at Koonja's rights department:
Tel: (82)-31-943-1888
Fax: (82)-31-955-9545
www.koonja.co.kr

Printed in South Korea
First Edition, © 2016 Koonja publishing
ISBN 979-11-5955-017-1
List Price USD 100

CCLMS

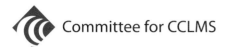 Committee for CCLMS

Conventional & Contemporary in Laser Medicine and Surgery

Conventional & Contemporary in Laser Medicine and Surgery (CCLMS) sponsored by Lutronic Corporation is a prestigious international symposium that will focus on meaningful applications of new and conventional treatments in laser medicine and surgery.

The CCLMS aspires to facilitate present insights into progressive challenges in conventional laser treatment methods and the potentials in achieving improved clinical laser applications. The CCLMS will be an opportunity to explore the expanding horizons of laser technology in the medical field.

About the Authors

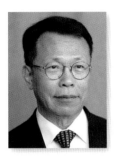

Soo Il Chun, MD, PhD

- Director, Chunsooil Skin Clinic
- Professor, Department of Dermatology, Yonsei University College of Medicine
- Visting Professor, Department of Dermatology, University of Munich, Germany
- Visiting Clinician, Department of Dermatology, Mayo Clinic. Rochester, U.S.A.
- Editorial Board, American Journal of Dermatopathology

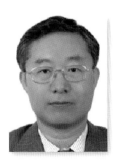

Il Hwan Kim, MD, PhD

- Graduated from Korea University College of Medicine
- Chief Professor of Korea University College of Medicine, Department of Dermatology
- Director & Board member of Korean Dermatological Association
- 36th Annual Meeting of the ISDS(2015, Seoul, COEX), organizing committee, vice-president
- President of Korean Society for Aesthetic and Dermatologic Surgery
- Inbong Award(2002), Stiefel Academic Award(2013), Korean Dermatological Association

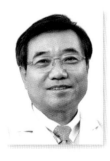

Jin Soo Kang, MD

- Graduated from Yonsei University College of Medicine
- Adjunct professor at Yonsei University
- (Former) Director, auditor, and vice chairman of Korean Dermatological Association
- (Former) Chairman of the Korean Society for Aesthetic and Dermatologic Surgery
- (Present) Chairman of Korean Socity Hair Restoration Treatment
- Book author of Textbook of chemical peels

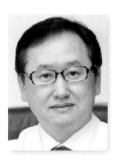

▶ Seung Ha Park, MD, PhD, MBA

— Professor, Director, Department of Plastic & Reconsctructive surgery, Korea University Hospital
— President of Korea University Hospital
— Chairman of Korean Society for Laser Medicine and Surgery
— President of Korean Society of Plastic and Reconstructive Surgery
— Author; Laser Dermatologic Plastic Surgery

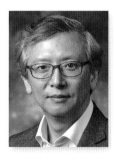

▶ Kee Yang Chung, MD, PhD

— Department of Dermatology
— Yonsei University College of Medicine
— Professor and Chairman
— President, Korean Skin Cancer Society
— International Traveling Mentor, ASDS

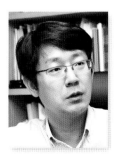

▶ Un Cheol Yeo, MD, PhD

— Graduated from Seoul National University Medical School
— Former Assistant Professor in Sungkyunkwan Unversity Medical School, Department of Dermatology
— Chief Director of S&U Dermatologic clinic
— Acacemic Director of Korean Dermatologic Society for Laser
— Academic Director of Korean Society for laser medicine and Surgery
— Book Author of Laser Dermatology and Plastic Surgery, RF in Dermatology

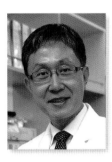

You Chan Kim, MD, PhD

- Graduated from Yonsei University School of Medicine
- Former Visiting Clinician, Dermatopathology Laboratory, Mayo Clinic, Rochester, Minnesota, USA
- Former Vice Dean for Research Affairs, Ajou University School of Medicine
- Professor and Chairman of Dermatology, Ajou University School of Medicine
- Director of Academic Affairs of Korean Dermatological Association
- President of Korean Society of Dermatopathology

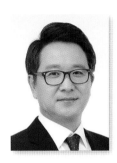

Jae-Woo Park, MD, PhD

- Chairman of 50th anniversary scientific meeting of KSPRS (Korean Society of Plastic and Reconstructive Surgery)
- Vice President of KSPS (Korean Society of Plastic Surgeons)
- Corresponding Member of American Society Of Plastic Surgeons
- Visiting Scholar IUPUI (Indiana university and Perdue university in Indianapolis)
- Chief of Dr.Park's Plastic Clinic, Seoul, Korea

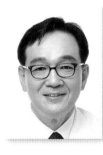

Woo Seok Koh, MD, PhD

- Graduate Seoul National University, Medical School
- Seoul National University Hospital, Department of Dermatology Resident
- Fellow of Harvard Medical School, Department of Dermatology
- Research Fellow of Wellman Center for Photomedicine
- Assistant Professor of Inje University Medical School Department of Dermatology
- Director of JMO Dermatology, Hair Removal Clinic

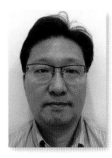

Won Serk Kim, MD, PhD

- Graduate School of Medicine, Seoul National University, Seoul, Korea
- Resident, Department of Dermatology, Samsung Medical Center, Seoul, Korea
- Associated Professor and Chairman, Department of Dermatology, Kangbuk Samsung Hospital, Sungkyunkwan University School of Medicine
- Visiting Professor of Beckman Laser Institute (BLI), University of California, Irvine
- Director of the Korean Society for Laser Medicine and Surgery

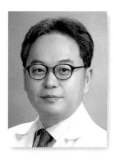

Sang Ju Lee, MD, PhD

- Yonsei University College of Medicine, Bachelor, Master, PhD
- Korean Medical Association, Executive Board Member, Health Insurance & Cooperation and Liaison
- Director of Starskin & Laser Clinic
- The association of Korean Dermatologists, Scientific Director
- The Korean Society for Acne Research, Inspection Commissioner
- Author and coauthor of books on Medical Skin Care, Aesthetic Dermatology, and over loo article in the peer-reviewed literature.

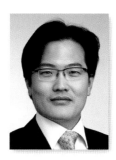

Chan Yeong Heo, MD, PhD

- Associate Professor: School of Medicine, Seoul National University
- Chairman: Department of Plastic Surgery, Seoul National University Bundang Hospital
- Visiting Researcher: Pharmaceutical Sciences, University of California Irvine
- Director: Medical Device Clinical Trial Center, Seoul National University Bundang Hospital
- Guest Editor: Advanced Drug Delivery Reviews Journal

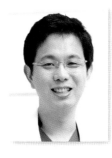

Jiehoon Kim, MD

- Education: Dermatology, Master of Medicine, Ajou University Medical School
- Director, Dr. Kim's Skin & Laser Clinic
- Board Member of the Korean Society for Dermatologic Laser Medicine and Surgery (KSDLS)
- Board Member of the Korean Society for Clinical Therapeutic Dermatology (KCD)
- Publication: HIFU (high Intensity Focused Ultrasound): technical basis and clinical applications, 2015

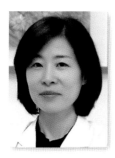

Hee Young Kang, MD, PhD

- Graduated from Ajou University School of Medicine
- Visiting Scholar (Enseignant-chercheur) in Department of Dermatology, University of Nice, France
- Professor in Department of Dermatology, Ajou University School of Medicine
- Coauthor of Books of Atlas of Pigmentary Disorder, Melasma: a monograph, and Pigmentary disorders: a comprehensive compendium

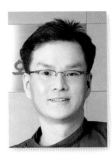

▶ Sung Jong Baek, MD

- Plastic Surgeon
- Graduated from Kyungbook National University School of Medicine graduate
- Member of Korean Society of Plastic and Reconstructive Surgeons
- Member of Korean Society for Aesthetic Plastic Surgery
- Member of International Society of Aesthetic Plastic Surgery (ISAPS)
- Director of Chungdam TIME Aesthetic Plastic Surgical Clinic

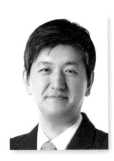

▶ Hyung Uk Choi, MD

- Graduated from Busan National University, School of Medicine
- Former Director in Maryknoll General Hospital, Department of Dermatology
- Chief Director of XEO Dermatologic Clinic
- Member of Organization Committee of 2015 WCD (World Congress of Dermatology) in Seoul, Korea

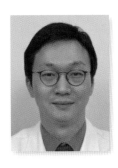

▶ Sung Bin Cho, MD, PhD

- Graduated from Yonsei University College of Medicine, Seoul, Korea
- Former Assistant Clinical Professor in Department of Dermatology and Cutaneous Biology Research Institute, Yonsei University College of Medicine, Seoul, Korea
- Post-doc in Department of Dermatology and Cutaneous Biology Research Institute, Yonsei University College of Medicine, Seoul, Korea
- Chief Director of Kangskin Sillim Clinic, Seoul, Korea

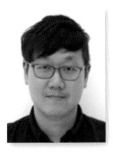

▶ Boncheol Leo Goo M.D., B.S.

- Graduated from Yonsei University College of Medicine / Graduate school
- Former Research Fellow in Seoul National University Hospital, Institiute of Clinical Reseatch / Department of Dermatology
- Director of Naeum Dermatology and Aesthetic Clinic
- Medical Director of R&D Center, Lutronic Corporation
- Korean Society for Laser Medicine and Surgery (Director)
- American Society for Laser Medicine and Surgery (Fellow)

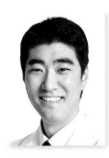

▶ Ji Hoon Kim, MD

- Kyung Hee University College of Medicine
- Fellow of Plastic and Reconstructive Surgery Seoul National University Hospital
- Clinical Professor of Plastic and Reconstructive Surgery Bundang Seoul National University Hospital
- Director of the Jae-Don Plastic Clinic

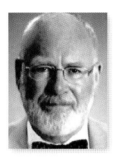

▶ R Glen Calderhead MSc PhD. DrMedSci FRSM

- University of Glasgow UK and Rocheville University USA
- Vice President, Medicoscientific Affairs, Lutronic Corporation
- Secretary-General, European Society for Laser Aesthetic Surgery
- Life Member and Fellow, International Society for Laser Surgery and Medicine
- International Research Fellow, Royal Society of Medicine (London)
- Author, coauthor and contributor to several text books on phototherapy and photosurgery, and over 30 articles in the peer-reviewed literature

Foreword

Dear Readers,

As the Chairman of the "Conventional & Contemporary in Laser Medicine and Surgery" (CCLMS) initiative, it is with great pleasure that I write to welcome you to this outstanding text book, ***Laser and Light Treatment in Asian Skin: Practical Approaches***, crystalizing the experience of Korea's leading laser and light practitioners in treating a vast range of cutaneous disorders in Asian skin. As we all know, the darker Asian skin types represent a special case when cutaneous lesions are targeted, simply because of the propensity of these skin types to form postinflammatory hyperpigmentation following any treatment causing undue inflammation, particularly at the dermoepidermal junction. Special care and precise techniques are therefore called for, based on a sound understanding of laser-tissue interaction in the darker skin type.

The CCLMS Committee is very proud to stand behind this keynote publication. Korea is renowned for her pool of expert surgeons, and the manufacture of some of the very best laser systems in the world for these experts to practice with. Sadly, the vast storehouse of knowledge remains often locked in Korea and her near environs, sometimes by the simple fact of publication in the Korean language, but often because Korean surgeons are very shy of their English language abilities, even though they may be fluent English speakers. It was because of this that the CCLMS Committee got together and this volume was discussed, then definitively planned, and now it has been published.

The range of topics herein has something for everyone. Furthermore, we all know that Asian skin is no longer limited to Asia, with a large diaspora of Asians in every major country worldwide. This spreading of the Asian skin gene brings problems for clinicians in these overseas regions whose patients are Asian, or of Asian descent, because of the inherent potential for PIH formation. A patient might present with melasma in Australia, for instance, who appears to be a Fitzpatrick skin type II. However, on history taking, it turns out she is third generation Asian. This means that the usual skin type II treatment regimens might well induce PIH, because the skin is basically still a type III or even IV. This excellent book is therefore not just intended for clinicians in Asia, although it will still find a place on the bookshelf here as a powerful treatment reference: the book is aimed more at those overseas surgeons who encounter Asian skin type patients in their practice, and may be at a loss as to how to treat them safely and effectively. I feel it will represent an invaluable guide for these circumstances, written as it is by the leading specialists here in Korea, whose expertise is freely shared with our brother and sister colleagues worldwide.

Please enjoy reading this wide-ranging textbook, either as a prelude to treating patients of one of the Asian skin types, as a reference volume, or simply just for pleasure, to enhance your knowledge and broaden your treatment techniques, even in non-Asian skin types. Thank you for purchasing *Laser and Light Treatment in Asian Skin: Practical Approaches*, and I am sure you will find it very useful.

Soo Il Chun, MD, PhD
Chairman, CCLMS

Contents

Pigmentary disorders

SECTION

01

C/O/N/T/E/N/T/S

General concept for pigmented target approach in the Asian skin: the character of pigmented lesions in Asians

▶ Hee Young Kang, MD, PhD, Boncheol Leo Goo M.D., B.S. & Sung Bin Cho, MD, PhD

The difference between Asian and Caucasian skin may be primarily attributed to pigmentation and melanocyte function. Indeed, pigmentary disease is the most common and troublesome condition in the Asian population. Moreover, in Asians, changes in pigmentation seem to be a more important feature of aging than wrinkling. The problem is that treatment of pigmentary disorders in Asian skin induces a higher incidence of postinflammatory hyperpigmentation (PIH). Treatment of pigmentary diseases in Asian skin is therefore more difficult than in Caucasians. This review explores the algorithmic approach in pigmentation treatment and current understanding of the etiopathogenesis of melasma, the most intractable pigmentary disorder in the Asian skin phenotype, and discusses the characteristics of Asian melasma.

Algorithmic approach in pigmentation treatment

Cutaneous pigmentary lesions can be classified into two categories. When phenotypical hyperpigmentation is due to an increase in the number of cells which contain melanosomes, this entity can be postulated as a tumorous condition. In contrast, physiologically activated melanocytes can cause a larger distribution of pigments or melanosomes, resulting in diffuse dyschromic features mostly in the epidermis. When pigmentary incontinence develops due to overt inflammation, melanophages can exist in the dermis in this type of lesion, resulting in a complex distribution of abnormal pigment in both the epidermis and in the dermis.

Such differences in pathophysiology need sophisticated approaches in treatment (Figures 01-1, 01-2). For tumorous conditions, complete removal or precise destruction should be performed. In contrast to lighter skin types, most of these lesions in the Asian skin contain an adequate amount of melanin. Certain lasers have melanin as their chromophore, so these lasers can be used to selectively remove such lesions. Once malingnancy or premalignancy has been

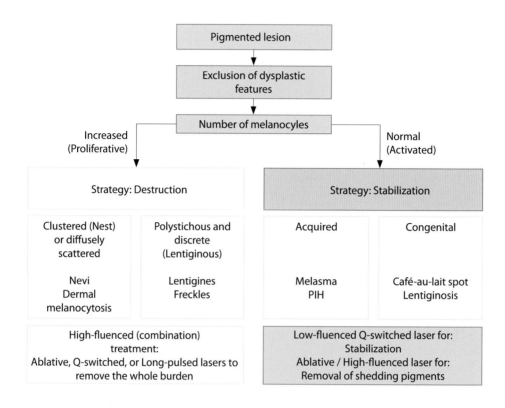

Figure 01-1   Algorithmic approach in pigmentation treatment

ruled out in a pigmented lesion, then the lesion with its pigmented nevus cells should be eradicated as completely as possible, to preclude recurrence from remnant nests of nevus cells.
In the case of recurrence in a previously laser-treated lesion, the presence of fibrotic scar
tissue could interfere with the efficacy of the laser treatment, possibly making such lesions
laser treatment-resistant. Precise and gentle removal of pigment is particularly important in
epidermal lesions with fine lines of horizontally-sited melanin pigmentation, because overtreatment could cause damage at the dermoepidermal junction, leading to inflammation with
the potential of PIH formation. For physiologically 'activated' lesions like melasma or PIH,
an over-aggressive and destructive approach could result in rebound or even exacerbation of
the lession through continuous overactivation of the already stimulated melanocytes. Specific
techniques have been developed using the Q-swithced Nd:YAG laser to maximise pigment
removal while minimizing damage-mediated inflammation. Because basal layer melanocyte
activity tends to be higher in darker Asian skin types, this has significant implications in treatment of pigmented lesions not only with lasers and energy-based devices, but also with other
approaches such as chemical or mechanical peels, or even topical cosmeceuticals.

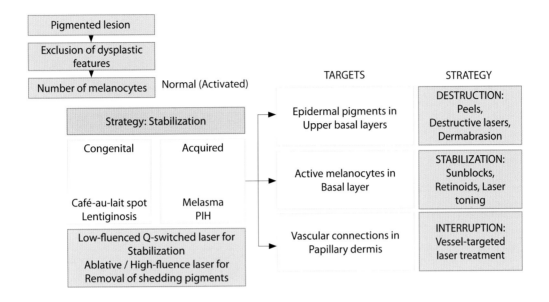

Algorithmic approach in pigmentation treatment (extended) - Strategy for acquired lesions with abnormally activated melanocytes.

Treatment of acquired lesions is especially important for dark or Asian skin, because PIH and melasma are often treatment-resistant. Shedding pigments can be gently removed, but stabilization should be mainstream in the treatment strategy. Laser toning with, for example, low-fluence Q-switched laser treatment which interrupts melanosome maturation and transfer to keratinocytes, plays a great role in this approach.

Pigmentary changes in melasma (Caucasian vs. Asian)

Increased epidermal pigmentation is the hallmark of melasma and must be the main target for melasma treatment. Based on the results of histological examinations of melasma, reports have consistently identified that lesional skin is characterized by increased melanin deposition in the epidermis. Melanin is concentrated at the basal layer but it is also distributed throughout the epidermis. A recent transcriptomics study of Korean melasma had showed upregulation of many melanin biosynthesis-related genes such as tyrosinase, tyrosinase-related protein (TYRP) 1, TYRP2 and Microphthalmia-associated transcription factor (MITF) in lesional skin compared to the perilesional normal skin of melasma patients. Immunohistochemical staining has also shown that the protein expression levels of these genes were

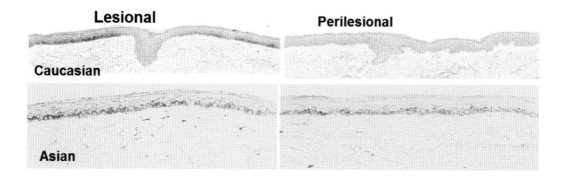

Figure 01-3 The pigmentation difference between Asian and Caucasian melasma is seen in the dermis.

higher in lesional skin. It is clear that increased melanogenesis from the melanocytes induces epidermal hyperpigmentation which results in hyperpigmented patches on the face.

The pigmentation difference between Asians and Caucasian melasma is seen in the dermis. In Caucasian melasma, dermal melanin levels are reportedly very low, in other word, there is no mixed type of melasma. On the other hand, dermal melanin is commonly found in melasma in skin types III to V. Some patients (36% in Korean, 45% in Indian) have dermal melanin as well as epidermal melanin in the lesional skin. However, the significance of the dermal melanin in melasma is doubtful. The amount of dermal melanin is not statistically significant and its distribution is heterogeneous throughout all of the lesional skin in melasma lesions. Moreover, dermal melanin deposition is commonly found in sun-exposed skin, and pigment particles can be found in the dermis in the normal facial skin of Koreans and Japanese. Therefore, it needs to be further studied if this small amount of dermal melanin in melasma lesional skin does really affect the therapeutic outcome of the treatment. Anyway, the existence of dermal melanin is a valuable finding in Asian skin compared to Caucasian skin.

Melanocytes in melasma

Melanocyte functions in Asians seem to differ from those of Caucasians. In melasma, it was shown that the melanocytes within the melasma lesional skin are larger, intensely NKI/beteb immunostained cells with prominent dendrites compared with melanocytes in the unaffected skin, suggesting that melasma-associated melanocytes are more active. Some melanocytes have shown the feature of protruding into the dermis, so called pendulous cells, in melasma. Regarding these protrusions of melanocytes, it had been reported that they are hyperactive

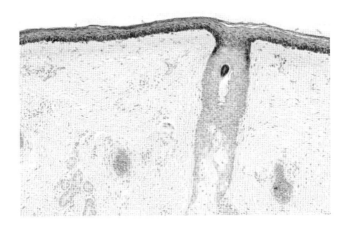

Figure 01-4　Some melanocytes have shown the feature of protruding into the dermis, so called pendulous cells, in melasma.

melanocytes related to epidermal hyperpigmentation. The feature seems more frequent in the darkly pigmented skin and skin more severely affected by melasma. Pendulous cells were found in 5 of 11 lesional skin and 1 of 11 perilesional normal skin specimens from Korean melasma patients. It was more frequently seen in the patients with skin type IV and V; 17 of 24 melasma lesions (70%) and in 9 of 24 (37.5%) of perilesional normal skin. The clinical significance of the pendulous melanocytes is unclear. However, it was suggested that the pendulous cells may easily drop into the dermis or become destroyed by trauma including laser treatment. When destroyed, these pendulous melanocytes would leave heavy pigmentation behind in the dermis resulting in hyperpigmentation or, sometimes hypopigmentation, after treatment.

　　How do the pendulous cells occur? Until recently, this was unclear but a more recent histological study of Korean melasma has suggested that impaired basement membrane-enhanced matrix metalloproteinase (MMP) 2 expression might be related to the pendulous changes of the melanocytes in melasma lesions. Weak staining for type IV collagen in the lesional skin suggested that the basement membrane structure in melasma was not intact and looked like it was somewhat disrupted. This study suggested that the increased MMP2 expression in lesional skin would be responsible for the pendulous change of melanocytes in melasma lesions. MMP2 expression was markedly increased in the lesional skin compared to the perilesional normal skin. A recent transcriptomics study of melasma also showed MMP2 mRNA levels were significantly up-regulated in melasma skin. Chronic ultraviolet (UV) irradiation may be responsible for the up-regulation of MMP2 expression in melasma because

MMP2 immunoreactivity was co-localized with elastotic materials. Treatment targeting the weak dermis associated with melasma would therefore probably be beneficial for melasma lesions.

Microvasculature in melasma

Recent histological and immunohistochemical studies have shown that melasma is associated with alterations in dermal structures in addition to pigmentation changes, suggesting a potential dermal role in melasma development. Melasma dermal tissue has been shown to be different from the perilesional normal tissue and showed features of prominent solar damaged skin. Increased solar elastosis in a study on lesional Indian skin was a predominant finding, suggesting implications of UV exposure in the pathogenesis of the disease.

Recently, it was shown both clinically and histologically that melasma is characterized by increased vasculature in the lesional skin. Melasma patients have additional features like telangiectatic erythema confined to hyperpigmented skin. The erythema index was significantly higher in the lesional skin than in the perilesional normal skin. Immunohistochemistry for vascular markers revealed increased numbers of vessels in the upper dermis. In addition, image analysis revealed a significant increase of both the size and numbers of blood vessels in the lesional skin. The number of vessels had a positive relationship with epidermal pigmentation in melasma lesional skin. Expression of vascular endothelial growth factor (VEGF), a major angiogenic factor of UV irradiated skin, was upregulated in melasma lesions compared to perilesional normal skin suggesting increased VEGF production during sun exposure may be responsible for the altered vessels in melasma. It is unclear whether the increased vasculature in melasma is just the result of chronic UV accumulation accompanying epidermal hyperpigmentation. However, recent studies have suggested that a connection between blood vessels and cutaneous pigmentation could exist. Normal human melanocytes in vitro were shown to express VEGF receptors and some of these receptors are functional, and these data suggest that VEGF may play a role in melanocyte behavior in skin. It is also shown that there is an increase in the inducible form of nitric oxide synthase (iNOS) expression in melasma lesions, providing further perspectives for the pathogenesis of increased vasculature in melasma lesional skin. Moreover, a recent study suggested that targeting blood vessels along with the melanin pigment is beneficial for the treatment of melasma. A prospective, controlled, comparative split- face study evaluating the effects of pulsed dye laser (PDL) therapy in association with triple combination cream, which contained 4% hydroquinone, 0.05% tretinoin, and 0.01% fluocinolone acetonide, in the treatment of melasma was performed.

The combination treatment induced a significant decrease in the pigmentation as compared to triple combination cream alone. Interestingly, the improvement induced by the combination of PDL and the cream remained significant even after one summer while relapses were observed in the group treated with only the cream. It would be tempting to think that the action of the PDL on the vascularization might have played an important role in preventing the relapses. By targeting vascularization and at least some part of elastosis in the melasma lesions we might decrease the stimulation of melanocytes, and thus decrease the incidence of relapse.

Barrier dysfunction in melasma or sensitive skin

It has been shown that darkly pigmented skin displays both a more resistant barrier and one that recovers more quickly after perturbation by tape stripping than does the skin of individuals with lighter pigmentation. However, in our study, it was found that melasma skin is characterized by impaired stratum corneum integrity and a delayed barrier recovery rate.

Biophysical measurements of lesional and perilesional normal skin of 16 Korean melasma patients demonstrated a tendency toward higher transepidermal water loss (TEWL) values after barrier perturbation and a* values (redness) although the skin hydration state and sebum contents in the subjects' skin were normal. Furthermore, a trend toward a thinned stratum corneum was observed for lesional skin, and this was correlated with the barrier recovery rate. All of above findings (reduced stratum corneum barrier function, increased skin redness due to enhanced vascular reaction and thinned stratum corneum) suggested that melasma skin displayed characteristics of subclinical, i.e., invisible, mild inflammation, so called sensitive skin. Improvement in epidermal barrier function might be another unrecognized factor to be considered in treating melasma.

Conclusions and perspectives

Successful and consistent treatment of melasma in the Asian skin phenotype continues to be a challenge for clinicians. Asian skin is likely to react differently than in Caucasians, perhaps due to differences in pigmentation, melanocyte function and barrier function. Hyperactive or labile melanocytes (pendulous melanocytes) may be responsible for the frequent PIH or dyschromia during treatment. It is commonly accepted that Asian skin is more prone than

Caucasian skin to develop irritation to retinoids. The role of the skin barrier is questionable. The significance of melanophages in treating melasma is also in doubt. It needs to be clearly addressed whether the therapeutic outcome is really dependent on dealing with dermal melanophages. Melasma is not a homogeneous disease and there are strong interindividual characteristics of patients with melasma. Future work is needed to answer the question as to why some patients respond differently to the standard melasma treatment compared to others.

REFERENCES

1. Chung JH. Photoaging in Asians. Photodermatol Photoimmunol Photomed 2003;19:109-121.
2. Kang HY, Bahadoran P, Suzuki I, Zugaj D, Khemis A, Passeron T, Andres P, Ortonne JP. In vivo reflectance confocal microscopy detects pigmentary changes in melasma at a cellular level resolution. Exp Dermatol 2010;19:e228-233.
3. Kang HY, Hwang JS, Lee JY, Ahn JH, Kim JY, Lee ES, Kang WH. The dermal stem cell factor and c-kit are overexpressed in melasma. Br J Dermatol 2006;154:1094-1099.
4. Kang HY, Suzuki I, Lee DJ, Ha J, Reiniche P, Aubert J, Deret S, Zugaj D, Voegel JJ, Ortonne JP. Transcriptional profiling shows altered expression of wnt pathway- and lipid metabolism-related genes as well as melanogenesis-related genes in melasma. J Invest Dermatol 2011;131:1692-1700.
5. Kang WH, Yoon KH, Lee ES, Kim J, Lee KB, Yim H, Sohn S, Im S. Melasma: histopathological characteristics in 56 Korean patients. Br J Dermatol 2002;146:228-237.
6. Kim EH, Kim YC, Lee ES, Kang HY. The vascular characteristics of melasma. J Dermatol Sci 2007;46:111-116.
7. Kligman AM, Sadiq I, Zhen Y, Crosby M. Experimental studies on the nature of sensitive skin. Skin Res Technol 2006;12:217-222.
8. Passeron T, Fontas E, Kang HY, Bahadoran P, Lacour JP, Ortonne JP. Melasma treatment with pulsed-dye laser and triple combination cream: a prospective, randomized, single-blind, split-face study. Arch Dermatol 2011;147:1106-1108.
9. Reed JT, Ghadially R, Elias PM. Skin type, but neither race nor gender, influence epidermal permeability barrier function. Arch Dermatol 1995;131:1134-1138.
10. Sarvjot V, Sharma S, Mishra S, Singh A. Melasma: A clinicopathological study of 43 cases. Indian J Pathol Microbiol 2009;52:357-359.
11. Torres-Álvarez B, Mesa-Garza IG, Castanedo-Cázares JP, Fuentes-Ahumada C, Oros-Ovalle C, Navarrete-Solis J, Moncada B. Histochemical and immunohistochemical study in melasma: evidence of damage in the basal membrane. Am J Dermatopathol 2011;33:291-295.

Melasma

▷ Il Hwan Kim, MD, PhD

Definition

Melasma is an acquired hyperpigmentation that occurs in an asymmetrical fashion particularly in middle-aged Asian women, mostly in skin areas exposed to sunlight. Although its etiology and symptom-aggravating factors are partly known, its root cause remains uncertain. Its known etiology and exacerbating factors include: (1) genes, (2) ultraviolet rays, (3) hormones (estrogen, pregnancy, and oral contraceptives: estrogen makes melanocytes hyperactive by combining with estrogen receptors in melanocytes), (4) anomalies in the dermal barrier due to chronic irritation such as by phototoxic agents, and (5) others (stem cell factors, c-kit, nerve growth factor (NGF), and vascular endothelial growth factor (VEGF)). From a therapeutic view point, melasma can be considered as a dark-brown hyperpigmentation which is a result of chronic irritation and inflammation.

Tips for diagnosis

Diagnostic criteria

Gross findings

- Women aged 16 or more, mostly with Fitzpatrick skin type III, IV or V
- Acquired facial pigmented macules that occur asymmetrically in the left and right sides of the zygoma area, frontal region, and lips. Melasma can be classified into 3 patterns as illustrated in Figure 02-1, the most common of which is the centrofacial pattern.
- Melasma is found as a diffuse brown-pigmented macule with unclear demarcation. If the margin of the melasma overlaps with the margin of the periorbital area of the margin of the zygoma area, the demarcation can be clear.

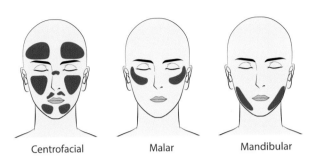

| Centrofacial | Malar | Mandibular |

Figure 02-1   Patterns of melasma based on gross findings (supplement from Lutronic Corp.).

Wood's light:

Wood's light is helpful in determining the distribution of pigments and the depth of the pigment in the affected skin. For epidermal melasma, a Wood's light test would reveal intensification of the color contrast, but would have difficulty in accurately assessing the dermal pigmentation.

Immunohistopathological examination

A characteristic of melasma is the increased concentration of melanin granules in the epidermal basal layer and the layer above the basal layer, the spiny-cell layer or stratum spinosum. The extent of the increase is proportional to the severity of the melasma. Melanophages and degenerated elastic fiber due to intradermal change are often observed, but are non-specific findings.

Melasma has been histopathologically classified into epidermal, dermal, and mixed type melasma. Recent studies on Asians, however, have suggested that the dermal melanophages seen in 'dermal type melasma' may be due to misdiagnosed acquired bilateral nevus of Ota-like macules (ABNOM).

Laboratory test

There is no need for screening for elevated hormone levels because there is not a clear causal link between elevated hormones and melasma in patients who are not pregnant. Serum levels of estradiol (17β-estradiol or E2) and β-melanocyte-stimulating hormone are often elevated in pregnant patients with melasma and may play a role in initiating or exacerbating melasma.

Differential diagnosis

A differential diagnosis must be made in the presence of acquired dermal melanocytosis (ADM), postinflammatory hyperpigmentation (PIH), lentigines, and lichen planus (Table

02-1 and Figures 02-2 and 02-3). To differentiate melasma from ADM, the particular features of these diseases must be understood by region (Table 02-1).

Table 02-1   Differential diagnosis of the facial pigmented lesions

	Melasma	ABNOM	Lentigines	PIH
Border and distribution	Irregular, geographical edge	Discrete	Discrete	Diffuse, irregular, distinct edge
Region	Lateral areas of cheek	Clusters on zygomas, upper eyelids, and lateral side of forehead	Scattered not found in clusters	Any place on previous inflammation site
Color	Light brown to grey-brown	Brown-blue or greyish	Brown to dark brown	Variable, depending on the stages

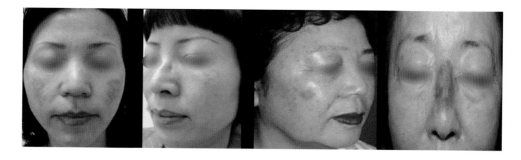

Figure 02-2   Differential diagnosis of facial pigmented lesions.

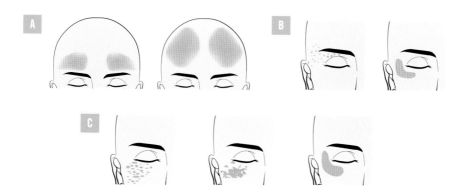

Figure 02-3   **A.** Left: melasma; Right: ABNOM. **B.** Left: ABNOM; Right: melasma. **C.** Left & Center: ABNOM; Right: melasma (supplement from Lutronic Corp.).

NOTE

Features of melasma in Asians: Clinically, differentiating melasma from ABNOM is most difficult. Melasma can be differentiated from ABNOM based on the clinical characteristics shown in Figure 02-3 and in particular, the histopathological findings.

Tips for treatment

Various treatment methods are being developed and tested, though none of them has been consistently successful enough yet to be established as a gold standard. The basis and effect of current melasma management strategies are shown in Table 02-2.

There have been attempts to treat refractory melasma using various types of laser. Pulsed dye laser, alexandrite laser, Q-switched neodymium-doped yttrium aluminium garnet (Nd:YAG) laser, Q-switched ruby laser, scanned superpulsed carbon dioxide laser, and Q-switched ruby lasers and erbium (Er):YAG lasers have been shown to worsen melasma. The

Table 02-2

Method	Action	Rationale and comments
Inhibition of the activity of melanocytes	Protection from sunlight and avoidance of precipitating factors	UV and shorter wavelength visible light can induce melanin formation
Inhibition of the synthesis of melanin	Topical bleaching agents	Hydroquinone, a tyrosinase inhibitor, has been extensively researched and found to be very effective in treating disorders of hyperpigmentation. A combination of hydroquinone, a retinoid, and a topical steroid appears to be highly effective for the treatment of melasma.
Removal of melanin	Chemical peeling	Glycolic acid peels should be used in conjunction with a depigmenting agent for maximal benefit and to minimize the risk of postinflammatory hyperpigmentation. Salicylic acid peels appear to be of minimal benefit in the treatment of melasma
Disruption of melanin granules	Light-based devices	In a recent study, an IPL-treated group achieved a significant improvement of 39.8% compared with 11.6% in the control group after four sessions of IPL and topical treatment. However, partial repigmentation was noted 24 weeks later, suggesting the need for repeated treatments for maintenance. Use of the lowest fluence is advised to achieve minimal erythema, a recommendation supported by the findings of Negishi et al. This avoids excessive thermal injury to labile melanocytes and reduces the risk of PIH.
Camouflage makeup	–	If the patient- and stage-specific treatments based on the aforementioned principles yield a poor outcome or fail to induce any treatment response, camouflage makeup is used as a last resort.

combination of the carbon dioxide laser with a Q-switched alexandrite laser does not appear to be beneficial for melasma and carries a significant risk of worsening hyperpigmentation in darker-skinned patients. Fractional resurfacing is approved by the FDA for the treatment of melasma and has been shown to have some benefit; however, additional controlled trials are needed to evaluate its efficacy for melasma.

Intense pulsed light (IPL) treatment may provide modest benefit as an adjunctive therapy for refractory patients. Copper bromide lasers may be of benefit for melasma, especially in patients with a visible vascular component, but require further study and are in any event very large and cumbersome systems, at least at present. Unfortunately, even when satisfactory results are obtained, they have been reported as being only temporary. Overall, with the current technology and approaches, the evidence for improvement with laser and IPL sources is mixed with a significant potential for worsening the condition.

A novel concept and approach are therefore currently required. To meet this need, the author has used the following approach.

1. The impaired barrier function and post-inflammatory melanosis is treated first.
- First, the damaged barrier should be repaired and the chronic physical hyperirritability relieved to treat the chronic pigmentation caused by hyperirritability. The patient should be educated on lifestyle improvement (e.g., should be told not to rub his/her face, apply good-quality moisturizers, daily UVA/B sunscreen application and so on).
- Correction of the chronic inflammation will lead to the discontinuation of the overproduction of melanin and will subsequently prevent the overproduced melanin from damaging the cells of the epidermal basal layer and the basement membrane, and thus from reaching the dermis.

2. A good grasp of the principles and action mechanism of current treatment methods is required. The turnover of the epithelial cells that contain overproduced melanin takes about 1 month. Chemical ablation can shorten the turnover time. For epidermal melasma accompanied by dermal inflammation and remarkable erythema, IPL or chemical ablation should not be performed.

3. Before the treatment, a bleaching agent and a UVA/B sunblock should be used for 6 weeks to 3 months to inhibit hyperactive melanocytes and reduce PIH risk. Combinations of hydroquinone with topical corticosteroids and tretinoin have been reported to be effective as a first-line treatment of melasma.

4. For Asians, in whom the risk of PIH is high, a stepwise approach should be used to minimize the damage. For refractory cases, laser should be used. For epidermal melasma in which the increase in the melanin level is obvious, chemical peeling to remove the epider-

mis is possible; but for dermal melasma, ablative lasers (e.g, carbon dioxide and Er:YAG lasers) and Q-switched alexandrite lasers should be used, as some success has been noted therewith, albeit with significant downtime and adverse effects. Although fractional skin resurfacing has been performed using a 1540 nm laser, it is not feasible for Asians because of the high risk of complications.

5. Thus, a treatment method that uses the low-fluence laser toning technique based on a new concept and background has been developed and used as follows. In a study in which an electron microscope was used, the author observed that the low-fluence Q-switched Nd:YAG laser toning technique destroyed the increased level of melanin in the dermis, and the destroyed melanin was subsequently removed by melanophages (see the illustrations comprising Figure 02-4). In the process, which the author has termed subcellular selective photothermolysis, Q-switched 1064 nm Nd:YAG laser energy is applied at very low fluences (typically <2 J/cm²) and multiple passes till gentle erythema is seen over the treated area. This is repeated for several sessions. As the author has proved with histological and electron-microscopical (Figure 02-4), this approach can destroy the melanin granules in the stratum spinosum cells and the melanosomes in the melanocyte dendrites, but leave the cells themselves intact so that the risk of PIH formation is dramatically reduced and the incidence of recurrence is lowered.

Table 02-3 Comparison between the treatment concepts of selective photothermolysis (SP) and the author's concept of subcellular selective photothermolysis (SSP)

| | QS Nd:Yag laser | | Published Methods versus Our Methods | |
	SP (SPTL)	SSP: Subcellular SPTL	Other Parameter	Our Parameter
1	primary target=melanosome 0.25 J, 1.0 J, 3.0 J animal data. >3.0 J 70 ns (TRT) → meoanosome lysis + cell death	targeting the melanin & melanosome itself 1.0 J~3.0 J human data. 2.0 J, & ns → melanosome lysis without cell death	Pass: 3~10	Pass: only 2~3
2	No data on 1.0 J~3.0 J	Evidence for SSP including TEM, 3D ultrastructural changes data	Fluence: 1.6~5.0 J/cm²	Fluence: 1.4~2.0 J/cm²
3	No data on human esp. Asian	Data on human esp. Asian melasma patients	Speed: >10 Hz	Speed: 5~10 Hz
4	No data on 3D changes		Spot size: 6~8 mm	Spot size: 7 mm
5			Intercals: variable	Intervals: 1~2 week
	JID 1989;93:28-32	JID 2010;130(9):2333-5	IH KIM Aesthatic Dermatology 2010. Vol(20):342-7	

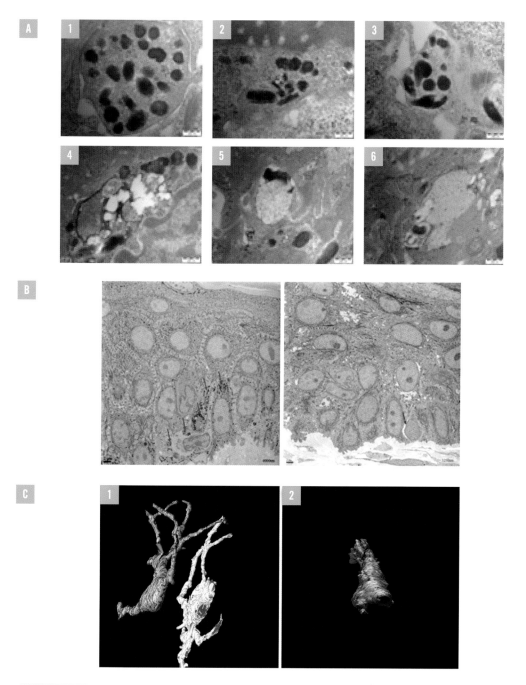

Figure 02-4   **A.** Transmission electron photomicrograph (x100,000) illustrating ultrastructural changes in melanosomes following subcellular photothermolysis treatment with the low-fluence Q-switched Nd:YAG laser toning technique, pulse width <5-7 ns, fluence 1.6-2.0 J/cm^2, 7 mm collimated beam, 2 passes. **1-3:** before treatment, fully developed stage IV melanosomes. **4-6:** after treatment, with internal electron lucency and disruption of internal contents. (Data originally presented as a poster at the 2009 ASLMS meeting) **B.** Epidermis of a melasma patient compared before (left) and after (right) laser toning. Red arrows, melanocyte; blue arrows, melanosomes. **C.** 3-dimensional view of melanocytes before (1) and after (2) Nd:YAG laser toning. The melanocyte in Figure 02-4B appears to have undergone a "dendrectomy", but is still alive. Note also the disappearance of the melanin granules from the daughter keratinocytes in B.

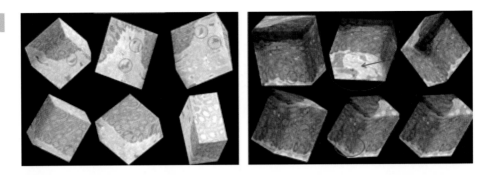

Figure 02-4 (continued) **D.** 3-dimensional changes seen in dermal melanophages before (left, blue circles) and after (right, red arrow) low fluence Q-switched Nd:YAG laser toning at the same parameters as given in Figure 02-4A.

NOTE

Laser treatment for Asians: Asians are susceptible to post-laser treatment exacerbation. A topical bleaching preparation and UVA/B sunscreen should be used for 2-3 months prior to laser treatment. If the topical application does not produce the desired treatment effect, the low-fluence laser toning technique can be performed.

Tips for post-treatment care and follow-up

Post-procedure treatment and F/U tips

Post-procedure treatment:

- Immediately after the laser toning procedure, Vitamin C iontophoresis (after the skin has sufficiently relaxed), or a whitening mask can be used as a post-procedure treatment. Vitamin C iontophoresis can also be applied 3 days post-treatment.
- Only on the day of the procedure, after the procedure, 1% hydrocortisone ointment can be applied evenly over the treated area, followed by a UVA/B sunblock, after which the patient can go home.
- It is recommended that patients use a moisturizer and a sunblock routinely.

1. Post-procedure treatment after laser toning: apply a soothing mask, then treat the skin with an 830-nm light-emitting diode (LED) phototherapy system (60 J/cm^2), and apply sunblock.

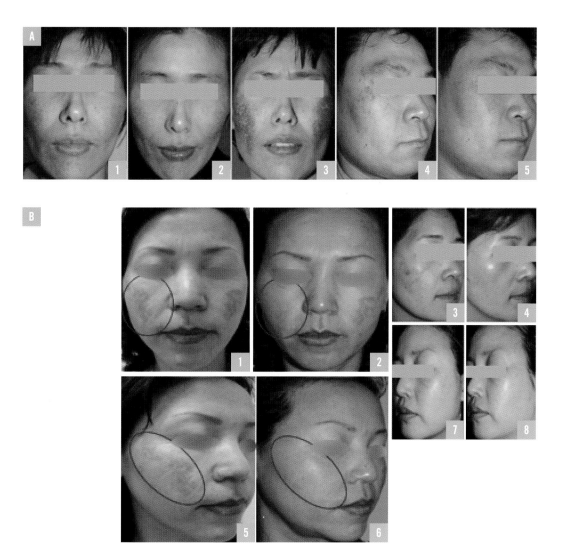

Figure 02-5 Side effects following high-fluence laser treatment (A, multiple passes, 2-2.5 J/cm^2) compared with the lack of side effects and good results after low-fluence laser toning (B, two passes, 1.6 = 2.0 J/cm^2). **A.** Baseline findings seen in (1); (2) is after treatment with distinct erythema, and exacerbation of the melasma is seen in (3). Baseline findings in (4), with mottled hyper- and hypo pigmentation in (5) as the unsatisfactory result. **B.** Good results after laser toning. (1) is baseline in a split-face laser toning study: only the right side (red oval) is to be treated. (2) is the result after the 7th session. The melasma on the treated side has cleared nicely. (3) shows baseline, and (4) shows typical mild erythema post-Tx. Two pairs of patients are seen at baseline in (5) and (6), and after the 7th session in (7) and (8).

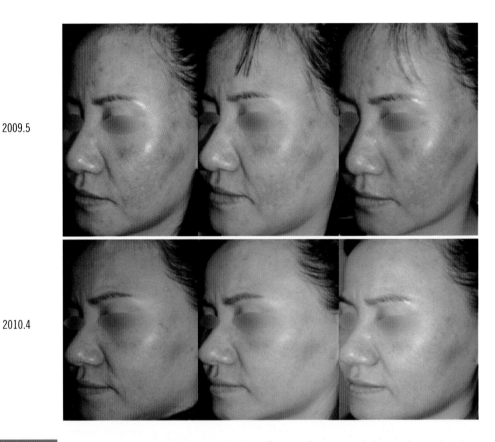

2009.5

2010.4

Figure 02-6   Topical maintenance application is useful for ineffective refractory case in laser toning treatment.

2. Treatment course: The treatment sessions should be performed every 1 or 2 weeks for a total of 6-12 sessions (illustrated above). Excessive attempts to treat residual pigmented lesions should be avoided, and a topical bleaching agent should be used from 7 days after the procedure. Antioxidants and a skin barrier repair cream can be added.

3. Side effects: During the repetition of the low-fluence irradiation, care must be taken to prevent overtreatment (overtoning). The skin condition and pigment response during and after the toning should be closely monitored. If hypopigmentation occurs, the toning treatment should be stopped, and topical application should be used. Excessive treatment should be avoided for areas not responsive to the treatment.

REFERENCES

1. Chan HHL. Effective and safe use of lasers, light sources, and radiofrequency devices in the clinical management of Asian patients with selected dermatoses. Lasers Surg Med 2005;37:179-185.

2. Ee HL, Goh CL, Khoo LS, Chan ES, Ang P. Treatment of acquired bilateral nevus of Ota-like macules (Hori's nevus) with a combination of the 532 nm Q-switched Nd:YAG followed by the 1064 nm Q-switched Nd:YAG is more effective: prospective study. Dermatol Surg 2006;32:34-40.

3. Ee HL, Wong HC, Goh CL, Ang P. Characteristics of Hori naevus: a prospective analysis. Br J Dermatol 2006;154:50-53.

4. Garcia A, Fulton JE Jr. The combination of glycolic acid and hydroquinone or kojic acid for the treatment of melasma and related conditions. Dermatol Surg 1996; 22: 443-447.

5. Glycolic acid, salicylic acid, and trichloroacetic acid peels are also useful adjuncts to topical treatments in the management of melasma in Asians.

6. Grekin RC, Shelton RM, Geisse JK, Frieden I. 510-nm pigmented lesion dye laser. Its characteristics and clinical uses. J Dermatol Surg Oncol 1993;19:380-387

7. Griffiths CE, Finkel LJ, Ditre CM, Hamilton TA, Ellis CN, Voorhees JJ. Topical tretinoin (retinoic acid) improves melasma. A vehicle-controlled, clinical trial. Br J Dermatol 1993;129:415-421.

8. Grimes PE, Yamada N, Bhawan J. Light microscopic, immunohistochemical, and ultrastructural alterations in patients with melasma. Am J Dermatopathol 2005;27:96-101.

9. Grimes PE. Melasma: etiologic and therapeutic considerations. Arch Dermatol 1995;131:1453-1457.

10. Grimes PE. The safety and efficacy of salicylic acid chemical peels in darker racial-ethnic groups. Dermatol Surg 1999;25:18-22.

11. Jeong SY, Chang SE, Park HN, Choi JH, Kim IH. New Melasma Treatment by Collimated Low Fluence Q-switched Nd:YAG Laser. Korean J Dermatol 2008;46:1163-1170.

12. Jeong SY, Shin JB, Yeo UC, Kim WS, Kim IH. Low-fluence Q-switched neodymium-doped yttrium aluminum garnet laser for melasma with pre- or post-treatment triple combination cream. Dermatol Surg 2010;36:909-918.

13. Kang WH, Yoon KH, Lee ES, Kim J, Lee KB, Yim H, Sohn S, Im S. Melasma: histopathological characteristics in 56 Korean patients. Br J Dermatol 2002;146:228-237.

14. Kim JH, Jeong SY, Shin JB, Park HC, Kim IH. Subcellular selective photothermolysis in zebrafish : an electron microscopic evidence after Q-switched Nd:YAG laser ablation. Korean J Dermatology 2008;46:S2, p187.

15. Kim JH, Kim H, Park HC, Kim IH. Subcellular selective photothermolysis of melanosomes in adult zebrafish skin following 1064-nm Q-switched Nd:YAG laser irradiation. J Invest Dermatol 2010;130:2333-2335.

16. Kunachak S, Leelaudomlipi P, Sirikulchayanonta V. Q-switched ruby laser therapy of acquired bilateral nevus of Ota-like macules. Dermatol Surg 1999;25:938-941.

17. Lam AY, Wong DS, Lam LK, Ho WS, Chan HH. A retrospective study on the efficacy and complications of Q-switched alexandrite laser in the treatment of acquired bilateral nevus of Ota-like macules. Dermatol Surg 2001;27:937-941.

18. Mun JY, Jeong SY, Kim JH, Han SS, Kim IH. A low fluence Q-switched Nd:YAG laser modifies the 3D structure of melanocyte and ultrastructure of melanosome by subcellular-selective photothermolysis. J Electron Microsc (Tokyo). 2011;60:11-18.

19. Negishi K, Kushikata N, Tezuka Y, Takeuchi K, Miyamoto E, Wakamatsu S. Study of the incidence and nature of "very subtle epidermal melasma" in relation to intense pulsed light treatment. Dermatol Surg 2004;30:881-886.

20. Polnikorn N, Tanrattanakorn S, Goldberg DJ. Treatment of Hori's nevus with the Q-switched Nd:YAG laser. Dermatol Surg 2000;26:477-480.

21. Rendon M, Berneburg M, Arellano I, Picardo M. Treatment of melasma. J Am Acad Dermatol 2006;54:S272-S281.

22. Rendon M, Cardona LM, Bussear EW, Benitez AL, Colón LE, Johnson LA. Successful treatment of moderate to severe melasma with triple-combination cream and glycolic acid peels: a pilot study. Cutis 2008;82:372-378.

23. Sanchez NP, Pathak MA, Sato S, Fitzpatrick TB, Sanchez JL, Mihm MC Jr. Melasma: a clinical, light microscopic, ultrastructural, and immunofluorescence study. J Am Acad Dermatol 1981;4:698-710.

24. Sarkar R, Kaur C, Bhalla M, Kanwar AJ. The combination of glycolic acid peels with a topical regimen in the treatment of melasma in dark-skinned patients: a comparative study. Dermatol Surg 2002;28:828-832.

25. Shin JB, Jeong SY, Ro KW, Seo SH, Son SW, Kim IH. Subcellular selective photothermolysis: an electron microscopic evidence in melasma patients treated with collimated low fluence Q-switched Nd:YAG laser. Korean J Dermatology 2008;46:S2, p187

26. Wang CC, Hui CY, Sue YM, Wong WR, Hong HS. Intense pulsed light for the treatment of refractory melasma in Asian persons. Dermatol Surg 2004;30:1196-1200.

27. Wanitphakdeedecha R, Manuskiatti W, Siriphukpong S, Chen TM. Treatment of melasma using variable square pulse Er:YAG laser resurfacing. Dermatol Surg 2009;35:475-481.

28. Yoshimura K, Harii K, Aoyama T, Iga T. Experience with a strong bleaching treatment for skin hyperpigmentation in Orientals. Plast Reconstr Surg 2000;105:1097-1108.

03

Freckles & lentigines

▶ Un Cheol Yeo, MD, PhD & Jin Soo Kang, MD

Definition

Freckles

Freckles, also known as ephelides (Greek, *ephelis* meaning a freckle), are clearly demarcated brown macules that are less than 5 mm in size. Unlike melasma, freckles are isolated from each other and appear in areas exposed to sunlight. Freckles occur easily when the skin is sunburnt in summer. Many freckles appear within a month after the skin in the affected area peels off.

Fair skin is more susceptible to freckles. Freckles can occur in both young and old people. They characteristically do not occur on areas of the skin that are unexposed to sunlight, and they darken when exposed to sunlight in summer. They occur mostly on the face, back, and arms. In some cases, freckles that formed in childhood multiply over time when exposed to sunlight, but tend to gradually decrease in size and number in adults. Freckles can occur in both men and women, and are the same in both. Freckles, however, involve genetic traits.

Lentigines

Lentigo simplex is a light brown to black macule that occurs anywhere on the body with no or little anatomic relationship to sun exposure. When compared to solar lentigines, lentigines simplex have more homogeneous pigmentation, a well-defined and regular border, and are smaller in size. However, some lentigines simplex cannot be clearly distinguished from solar lentigines without histologic examination. Lentigines simplex occurring on the mucous membrane have the clinical features of a relatively irregular border and non-homogeneous pigmentation and can slowly increase in size.

Lentigines simplex can present at birth and increase in number during childhood or puberty. Lentiginosis, which refers to an eruptive form of lentigines simplex, may develop with or without associated syndromes, including LEOPARD (lentigines, electrocardiographic conduction defects, ocular hypertelorism, pulmonary stenosis, abnormalities of the genitalia, retardation of growth, and deafness) syndrome, Peutz-Jeghers syndrome, LAMB (lentigines, atrial myxomas, mucocutaneous myxomas, and blue nevi) syndrome, and Cronkhite-Canada syndrome.

Blemishes

'Blemish' is not a medical term. In South Korea, 'blemish' generally has two meanings. In a broad sense, blemishes include melasma, freckles, age spots, and other pigment diseases. In a narrow sense, blemishes indicate brown pigmented lesions that are hard to diagnose, excluding melasma, freckles, and age spots. Generally, the clinical manifestation, treatment response, and prognosis of blemishes are closest to those of freckles. Blemishes appear in relatively older people than do freckles, and are bigger and are relatively darker in color.

Tips for diagnosis

The number of melanocytes in freckles is not greater than that in normal skin. In freckles, however, melanocytes are bigger and melanosomes are larger and more mature than in the melanocytes in the neighboring normal skin, which are smaller, producing round melanosomes. Meanwhile, the histologic features of lentigo simplex include elongated epidermal rete ridges and the increased number of melanocytes. Thus, freckles must be differentiated from various types of lentigo. Although the distribution of lesions and their relationship with exposure to sunlight are helpful in their differentiation, histological examination is required for their definitive diagnosis.

Tips for treatment

Comparison of Q-switched Nd: YAG laser and intense pulsed light in the treatment of pigmented lesions

In this section, the basic characteristics of Q-switched lasers and intense pulsed light (IPL) systems will be explored, especially regarding their use in the treatment of freckles and lentigines.

Table 03-1   Impact of short-pulsed (<1 ms) laser – immediate endpoints and and subsequent events

Timing	Reaction	Comments
Immediate reaction	Immediate but temporary whitening	
5-20 min	Appearance of ring cell phenomenon	Dispersion of pigment to the periphery of pigmented keratinocytes, melanocytes, nevus cells, etc.
1-2 days	Scab or crust formation and epidermal death caused by release of melanin from the melanosome	Lasts for several days
Post-healing endpoint	Ideal situation: lesion removed	Unwanted pigment is eliminated, whereas the surrounding skin maintains its normal pigmentation level

Q-switched laser systems

The Q-switched laser delivers ultrashort pulses in the nanosecond domain with extremely high peak powers, and is an ideal laser for pigmented lesion treatment. There are 3 types of Q-switched laser: the Q-switched ruby laser (wavelength 694.3 nm), Q-switched alexandrite laser (755 nm), and the Q-switched neodymium-doped yttrium aluminium garnet (Nd:YAG) laser (1064 nm). Immediately after treatment with these lasers, the lesions appear white for about 20 minutes (so-called 'frosting') and then crusts form which fall off a few days later. Table 03-1 describes some aspects of the short-pulsed laser (i.e., pulsewidth < 1 ms) treatment of pigmented lesions.

Laser Fluence

Selection of the most appropriate fluence per pulse is essential, and although general guidelines exist for each laser wavelength, optimum results require assessment of lesions on a case-by-case basis. Whereas excessive fluence could clearly be understood to give rise to unwanted side effects, undertreatment could also give unexpected results. The three cases for fluence are as follows:

- **Subthreshold fluence:** Can result in hyperpigmentation.
- **Threshold fluence:** Uniform whitening immediately after treatment. Lower the fluence to a level that produces uniform but faint whitening. Healing is more rapid. Note that darker skin types, such as Asian types III-IV, have a lower threshold.
- **Suprathreshold fluence:** Tissue sloughing, prolonged healing, greater risk of postinflammatory hyperpigmentation (PIH), hypopigmentation or textural change.

A suitable level of laser fluence results in the formation and natural falling off of the crust, which indicates a good outcome; on the other hand, a fluence level that is lower or higher than the suitable level increases the risk of pigmentation. A high fluence level may appear to make treatment easier but actually increases the risk of pigmentation. A low fluence level results in poor formation of crusts, and even after the falling-off of the crust, lesions may still remain and even become darker. Thus, optimal treatment should be performed and should be varied according to the lesion. Optimal treatment requires that the fluence level be adjusted so that the lesions would not be too white after the treatment. Lasers which are appropriate for the treatment of pigmented lesions (namely the Q-switched Nd:YAG, alexandrite, and ruby lasers) can remove almost all the lesions with one treatment session. Due to the characteristics of the lasers, however, some parts of the lesions may be skipped in the treatment; uneven discoloration may result; or the treated skin may look mottled due to excessive discoloration. In many cases, erythema remains after the crust falls off. These phenomena are resolved over time. The main disadvantage is the high frequency of relapses immediately after the treatment. In some cases, the recurring lesion may become larger than the original lesion and as large as the crust that formed immediately after the treatment. A relapse occurs most often within 1-2 weeks after the crust falls off. Laser treatment removes lesions more effectively than treatment with IPL but has the disadvantage of frequent relapses. Besides, laser treatment is more painful than IPL.

Long-pulsed laser systems

The long-pulsed lasers, including 755-nm long-pulsed alexandrite laser, 595-nm pulsed dye laser, and 532-nm potassium titanyl phosphate (KTP) laser, deliver pulse widths of microseconds to milliseconds. Although Q-switched lasers are the most widely used devices, long-pulsed lasers also have been effectively used in the treatment of epidermal pigmentary lesions, including freckles, lentigines, and seborrheic keratoses with satisfactory therapeutic outcomes. Additionally, long-pulsed lasers reportedly can reduce the risk of PIH compared to Q-switched lasers. The longer pulse width of these laser devices treat the target pigments through only photothermolysis, whereas the Q-switched lasers, delivering as they do high energy with ultrashort pulses in the nanosecond domain, produce both photothermal and photomechanical effects on both target pigments and adjacent vascular structures.

IPL systems

IPL systems deliver a much longer pulse duration than the laser. The laser energy emitted from the nanosecond-domain Q-switched laser is delivered to the melanosome within an exposure time which is shorter than the melanosome thermal relaxation time (TRT), as a result of which the melanosomes are destroyed and the debris is dispersed to the peripheral cells without any thermal damage to surrounding cells. This explosive reaction can cause photoosmotic and photoacoustic shock waves within the target cell, resulting in the formation of empty spaces within the cell and consequently inducing the whitening effect.

With IPL systems, however, light is emitted in the millisecond domain and thus conducted heat is delivered to the areas surrounding the target pigment: consequently not only the basal layer of the epidermis but also the full thickness of the epidermis is heated before the melanosomes can be destroyed. In this case, a whitening effect is not observed but only a slight darkening of the treated lesion. The advantage of IPL systems with their much larger spot size than lasers, is that all the lesions can be treated without skipping any lesion, and a uniform skin tone can be achieved as entire lesions are treated at once due to the large spot size.

The secondary effects after IPL treatment are mild, compared with the Q-switched laser. Thus, the redness or erythema that occurs immediately after the treatment disappears within several hours or in a day. The freckles and lentigines simplex can still be visible and, about after about 5-7 days they will slightly darken. The face can already be washed and make-up can already be worn. The entire treated area then tends to become brighter. The most important advantage is the occurrence of fewer relapses after IPL treatment compared with the Q-switched laser. In addition, IPL is less painful during the treatment.

A disadvantage of IPL, however, is its ineffectiveness with some cases of freckles and relatively many cases of lentigines simplex, especially those with lighter pigmentation, which cannot be readily distinguished from the surrounding normal skin. In the ideal Q-switched laser treatment of freckles and lentigines simplex, the crust on the treated area will usually fall off almost completely within a few days revealing normal pigmentation, but this is not the case with IPL treatment. Thus, with IPL, retreatment is normally repeated at an interval of about a month.

Treatment with the Q-switched Nd:YAG Laser

The Q-switched Nd:YAG laser effectively removes freckles, lentigines simplex and solar lentigines, and it is recommended that treatment be performed until a slight frosting forms on the lesion (Figure 03-1). A high fluence level may result in severe frosting and epidermal detachment, and may even cause oozing or bleeding that requires a biological dressing (Table 03-2). In most of these cases, PIH will almost certainly develop, especially in the Asian skin phenotype, or a scar may form, all of which degrades the treatment effect. Thus, an energy level of 0.8-1.5 J/cm^2 and a beam diameter of 2-3 mm (to suit the freckle size) are desirable, and a collimated beam is essential so that laser energy is matched precisely to the lesion to be treated. The importance of collimation is that the same irradiance or power density is maintained more or less irrespective of the distance between the handpiece and the target lesion. With an uncollimated (focused or defocused) beam on the other hand, small changes in the distance between the handpiece and the target tissue can result in dramatic changes in the

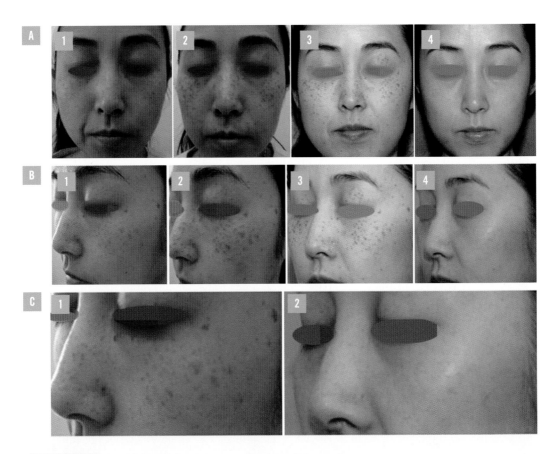

Figure 03-1 **Freckle treatment with the Q-switched Nd:YAG Laser (532 nm). A. (1)** before treatment. **(2)** Immediately after treatment. **(3)** 3 days after treatment. **(4)** 10 days after treatment. **B. (1)** before treatment. **(2)** Immediately after treatment. **(3)** 3 days after treatment. **(4)** 10 days after treatment. **C. (1)** before treatment. **(2)** 10 days after treatment.

Table 03-2 **Endpoint for pigmentation treatment by laser**

Impact of short-pulsed(<1 ms) laser **Immediate and temporary whitening:**
5-20min "Ring cell ; dispersion of pigment in pigmented keratinocyte, melanocyte, nevus cell to the periphery of cell"
Scab or crust:
"Forms over 1 to 2 days, lasts for several days" Epidermal death caused by release of melanin from melanosome
Ideal situation:
"Unwanted pigment is eliminated, surrounding skin maintains constitutive pigment"

irradiance and therefore the treatment effect. Immediately after irradiation with the laser, a whitish frosting will develop over the target lesion but will disappear fairly quickly. Within 1-2 days, a crust will form at the site of the frosting and it will become brown or black. After the crust naturally falls off, in the ideal situation the lesion completely disappears. As for the Q-switched ruby and Q-switched alexandrite lasers, treatment should be performed until this slight frosting develops, and the treatment procedure is similar.

Treatment using long-pulsed lasers

Long-pulsed lasers have been increasingly used for the treatment of freckles and lentigines simplex (Figure 03-2). Comparison studies using Q-switched and long-pulsed alexandrite lasers in Asian patients demonstrated significant improvement in freckle lesions after both Q-switched and long-pulsed alexandrite lasers. However, long-pulsed alexandrite laser reduced the procedure time and also carried a lower risk of adverse effects. When using a 755-nm long-pulsed alexandrite laser, the use of a 3-5-msec or shorter pulse width compared to the 20-, 40-, and 60-msec pulsewidths and laser fluences of 35 to 50 J/cm^2 are generally recommended. When using a 532-nm long-pulsed KTP laser, a pulse duration of 2 msec and a fluence of 9-12 J/cm^2 or a pulse duration of 10-12 msec and a fluence of 15-18 J/cm^2 can

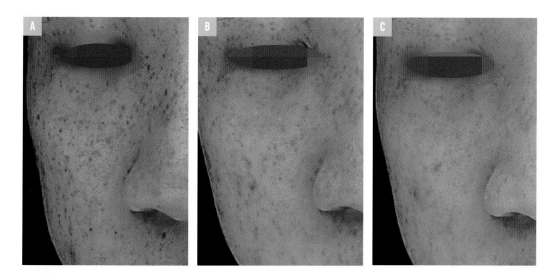

Figure 03-2   **Centrofacial lentiginosis.** A 22-year-old male patient with centrofacial lentiginosis. **A.** Before. **B.** one week after one session of long-pulsed 755-nm alexandrite laser and four sessions of Q-switched low-fluenced Nd:YAG laser treatment, and C. one month after an additional two sessions of wavelength-converted 660-nm Q-switched ruby-like versatile YAG treatment and eight sessions of QS low-fluenced Nd:YAG laser treatment. (Figures were adapted from "Goo B, Kang JS, Cho SB. Therapeutic efficacy and safety of wavelength-converted 660-nm Q-switched ruby-like versatile YAG treatment on various skin pigmentation disorders. Med Laser 2014;3:48-54" with permission and modified.)

be used for the treatment of epidermal pigmented lesions. However, adjustment of treatment parameters should be made according to the individual device. Q-switched laser treatment causes the immediate white-colored frosting on the epidermal pigmented lesions, whereas the long-pulsed laser often produces a delayed response after treatment on the pigmented lesions for up to 10 minutes. However, as shown in Q-switched lasers, crusts spontaneously fall off a few days to one week later.

The protection of the epidermis using an integrated air-cooling or a cryogen spray cooling with spray pattern enables delivery of high fluence laser energy on the target pigments. However, when using the larger spot sizes associated with long-pulsed lasers, the cyrogen spray cooling approach may not uniformly protect the epidermis. Therefore, air-cooling or post-irradiation epidermal cooling rather than pre-irradiation cooling is preferred, however, the optimal laser setting with or without cyrogen spray cooling remains to be evaluated in Asian skin.

Treatment using IPL systems

As with Q-switched lasers, determination of the most appropriate parameters is of paramount importance when treating freckles and lentigines simplex with IPL energy. With the Q-switched laser and long-pulsed laser, the wavelength is fixed, but with IPL, the waveband of the treatment beam is selectable using interchangeable cut-off filters.

Adjustment of the waveband for the treatment of pigmented lesions
Pigmented lesions - guidelines
- Shorter cut-off filter
    - Light skin
    - Light lesion
    - Shallow lesion
- Longer cut-off filter
    - Dark skin
    - Dark lesion
    - Deep lesion
- Filters used: 500-600 nm cut-off filter
    - For the treatment of a pigment lesion, cut-off filters in the shorter 500 nm to the mid 600 nm waveband can be used. This provides semi-selective pigment selectivity depending on the cut-off value, because it must be remembered that IPL energy is polychromatic with a waveband extending from the near infrared (IR) down to the cut-off value, and the cut-off filters simply remove unwanted shorter wavelengths. By careful selection of the most appropriate cut-off filter, however, effective treatment of pigmented lesions can be achieved with an IPL system, taking patient skin type into consideration.

Use of cut-off filters with shorter wavelengths

With cut-off filters in the short to mid 500 nm range (green-yellow), IPL systems can deliver all wavelengths of light energy in the waveband from near infrared (1200 nm to around 960 nm, depending on the system) to the selected cut-off value. In other words, a portion of the total emitted light energy is in the shorter green-yellow waveband. Light energy at these wavelengths is highly absorbed in melanin, and reacts intensively with the epidermal melanin. Thus, a cut-off filter with a shorter wavelength is suitable for skin types I-III, and for lighter and shallower lesions. If the shorter cut-off filters were to be used for skin type IV, V or higher with a much higher intrinsic overall melanin content, the strong reaction of the melanin content with the shorter green-yellow wavelengths can lead to burn formation, resulting in blistering and crusting with the potential for hyper- or hypopigmentation and textural changes, or even some scarring.

Use of a longer cut-off filter

With cut-off filters in the mid-600 nm range (visible red), the emitted waveband now includes the near IR component but stops in the visible red waveband at the cut-off value, in other words, the filter has cut-off the shorter yellow and green components. Visible red light in the mid 600 nm range is less well-absorbed in melanin, and is therefore safe for treatment of pigmented lesions in skin type IV, V or higher, as the reaction of the light with the melanin pigment is gentler. Longer cut-off filters can also allow IPL systems to be used in the treatment of melasma. Although only two specific cut-off filters have been discussed, typically 520 nm and 670 nm, depending on the IPL manufacturer, a range of five or six cut-off filters is usually available to fine tune the appropriate waveband to both skin type and lesion to be treated. Although not of interest in the treatment of freckles, a near-IR cut-off filter is also usually provided for skin rejuvenation or hair removal.

Figure 03-3 shows the absorption curve of biological pigments by wavelength. Hemoglobin has absorption peaks around 520 nm (green), and also around 585 nm, and melanin is also a strong absorber at these wavelengths. Absorption in both hemoglobin and melanin decreases as wavelengths enter the red waveband (from 600 nm upwards), and with progressively longer wavelengths, absorption in melanin decreases. As a general rule, we could therefore state that treatment of pigmented lesions with longer wavelengths from 630 nm or so will give a mild reaction and a more gentle treatment effect, whereas the use of the wavelengths in the 500 nm waveband will result in very high absorption in melanin, giving a much stronger treatment with a more extensive reaction.

Treatment of freckles with IPL

In the past, before laser was developed, an ablative technique was used widely for the

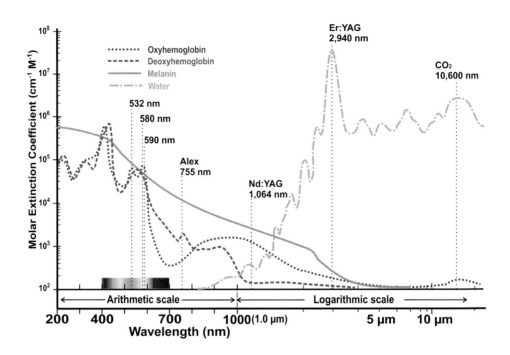

Figure 03-3   **Wavelength-related absorption curve of biological pigments.** Biological pigment absorption curves by wavelength.

treatment of freckles, whereby the epidermis was fully ablated off the epidermis, and with more aggressive approaches, ablation of even the dermis occurred. With ablation, although freckles can be removed, the side effects are more pronounced: erythema, for example, can persist for as long as 3 months after the ablative procedure, with a very strong potential for pigmentary and textural changes. PIH was almost certainly the outcome of these more aggressive approaches in the Asian skin types III-IV. Due to these unwanted side effects and long patient downtime, the ablative technique is not commonly used nowadays. With the development of more versatile laser systems in the late 1990s coupled with a more comprehensive understanding of laser/tissue interaction, it has become possible to remove freckles more safely and effectively; ablation is therefore rarely used at present. Shallow ablation or treatment with a whitening agent, which is still widely used nowadays, cannot completely remove freckles. To completely remove freckles, a pigment-specific treatment should be used. IPL systems are now also being used to treat freckles successfully. IPL treatment generally results in milder sequelae compared with the use of Q-switched lasers for pigmented lesions. The erythema that develops immediately after an IPL procedure will usually disappear within about an hour, though lesions may require more treatment sessions to ensure total removal of the freckles or other pigmented lesions, depending also on the intensity of the treatment. The skin over the freckles then forms very mild 'microcrusts', which darken and fall off after about 5-7 days. As a result, the treated freckles do not stand out clearly against the surrounding normal skin, becoming more natural-looking with subsequent treatments.

As already stated, after an IPL treatment, provided the correct cut-off filter has been selected and appropriate energy densities have been chosen, the sequalae are milder than with the laser but the prognosis is good. The overall facial skin tone becomes lighter as the entire face is treated, unlike laser treatment where small spot sizes can result in uneven pigmentation. After IPL treatment, the skin becomes slightly darker but returns to normal soon. Then the next day, the skin appears to become as dark as the original lesion. This phenomenon is called microcrusting, as already mentioned above. The microcrust falls off naturally several days later and erythema at the microcrust site is not usually a problem. Despite this advantage, IPL is not effective for mildly pigmented freckles or melasma with overall pigmentation similar to that of the surrounding skin, in which case laser treatment is required.

Tips for post-treatment care and follow-up

Apply a water-based moisturizer to the crust or microcrust. As the crust from Q-switched laser treatment or long-pulsed laser treatment and microcrust following IPL treatment will fall off naturally in about 5-10 days later in most cases, inform the patient not to attempt to remove the crust by picking at it; delayed healing and adverse side effects may result. Once the crust falls off, instruct the patient to apply a daily UVA/B sunblock to prevent PIH and to help prolong the treatment efficacy, as freckles are genetic in nature and UV-mediated recurrence is common.

REFERENCES

1. Goo B, Kang JS, Cho SB. Therapeutic efficacy and safety of wavelength-converted 660-nm Q-switched ruby-like versatile YAG treatment on various skin pigmentation disorders. Med Laser 2014;3:48-54.
2. Ho SG, Chan NP, Yeung CK, Shek SY, Kono T, Chan HH. A retrospective analysis of the management of freckles and lentigines using four different pigment lasers on Asian skin. J Cosmet Laser Ther 2012;14:74-80.
3. Ho SG, Yeung CK, Chan NP, Shek SY, Chan HH. A comparison of Q-switched and long-pulsed alexandrite laser for the treatment of freckles and lentigines in oriental patients. Lasers Surg Med 2011;43:108-113.
4. Korean Dermatological Association. Dermatology: 3rd Revision. Text Publishing Committee;444-445.
5. Trafeli JP, Kwan JM, Meehan KJ, Domankevitz Y, Gilbert S, Malomo K, Ross EV. Use of a long-pulse alexandrite laser in the treatment of superficial pigmented lesions. Dermatol Surg 2007;33:1477-1482.
6. Vejjabhinanta V, Elsaie ML, Patel SS, Patel A, Caperton C, Nouri K. Comparison of short-pulsed and long-pulsed 532 nm lasers in the removal of freckles. Lasers Med Sci 2010;25:901-906.

Nevus of Ota

▶ Jiehoon Kim, MD

Definition

Nevus of Ota (also known as oculodermal melanocytosis) is a form of benign melanocytosis that involves areas innervated by the first (ophthalmic) and second (maxillary) branches of the trigeminal nerve. It was first referred to by Ota and Tanino (1939, Japan) as "naevus fusco-caeruleus ophthalmomaxillaris." Nevus of Ota appears as a blue-black or gray-brown dermal melanocytic pigmentation. It develops at birth or soon after as well as at puberty and shows a female predominance with a female-to-male ratio of 4-5:1, and here are no reports of spontaneous regression.

Nevus of Ota may develop mucosal pigmentation in the conjunctiva, sclera, and tympanic membranes. Most cases of nevus of Ota have been reported in Asia, including Japan and South Korea, and there has been no study thus far on its global incidence. It was reported that one in 500 people develops nevus of Ota in Japan, and that it is a common pigmentary disease in Asian skin.

Tips for diagnosis

The skin diseases with acquired spindle-shaped dermal melanocytes include Mongolian spot, blue nevus, nevus of Ota, acquired bilateral nevus-of-Ota-like macules (ABNOM), and nevus of Ito. Clinically, nevus of Ota, which is characterized by ill-defined brown-gray or blue-black patchy areas of hyperpigmentation intermingled with small, flat, brown spots, is observed on the maxillary and ophthalmic branches of the trigeminal nerve (5th cranial nerve) (Figure 04-1).

Occular involvement in nevus of Ota occurs approximately in two-thirds of the patients. Nevus of Ota has been classified into four types based on the extent of the anomaly (Figure

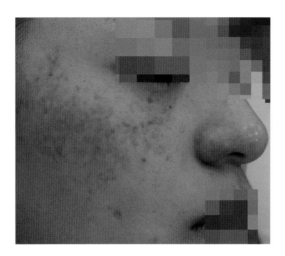

Figure 04-1 **Typical case of nevus of Ota.** Note blue-black or gray-brown colored macules on areas innervated by the second branches of the trigeminal nerve.

04-2). For a confirmatory diagnosis, the histopathological features are observed from skin biopsy (Figure 04-3). When melanocytosis is observed in the whole papillary dermis and the upper part of the reticular dermis while the epidermis exhibits normal features, as in Figure 04-3, a confirmatory diagnosis of nevus of Ota is made.

If skin biopsy is not available, a diagnosis can be made clinically. In most cases, nevus of Ota can be easily identified based on the clinical features described above. In darker skins such as Asian skin, however, it is important to make a differential diagnosis from other pigmentary diseases. As nevus of Ota shows unilateral features, it can be easily distinguished from ABNOM, which shows bilateral symmetrical features. Nevus of Ota can also be differentiated from other pigmentary diseases with dermal melanocytosis, such as Mongolian spot and nevus of Ito, because its pigmentation distribution is different. Occasionally, a differential diagnosis of nevus of Ota is difficult in Asian skins when it is observed in patch form rather than in macular form, as shown in Figure 04-4. In this figure, the patient exhibits a patch-form nevus of Ota instead of the commonly observed macular form, which makes it difficult to make a differential diagnosis of nevus of Ota from other epidermal pigmentations with patch forms, such as café-au-lait macule or lentigo simplex. In this case, Wood's light (320- to 400-nm ultraviolet light) can be used to make a differential diagnosis. The illumination of Wood's light on the lesions accentuates the epidermal pigments and does not accentuate the dermal pigments, a characteristic of nevus of Ota. For a clinician to make an accurate clinical diagnosis, the clinical features of the lesions, the patient's history, and the results of Wood's light illumination should all be considered. A definitive diagnosis is very important because it is essential not only for identifying the disease but also for selecting a treatment modality.

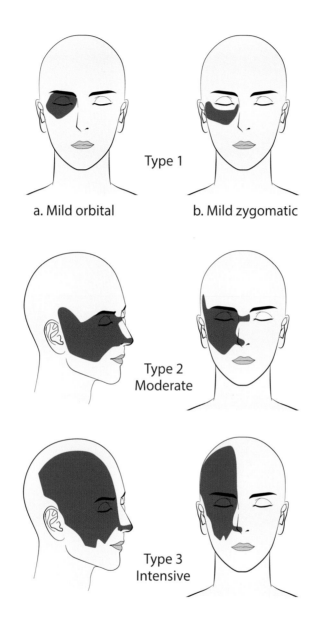

Figure 04-2   **The 4 types of nevus of Ota.** (cf reference: Tanino H. Nevus fuscoceruleus ophthalmomaxillaris Ota. Jpn J Dermatol 1939;46:435-451) (Supplement from Lutronic Corp.)

Type I. Subdivided into types Ia, Ib, 1c and Id. Type Ia Mild orbital type: distribution over the upper and lower eyelids, periocular and temple region. Type Ib: Mild zygomatic type: pigmentation is found in the infrapalpebral fold, nasolabial fold and the zygomatic region. Type Ic: Mild forehead type: involvement of the forehead alone. Type Id: Involvement of ala nasi alone.

Type II. Moderate type: Distribution over the upper and lower eyelids, periocular, zygomatic, cheek and temple regions.

Type III. Severe type: The lesion involves the scalp, forehead, eyebrow and nose.

Type IV. Bilateral type: Both sides are involved.

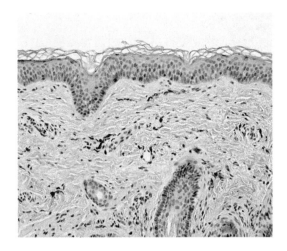

Figure 04-3 Histopathology of nevus of Ota, in which dermal melanocytes are present under a normal epidermis. Dermal melanocytes (in red) are distributed in the dermis. (Pmel/gp100 stain, original magnification x200)

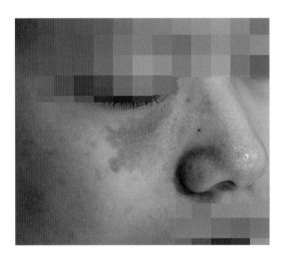

Figure 04-4 A case of the patch form of nevus of Ota. It should be differentiated from other epidermal pigmented lesions such as lentigines or café-au-lait macules.

A histopathologic diagnosis from skin biopsy leads to a confirmative diagnosis of nevus of Ota. In addition, the histopathologic findings are used to determine the parameters for laser treatments and to make a treatment prognosis because the depth of the dermal melanocytes within the dermis can be identified. For example, when the dermal melanocytes are distributed sparsely in the superficial portion of the upper dermis, a good prognosis can be made after a few treatment sessions using low laser fluences with small overlaps. On the other hand, when the dermal melanocytes are distributed densely from a superficial to a deeper portion, and in severe cases, to the hair bulbs, a poor prognosis is expected if the same laser parameters are applied as above. In this case, more treatment sessions using higher laser fluences might be required.

Tips for treatment

In the past, when laser treatments had not yet been introduced, surgical approaches such as dermabrasion and skin grafts were used to treat nevus of Ota. As these surgical treatments cause scarring in almost all cases, however, they are no longer used at present. Cryosurgery was also used in the past, depending on the location of the lesions, but this method is no longer used at present because its results are unreliable and because it is frequently accompanied by complications such as atrophy and scarring in addition to cold injuries.

The treatment of choice for nevus of Ota is Q-switched laser irradiation with nanosecond pulses. The Q-switched laser treats nevus of Ota by emitting laser energy with pulse durations that are shorter than the thermal relaxation time (TRT) of melanosomes (0.5-1 μsec) and melanocytes (7 μsec), and by selectively photothermolyzing melanosomes and melanosome-containing melanocytes. For the treatment of nevus of Ota, Q-switched ruby laser (wavelength 694 nm), Q-switched alexandrite laser (755 nm), and Q-switched neodymium-doped yttrium aluminium garnet (Nd:YAG) laser (1064 nm) have been frequently used. Although the use of the Q-switched ruby laser and Q-switched alexandrite laser was preferred in the past, Q-switched Nd:YAG lasers have been increasingly used for the treatment of nevus of Ota. Comparison studies among Q-switched lasers demonstrated better or equivalent clinical outcomes with Q-switched ruby laser or Q-switched alexandrite laser treatment than Q-switched Nd:YAG laser treatment. However, the Q-switched Nd:YAG laser has various advantages for the treatment of nevus of Ota compared to the other Q-switched lasers. First of all, because it can penetrate deeper than the other Q-switched lasers due to its longer wavelength, it effectively treats deeply located dermal melanocytes, which are usually resistant to treatment. Second, the risk of epidermal injury is relatively lower in Q-switched Nd:YAG laser treatment compared to the other Q-switched lasers as the epidermis absorbs minimal light at the wavelength of 1064 nm. Higher epidermal melanin content in Asian skin is associated with a higher risk of laser and light treatment-induced complications. Third, the Nd:YAG laser equipment is sturdy, malfunction-free, and more practical than the other Q-switched laser systems. In addition, treatments using the Nd:YAG laser can usually be completed quickly.

According to the previous reports, the recommended laser settings for the 694-nm Q-switched ruby laser include a 4 mm spot size and a fluence of 5.0-7.0 J/cm^2; those of the 755-nm Q-switched alexandrite laser include a 2-4 mm spot size and a fluence of 5.5-8.0 J/cm^2; and those of the 1064-nm Q-switched Nd:YAG laser include a 2-4 mm spot size and a fluence of 6.0-12.0 J/cm^2. The treatment intervals vary from 1 to 3 months according to the patients' response to the laser treatment. However, adjustment of treatment parameters should be made according to the individual device and each individual patient.

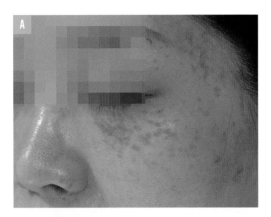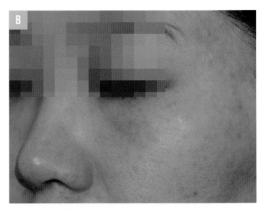

Figure 04-5 **28 years old Korean female patient with nevus of Ota. A.** before treatment. **B.** 3 months after 1 treatment. (Note: Some partial pigmentation persists after the 1st treatment.)

Case 1

A 28-year-old female Korean patient presented with discrete brownish macules distributed on the left periorbital area, left nostril, and left temple and was clinically diagnosed as having nevus of Ota (Figure 04-5A). After obtaining a written informed consent, we treated the patient with the 1064-nm Q-switched Nd:YAG laser. In the first session the laser settings selected were a 3-4-mm spot size and a fluence of 6.5 J/cm^2. Three months after the first session, overall improvement of the pigmented lesions in the skin was observed (Figure 04-5B). In the second 1064-nm Q-switched Nd:YAG laser session, the laser settings were a 3-4-mm spot size and a fluence of 7.5 J/cm^2 for the treatment of the residual pigmented lesions, which were suggested to result from melanocytes and melanophages in the deeper portions of the dermis. A satisfactory outcome was subsequently obtained.

Case 2

A 31-year-old female Korean patient presented with discrete brownish macules distributed on the left periorbital area and was clinically diagnosed as having nevus of Ota (Figure 04-6A). After obtaining a written informed consent, we treated the patient with the 1064-nm Q-switched Nd:YAG laser. In the first session the laser settings used were a 3-4-mm spot size and a fluence of 7.0 J/cm^2. Three months after the first session the second session of the 1064-nm Q-switched Nd:YAG laser used a 3-4-mm spot size and a fluence of 7.5 J/cm^2 for the treatment of residual pigmented lesions. Marked improvement of the pigmented skin lesions was subsequently observed (Figure 04-6B).

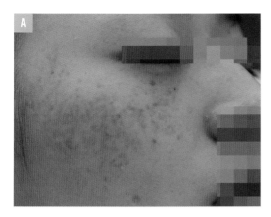 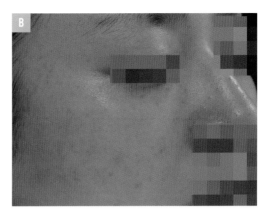

Figure 04-6   **31 years old Korean female patient with nevus of Ota. A.** before treatment. **B.** After treatment.

Case 3

A middle-aged female Korean patient, who originally had lesions on her right forhead and cheeks, was clinically diagnosed as having nevus of Ota. She had previously undergone multiple treatments for the cheek lesions using the Q-switched ruby laser some 15 years previously. When the target chromophores are densely packed, as shown in this picture, treatment using a relatively high fluence of 7.0~8.0 J/cm^2 can cause heavy bleeding during the treatment, and can leave scars. It was explained to the patient that more than three treatment sessions might thus be needed. The first treatment session was given with the Q-switched Nd:YAG laser at a fluence of 6.5 J/cm^2 and a 4 mm spot size, and the second treatment session was scheduled 6 months after the first treatment session. In the second treatment session, laser treatment was delivered at a fluence of 7.0 J/cm^2 and a 4 mm spot size. The lesions significantly improved after the second treatment session, but the patient received one more treatment after three months. Figure 04-7A shows the patient before treatment, and Figure 04-7B shows the same patient after undergoing three treatment sessions. The treatment was deemed finished after the three sessions because the lesions were almost undetectable and the patient was satisfied with the outcome.

Tips for post-treatment care and follow up

Most cases diagnosed as nevus of Ota develop in early childhood and puberty. Therefore, the most frequently asked question regarding the laser treatments of infants or children is the

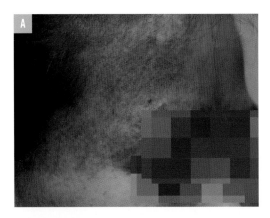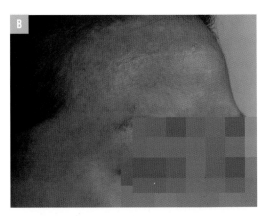

Figure 04-7   **Middle aged Korean female patient with nevus of Ota. A.** before treatment. **B.** After treatment

timing of such treatments. In theory, the Q-switched laser should not leave scars because it selectively photothermolyzes melanosomes, destroying the dermal melanocytes and melanophages. However, unwanted damage can occur in the neighboring keratinocytes in the epidermis or to the extracellular matrix in the upper dermis while the dermal melanocytes are being targeted by laser irradiation. The damaged keratinocytes release various cytokines with wound-healing effects, but these cytokines can also cause reactive hyperpigmentation and scar development. As a result, complications such as postinflammatory hyperpigmentation (PIH) and hypertrophic scar can arise. Pre-puberty children in particular carry a higher risk of scar development during the wound-healing process because the pilosebaceous units are not yet fully developed in this age group. Therefore, the best times for the laser treatments are as follows:

(1) after the dermal melanocytes are completely positioned (when nevus of Ota stops to progress); and

(2) after puberty, when the pilosebaceous units have already fully developed.

Despite the risk of scarring, either the patient or the patient's parents sometimes want to obtain treatment. In this case, it is very important to address the risk of scar development and to use the laser at a low fluence (20-30% lower fluence than that used for adults). Children's skin is much thinner than adults' skin, and relatively-low-fluence lasers can be effective in treating nevus of Ota in children.

The potential complications associated with nevus of Ota are similar to those associated with other laser treatments. As the Q-switched Nd:YAG laser has a long wavelength, it only occasionally causes scarring or PIH by injuring the epidermis. When PIH occurs after a laser treatment, laser toning using a Q-switched Nd:YAG laser at a low fluence can be useful for the treatment.

REFERENCES

1. Chan HH, Ying SY, Ho WS, Kono T, King WW. An in vivo trial comparing the clinical efficacy and complications of Q-switched 755 nm Alexandrite and Q-switched 1064 nm Nd:YAG lasers in the treatment of nevus of Ota. Dermatol Surg 2000;26:919-922.
2. Choi JE, Lee JB, Park KB, Kim BS, Yeo UC, Huh CH, Kim JH, Kye YC. A retrospective analysis of the clinical efficacies of Q-switched alexandrite and Q-switched Nd:YAG lasers in the treatment of nevus of Ota in Korean patients. J Dermatolog Treat 2014;9:1-6.
3. Fitzpatrick TB, Zeller R, Kukita A, Kitamura H. Ocular and dermal melanocytosis. Arch Ophthalmol 1956;56:830-832.
4. Kono T, Nozaki M, Chan HH, Mikashima Y. A retrospective study looking at the long-term complications of Q-switched ruby laser in the treatment of nevus of Ota. Lasers Surg Med 2001;29:156-159.
5. Nordlund JJ, Boissy RE, Hearing VJ, King RA, Oetting WS, Ortonne JP. The Pigmentary System (2nd edition), Chapter 52: Acquired and congenital dermal hypermelanosis. USA: Blackwell Publishing; 2006:1006-1011.
6. Patel BC, CA. Egan CA, Lucius RW, Gerwels JW, Mamalis N, Anderson RL. Cutaneous malignant melanoma and oculodermal melanocytosis (nevus of Ota): report of a case and review of the literature. J Am Acad Dermatol 1998;38:862-865.
7. Tanino H. Nevus fuscocaeruleus ophthalmomaxillaris Ota. Jpn J Dermatol 1939;46:435-451.

Acquired bilateral nevus of Ota-like macules

🔹 Jiehoon Kim, MD

Definition and etiopathogenesis

Acquired bilateral nevus of Ota-like macules (ABNOM; Hori's nevus) is an acquired facial dermal melanocytosis, which is characterized by the development of bilateral blue-brown or slate-gray discrete macules on the face (Figure 05-1). These macules are typically found on the malar areas, lateral sides of the forehead, temples, eyelids, and root and alae of the nose. However, the ocular and mucosal membranes are usually spared. The color of ABNOM was categorized into one of four groups 1) brown, 2) slate-gray, 3) brown–blue, and 4) blue. Women are more commonly affected than men with the estimated female to male ratio of approximately 9:1. The prevalence of ABNOM rises after the age of 15-20 years and significantly decreases after the age of 50. Histopathologic findings have been revealed that weakly DOPA-positive bipolar or oval-shaped dermal melanocytes appear scattered in the upper and middle portions of the dermis, particularly subpapillary dermis, in a perivascular distribution. However, the skin architecture is well preserved and in contrast to melasma lesions, epidermal pigmentation in ABNOM lesions is not significantly increased compared to non-lesional skin. Additionally, stem cell factor and c-kit, one of the dermal melanogenic paracrine networks, is upregulated in the dermis of ABNOM lesions, but not in the epidermis.

Tips for diagnosis

ABNOM is one of the common pigmentation disorders in the Asian and Hispanic populations, with Fitzpatrick skin types of VI-V. The overall prevalence of ABNOM was reported as 0.8-2.5% and in the female population, the prevalence was estimated up to 4.2% in Asian skin. The definitive diagnosis of ABNOM is very important for a proper treatment. Although a definitive

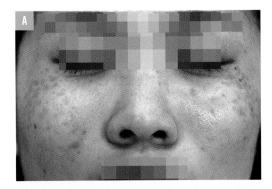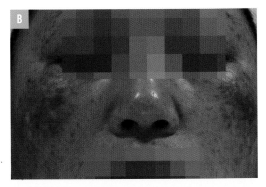

Figure 05-1   **Typical clinical features of ABNOM. A.** 28 years old Korean patient with ABNOM. A moderate case where involvement is noted of both the malar area and nose. **B.** 45 years old Korean patient with ABNOM. A severe case, where involvement of the malar area, nose and temple can be seen.

diagnosis can be made based on the histopathologic features, skin biopsies are not always available in patients with pigmentation disorders, who have visited hospitals or clinics for cosmetic purposes. Additionally, because the clinical features of ABNOM are variable and are frequently combined with those of other pigmentary diseases, it is often difficult to make a definitive diagnosis.

Both nevus of Ota and ABNOM present facial dermal melanocytosis, and ABNOM (see Table 05-1) was named by its histologic similarities to nevus of Ota. Therefore, ABNOM is regarded by some clinicians as an "symmetrical variety of bilateral nevus of Ota" rather than as a completely different disease entity. However, the differences in the clinical and histological features between these two entities can be summarized as seen in Table 05-1. Briefly, most of their prominent differences lie in the distribution of the lesions and in the time of disease onset: ABNOM is a late-onset disease that exhibits bilateral distribution whereas nevus of Ota is an early-onset disease that usually exhibits unilateral distribution. The typical histological findings in ABNOM feature randomly shaped bipolar melanocytes that are located densely in the subepidermal papilla while nevus of Ota features dermal melanocytes that are irregularly distributed from the upper to the deep dermis. To summarize, the most prominent clinical features of ABNOM that are different from those of nevus of Ota include the following:

(1) Late onset in adulthood;

(2) Bilateral presentation;

(3) Speckled, discrete, or confluent distribution; and

(4) Lack of mucosal involvement.

Table 05-1   **ABNOM vs. Nevus of Ota**

	ABNOM	Nevus of Ota
Clinical features		
shapes	scattered speckled macules	confluent patches and macules
symmetry	"symmetrical, bilateral"	unilateral
distribution	zygomatic areas	ophthalmo-maxillary areas
sex ratio (M:F)	1:6	1:4
onset	95% after 1st decade	> 50% at birth
occular pigmentation	none	60~70% of cases
Palatal pigmentation	none	10~18% of cases
Familial incidence	high (18%)	low (1%)
Recorded incidence	high	low
Histologic features		
Epidermis	normal	normal
Dermal melanocytes	positive	positive
Pigment-bearing cells	"upper dermis, relatively sparse"	"upper to deep dermis, relatively abundant"

In Asian skin, ABNOM frequently requires a differential diagnosis from melasma. Melasma, an epidermal melanosis or melanocytosis disease, and ABNOM, a dermal melanocytosis disease, are commonly confused with each other even though they are categorized into clearly different disease entities. Actually, the coexistence of ABNOM and melasma can be observed in some cases. Suggested reasons for diagnostic confusion between them may include 1) both ABNOM and melasma are late-onset diseases, 2) both pigmentation disorders frequently occur in the malar areas, 3) Some Asian patients with melasma histopathologically present with dermal melanin components, which result in clinical similarity with ABNOM lesions, and 4) dermal melanocytes, which are located in the upper papillary dermis of ABNOM lesions can be clinically indistinguishable from the epidermal melanosis of melasma lesions.

The differences of the clinical and histological features between these two diseases can be summarized as seen in Table 05-2. For example, when the disease develops after puberty and there is neither disease progression nor regression, a diagnosis of ABNOM is more favored than melasma. On the other hand, when the disease develops during or after pregnancy and keeps progressing, a diagnosis of melasma is more favored than ABNOM. When facial pigmentation is found on the malar area as well as the forehead with similar pigment densities or pigment lesions occur on the alae nasi, the diagnosis of ABNOM is preferred to melasma. Melasma is more prevalent in patients who, through their occupation, are at higher risk of high ultraviolet exposure or who have a history of pregnancy, oral-contraceptive medication,

Table 05-2 **ABNOM vs. Melasma**

	ABNOM	Melasma
Clinical features		
distribution	not related to UV exposed area	UV exposred area more common (ex malar area)
nose and forehead involvement	common	rare
onset	after puberty	middle age
predisposing factors	negative	"related to pregnancy, oral contraceptives, UV exposure"
aggravated by UV exposure	negative	commonly related
wood's light illumination	not accentuated	accentuated
Histologic features		
Epidermis	normal	hyperpigmentation
Dermal melanocytes	positive (upper portion of dermis)	negative (positive in some dermal melanophages)

hormone replacement therapy, or hyperthyroidism. Wood's light examination can provide very useful information in distinguishing ABNOM lesions from melasma. Under Wood's light, no or slight accentuation of the pigmented lesions is found in ABNOM, whereas re- markable accentuation is noted in the epidermal melanosis lesions of melasma.

Tips for treatment

Many treatment modalities have been used for treating ABNOM. In the past, topical bleach- ing agents and superficial- to medium-depth chemical peels have been utilized as a mono- therapy or a combination therapy, however, satisfactory clinical outcomes could not be ob- tained in most of the patients. At present, Q-switched lasers with nanosecond pulse widths, including the Q-switched ruby laser (wavelength 694 nm), Q-switched alexandrite laser (755 nm), and Q-switched neodymium-doped yttrium aluminum garnet (Nd:YAG) laser (1064 nm), are most frequently chosen to destroy the dermal melanocytosis of ABNOM lesions. Compared to nevus of Ota, because target pigments and melanocytes are mainly located in the upper dermis, ABNOM lesions generally respond well to Q-switched lasers. ABNOM can be treated with Q-switch lasers as a monotherapy. However, because many patients with ABNOM also present with other pigmentary disorders, such as melasma, lentigines, and postinflammatory hyperpigmentation (PIH), combination treatment with other laser or light devices is frequently required.

According to a previous report, recommended laser settings for the treatment of ABNOM lesions with the 1064-nm Q-switched Nd:YAG laser include a 3-mm spot size, a pulse width of 5-7 nsec, energy densities ranging from 4.2 to 9.9 J/cm^2 with a mean fluence of 7.8 J/cm^2, and a repetition rate of 10 Hz. The treatment interval was 3 months and the average number of treatments to achieve excellent results was 5.3. Another report suggested that the ideal settings of the 1064-nm Q-switched Nd:YAG laser were a 3-4 mm spot size, a fluence of 4.0-6.0 J/cm^2, and two or three passes with the appearance of fine petechiae as a clinical end-point. When combined with laser toning, the entire face or both cheeks, including the ABNOM lesions. is firstly treated at a setting of 2.2-2.6 J/cm^2 using a 6-mm spot size, and two to three passes. Then, additional treatment can be given directly at a setting of 4-6 J/cm^2 using a 3-4-mm spot size on the ABNOM lesions. Treatment intervals are reportedly recommended from 1-4 weeks and the estimated mean number of treatment sessions at which clinical improvement starts to become apparent is 4-5 sessions. However, adjustment of treatment parameters should be made according to the individual device and depending on the characteristics of the individual patient.

Case 1

A 23-year-old female Korean patient presented with ABNOM lesions involving both malar areas, which were not combined with other pigmentary diseases (Figure 05-2A). At the first treatment session, the patient was treated using the 1064-nm Q-switched Nd:YAG laser with a 4-mm spot size and a fluence of 6.0 J/cm^2. Because the dermal melanocytes of ABNOM lesions are generally located more superficially in the dermis compared to those associated with nevus of Ota, ABNOM lesions are usually treated at a laser fluence 10-20% lower than that used for treating nevus of Ota. At five months after the first treatment session, the skin lesions had improved, but remnant pigmentation was still observed (Figure 05-2B). In the second treatment session, the Q-switched Nd:YAG laser (1064 nm, 4 mm spot size) was used a slightly higher fluence of 6.5 J/cm^2. Four months after the second treatment session, most of the ABNOM lesions were almost completely cleared.

Case 2

A 41-year-old Korean patient with ABNOM wanted her pigmentary skin lesions treated without the formation of any crusts or purpura (Figure 05-3A). Therefore, a 1064-nm Q-switched Nd:YAG laser treatment at low fluence (8-mm spot size and 1.5-2.1 J/cm^2) was delivered at one- to two-week intervals for three months. However, noticeable clinical improve-

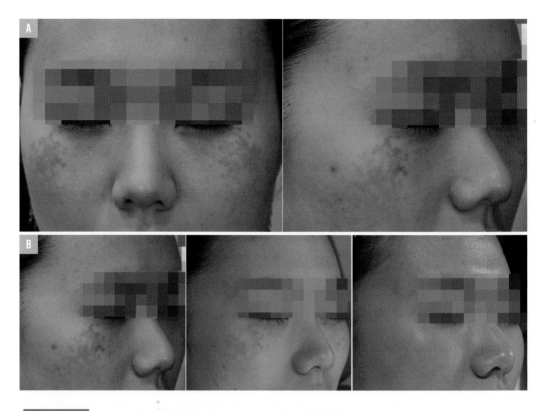

Figure 05-2 **Conventional ABNOM treatment with Q-switched Nd:YAG laser. A.** 23 years old Korean patient with ABNOM. A typical case with bilateral involvement of the malar areas, before treatment. **B.** Left: before treatment, Center: 5 months after the 1st treatment, Right: some recurrence is seen 4 months after the 2nd treatment.

ment could not be obtained. Therefore, the patient was treated with a 1064-nm Q-switched Nd:YAG laser treatment at the laser settings of 4-mm spot size, 7.0 J/cm^2 and satisfactory clinical outcomes were observed (Figure 05-3B, right). As shown in the previous report and this case, when treating the ABNOM patients with the 1064-nm Q-switched Nd:YAG laser treatment at low fluence, additional treatment at a setting of 4-7 J/cm^2 using a 3-4-mm spot size on the ABNOM lesions seems to be necessary which can be delivered in the same session or in a separate session.

Case 3

A 39-year-old Korean patient was clinically diagnosed as having freckles and pigmented nevi (Figure 05-4A). The patient was treated with intense pulsed light to deal with the epidermal pigmentary lesions of freckles and the carbon dioxide laser to treat the pigmented nevi. Most of the epidermal lesions were effectively treated after two sessions of combination treat-

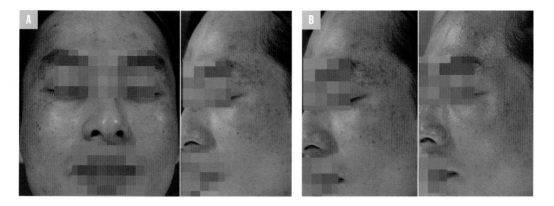

Figure 05-3 **41 years old Korean patient with ABNOM. A.** Before treatment. A typical case of ABNOM with involvement seen of the temple and nose areas. **B.** Left: before treatment, Right: 3 months after high fluence (7.0 J/cm²) Q-switched Nd:YAG laser treatment.

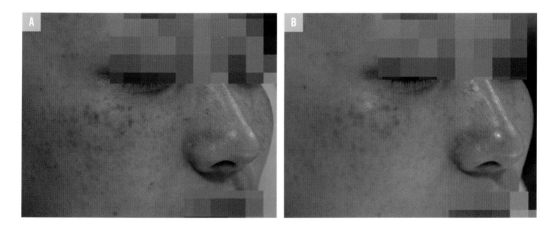

Figure 05-4 **ABNOM accompanied and masked by freckles (epidermal pigmentation). A.** 39 years old Korean patient with complex pigmentation. **B.** after 2 treatment sessions with IPL (1 month interval), the ABNOM lesions can be clearly differentiated.

ment. However, ABNOM lesions, which had been somewhat hidden by the freckles, were noticed (Figure 05-4A). The patient was subsequently treated with two sessions of 1064-nm Q-switched Nd:YAG laser at the settings of 3-mm spot size and 6.5-7.0 J/cm² fluence with satisfactory clinical outcomes (Figure 05-4B). In Asian patients with ABNOM, however, ABNOM often accompanies melasma and other pigmentary disorders. In these cases, AB-NOM lesions can be resistant to conventional treatments, and unwanted and/or unexpected outcomes often result from such treatment approaches. Therefore, a correct diagnosis is necessary to plan the proper treatment and to make an accurate prognosis.

Tips for post-treatment care and follow up

The treatment of ABNOM using the Q-switched Nd:YAG laser is accompanied by downtime due to purpura and crust formation, as is the case in the treatment of nevus of Ota. During this time, careful wound care is as important as the treatment itself. PIH and erythema are usually and particulalry more severe and last longer in Asian skin than in Caucasian skin. A previous report has suggested that more than 70% of patients with ABNOM developed transient PIH after the treatment with the 1064-nm Q-switched Nd:YAG laser with a fluence ranging from 4 to 6 J/cm^2. Another study reported that nearly all of the patients who underwent treatment of their ABNOM lesions with the 1064-nm Q-switched Nd:YAG laser with a 3-mm spot size, a pulse width of 5-7 nsec, and energy densities ranging from 4.2 to 9.9 J/cm^2 experienced transient PIH after the laser treatment. The PIH usually gradually faded in 2-6 months after 1064-nm Q-switched Nd:YAG laser treatment.

The higher risk of PIH in ABNOM patients has been suggested to be associated with epidermal hyperreactivity in the ABNOM lesions or dermal melanocytes which can be identified histologically in the upper papillary dermis. To reduce the risk of PIH, supplementary treatments, including short-term usage of topical and systemic steroids and long-term usage of bleaching agents, can be helpful. It is also important to help normalize damaged skin by rendering proper wound care and preventing secondary infection while crusts exist in the first week following the laser treatment. In cases of laser-induced PIH, combination treatment with topical bleaching agents and 1064-nm Q-switched laser treatment with low fluence (laser toning) can be effectively used for treating PIH. However, there have been no cases of persistent postinflammatory hypopigmentation, textural changes, persistent erythema, or hypertrophic scarring.

REFERENCES

1. Cho SB, Park SJ, Kim MJ, Bu TS. Treatment of acquired bilateral nevus of Ota-like macules (Hori's nevus) using 1064-nm Q-switched Nd:YAG laser with low fluence. Int J Dermatol 2009;48:1308-1312.
2. Hori Y, Kawashima K, Oohara K. Acquired, bilateral nevus of Ota-like macules. J Am Acad Dermatol 1984;10;961-964.
3. Hori Y, Oohara K, and Niimura M. Electron microscopy: ultra-structural observations of the extracellular sheath of dermal melanocytes in nevus of Ota. Am J Dermatopathol 1982;4:245-251.
4. Lee B, Kim YC, Kang WH, Lee ES. Comparison of characteristics of acquired bilateral nevus of Ota-like macules and nevus of Ota according to theraputic outcome. J Korean Med Sci 2004;19:554-559.
5. Lee JY, Kim EH, Kim KH, Kang HY, Lee ES, Kim YC. Acquired bilateral naevus of Ota-like macules: an immunohistological analysis of dermal melanogenic paracrine cytokine networks. Br J Dermatol 2011;164:580-585.

6. Nordlund JJ, Boissy RE, Hearing VJ, King RA, Oetting WS, Ortonne JP. Acquired and congenital dermal hypermelanosis. In: The Pigmentary System. 2nd ed., pp.1017-1019.

7. Park JM, Tsao H, Tsao S. Acquired bilateral nevus of Ota-like macules (Hori nevus): etiologic and therapeutic considerations. J Am Acad Dermatol 2009;61:88-93.

8. Polnikorn N, Tanrattanakorn S, Goldberg DJ. Treatment of Hori's nevus with the Q-switched Nd:YAG laser. Dermatol Surg 2000;26:477-480.

9. Suh DH,Han KH,Chung JH. Clinical use of the Q-switched Nd:YAG laser for the treatment of acquired bilateral nevus of Ota-like macules (ABNOMs) in Koreans. J Dermatol Treat 2001;12:163-166.

10. Wang BQ, Shen ZY, Fei Y, Li H, Liu JH, Xu H, Zhang Z, Yu XH, Chen XD. A population-based study of acquired bilateral nevus-of-Ota-like macules in Shanghai, China. J Invest Dermatol 2011;131:358-362.

Postinflammatory hyperpigmentation

Il Hwan Kim, MD, PhD & Sung Bin Cho, MD, PhD

Definition and etiopathogenesis of postinflammatory hyperpigmentation

Postinflammatory hyperpigmentation (PIH) is a common acquired epidermal and dermal melanotic hypermelanosis, which results from exo- and endogenous cutaneous inflammatory reactions, including infections, acute and chronic inflammatory dermatoses, traumatic mechanical injuries, adverse reactions against medications and treatments with various energy-based systems. Darker skinned types, especially Fitzpatrick skin types IV-VI, containing larger amounts of eumelanin in the epidermis are at higher risk of developing PIH.

The precise etiopathogenesis of PIH has not yet been determined. The severity of PIH is related to the extent of the causative skin inflammation and associated injury to the dermoepidermal junction. During the wound healing process PIH can develop as a biologic response against cutaneous inflammatory reactions through the affected keratinocytes and/or melanocytes. Additionally, inflammatory processes, which can be mediated by arachidonic acid metabolites, including prostaglandin (PG) E2, PGF2α, thromboxane B2, leukotriene (LT) C4, and LTD4, stimulate melanocytes to over-produce melanin by enhancing tyrosinase activity and the transfer of melanosomes to keratinocytes. For these reasons, the histologic features of increased and abnormally distributed melanin as well as dermal melanophages and hemosiderin deposition can be found.

Intrinsic pigment regulators are controlled by the crosstalk among keratinocytes, fibroblasts, endothelial cells, and inflammatory cells. The risk of PIH has therefore been implicated and associated with trauma or post-procedure vascular damage. When treating pigmentary lesions using Q-switched lasers a burst of high peak power laser energy in an ultrashort pulse duration in the nanosecond domain induces both photothermal and photomechanical effects on the target melanin. However, it can also induce undesirable damage to superficial vessels and as a result, inflammatory mediators from endothelial cells and inflammatory cells regulate the activity of melanocytes. Nitric oxide, which is secreted from endothelial cells, has been shown to initiate and enhance melanogenesis after UV radiation. Additionally, when treating pigmentary lesions with large spot sizes, the risk of PIH can be increased in cases of skin lesions having an area smaller than the spot size and with low contrast between the lesion and surrounding skin.

Tips for diagnosis

PIH clinically presents as a light brown to black skin lesion, which varies in size and shape, and appears in accordance with the distribution of the primary inflammatory skin lesion. When the PIH lesions are mainly composed of epidermal melanosis, clinical features of well-circumscribed lighter brown macules or patches can be found. However, PIH lesions, which mainly have histologic features of dermal melanosis, clinically present with a poorly circumscribed darker gray appearance.

Differentiation of epidermal lesions from dermal lesions in PIH can be clearly determined by a Wood's lamp examination. This lamp accentuates increased melanin pigments in the epidermis, but not dermal pigments or melanophages. However, epidermal melanosis in patients with PIH does not mean that the pigmentation is only limited to the epidermis. For the evaluation of dermal pigments in cases of PIH with both epidermal and dermal melanosis, the skin stretch test may be helpful. If the pigment appears lighter, it is epidermal melasam; if not, it is dermal.

For the diagnosis of PIH, a histological test is generally unnecessary because the reason for the induction of PIH is usually clear: overtreatment with laser or intense pulsed light (IPL) energy, for example. However, if any doubt exists that the entity is, in fact, PIH, then a histological test can certainly be performed. Histological criteria associated with PIH include a thicker epidermis, bigger melanocytes, and increased amounts of melanin in the epidermis and dermis. Furthermore the number of dermal giant melanosomes or melanophages may also increase, and a larger number of mast cells might also be demonstrated. Fontana-Masson silver stain can be used for identifying melanin pigments in the epidermis and dermis.

Prediction of postprocedure pigmentation in Asian patients

Physical examination of past traumatic wounds or postprocedure scars can be helpful to predict the risk of PIH. Additionally, the risk of PIH can be evaluated by comparing the skin tone of finger joints with that of surrounding skin. Because the various degrees of inflammatory reactions can be developed on the finger joints by continuous movements or frequent friction and trauma, tone difference is suggested to implicate the higher risk of postprocedure hyperpigmentation.

Natural course of PIH

PIH commonly occurs during the first 1-2 months after the inflammatory tissue reaction. However, most of the PIH lesions resolve naturally even if untreated. They generally resolve over a period of 6 months on the face, 1-2 years in the trunk and upper extremities, and 3-4 years in the lower extremities. Though quite rare, PIH lesions may be accompanied by freckle-like irregular pigmented macules or vitiliginous lesions in cases of a very severe inflammatory reaction, which result in excessive damage to the component cells of the basal layer and possibly the dermal vasculature.

Tips for treatment

Prevention of PIH

Despite predictions and precautions, even when using the same laser parameters, the development of PIH is still unpredictable and reportedly occurs in some 10-25% of patients treated with Q-switched lasers and in 30% of patients treated with ablative resurfacing lasers or nonablative long-pulsed lasers. To prevent PIH after trauma or procedures, patients are instructed to avoid excessive exposure to sunlight and after the crusting falls off, the use a broad-spectrum sunscreen is also recommended. During the inflammatory stage of skin wounds, efforts should be focused on minimizing the inflammation, and then on protecting the skin against factors that induce hyperpigmentation, and encouraging those that promote recovery and stabilization of the epithelial barrier function. Previous clinical investigations demonstrated that the short-term use of systemic and/or topical corticosteroids after the treatment with ablative fractional resurfacing decreased the risk of PIH. This is believed to work because corticosteroids theoretically inhibit the release of arachidonate-derived inflammatory mediators, including PGs and LTs.

Topical treatment

Topical bleaching agents are the first-line therapy for PIH by targeting different steps in melanogenesis. Hydroquinone is the gold-standard topical agent, though kojic acid, azelaic acid, mequinol, and retinoids are also used, besides cosmeceutical agents such as licorice, arbutin, soy, N-acetyl glucosamine, and niacinamide. Additionally, the iontophoretic penetration of vitamin C can be effectively used alone or in combination with topical bleaching agents for treating PIH.

Laser or light therapies

Topical treatment is mainly effective for the epidermal pigmentary component of PIH lesions. Laser or light therapies are also available but should be used with caution, as they are very dangerous if used inappropriately. These treatment methods are highly effective when used at appropriate parameters in combination with bleaching agents.

Treatment of PIH lesions using low-fluence 1,064-nm Q-switched neodymium-doped yttrium aluminium garnet (Nd:YAG) laser, known as laser toning, has been effectively used without remarkable side effects. The parameter settings of laser toning comprise a spot size of 6-8 mm, a pulse duration of 5-10 ns, and a fluence of 1.6-2.6 J/cm^2. Treatments are usually delivered with 3-5 passes/session over the skin lesions with 5 to 20 sessions at one or two-week intervals. However, adjustment of treatment parameters should be made according to the individual device and each patient's respentive condition.

Dual pulse mode or quick pulse-to-pulse (Q-PTP) mode refers to the treatment mode of the Q-switched Nd:YAG laser whereby laser energy is emitted as a split fluence in a double pulse with an interpulse interval of 80 to 100-μsec. Therefore, when PIH lesions are treated with the 1,064-nm Q-switched Nd:YAG laser at 1.6-2.0 J/cm^2 in the Q-PTP mode, dual pulses of 0.8-1.0 J/cm^2 at pulse intervals of 80-100 μs are actually delivered to the lesions. Shorter intervals (80-100 μs) between the double pulse train increase the chance of delivering laser energies to approximately identical target chromophores. A comparison study between Q-switched single pulse Nd:YAG and Q-switched Q-PTP Nd:YAG treatments demonstrated that laser treatment with Q-PTP mode resulted in better clinical outcomes for treating PIH lesions on the forearm without remarkable post-treatment hypopigmentation than with the single pulse mode.

PIH lesions refractory to the various treatments, including topical bleaching agents, vitamin C iontophoresis, and laser toning, can be treated with a nonablative 1,540-nm fractional photothermolysis system. Additionally, the 578 and 511 nm copper bromide laser alone or in combination with other treatment modalities can be effectively used for treating PIH. The

511 nm beam is in the green waveband and mainly targets pigmentary lesions, whereas the 578 nm yellow beam mainly targets vascular lesions. As the endothelial cell is one of the important sources of intrinsic pigment regulators as described above, the use of the yellow beam to target vascular structures can be effectively used especially for treating early PIH lesions.

Clinical cases of PIH

Hyperpigmentation related to chronic inflammation such as acne: treatment of the inflammation should be prioritized in the 24-year-old(A) and 21-year-old(B) female seen in Figure 06-1.

Chronic refractory PIH was caused by several cosmetics, ointments and so on.: We should treat the underlying inflammation first, and any vascular and pigmentary skin changes. The

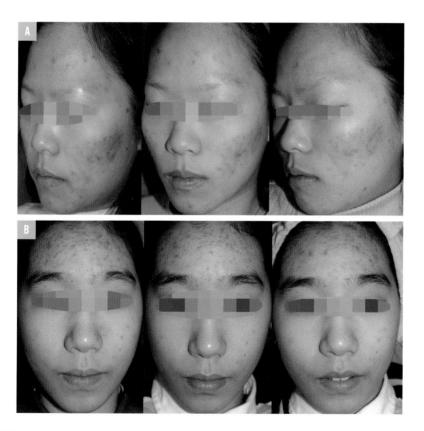

Figure 06-1 **Hyperpigmentation related to acne: Effect of whitening ablation treatment.** With the resolution of the inflammation, the pigmentation decreased.

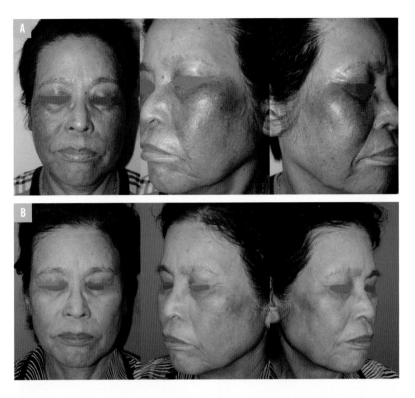

Figure 06-2 **Laser treatment of chronic refractory PIH.** PIH was caused by several cosmetics, ointments and so on.: The patient was satisfied with the combination of the treatment for inflammation, 595-nm pulsed dye laser treatment, triple combination cream treatment and laser toning.

V-beam laser for ecstatic superficial vessels, triple combination cream for hyperpigmentation, laser toning for melanocyte stabilization and dermal rejuvenation, etc (Figure 06-2, 06-3). As high fluence laser treatment for removing the pigment deposited in the PIH lesion involves a high rate of recurrence, it should be used sparingly. In our experience, conventional high fluence treatment should first be used, and then a topical bleaching agent should be applied for at least 2 months. Though the hyperpigmentation can be removed via laser treatment, pigmentation may reoccur rapidly once the epithelization is completed. The recurrence of pigmentation can be considered as being due to the rapid recurrence of inflammation during the healing process. The treatment success depends on the control of this stage. External irritation should be reduced and a skin moisturizer should be used. Any topical preparation that contains steroids should be used only up to 3-7 days.

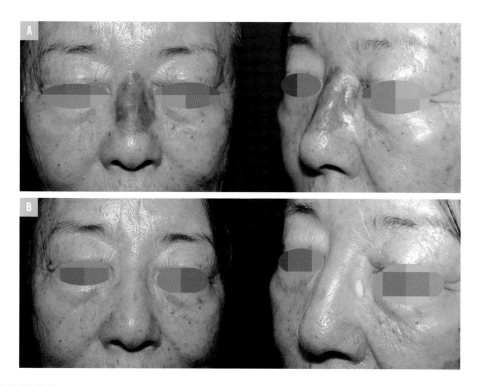

Figure 06-3 **This patient had suffered from PIH of unknown etiology for 20 years.** First, she was treated 8 times with laser toning. After 3 months, 2 treatments were performed with a Q-switched 532 nm laser. A successful result was obtained without recurrence at 1 year.

NOTE

Pigmentation in exposed areas such as the face, or other areas exposed to UV energy, is more severe in summer.

- Points to note with sunscreen: It is important to select a preparation, which will not only block UVA but will also block UVB.
- Some Asian people have very sensitive skin, and need to exercise caution when using a topical preparation that contains hydroquinone. In other words, patients who show symptoms of inflammation due to irritation should stop using the topical preparation, and should use other methods that can reduce inflammation and restore the dermal barrier.
- A silicon gel sheet or spray can be used. The use of these may help protect the skin and remodel the structure of the tissue during the healing process, though the mechanisms of action of this approach have not yet been established.

REFERENCES

1. Ahn HH, Kim IH. Whitening effect of salicylic acid peels in Asian patients. Dermatol Surg 2006;32:372-375.
2. Callender VD, St Surin-Lord S, Davis EC, Maclin M. Postinflammatory hyperpigmentation: etiologic and therapeutic considerations. Am J Clin Dermatol 2011;12:87-99.
3. Chan HH, Manstein D, Yu CS, Shek S, Kono T, Wei WI. The prevalence and risk factors of post-inflammatory hyperpigmentation after fractional resurfacing in Asians. Lasers Surg Med 2007;39:381-385.
4. Cheyasak N, Manuskiatti W, Maneeprasopchoke P, Wanitphakdeedecha R. Topical corticosteroids minimise the risk of postinflammatory hyper-pigmentation after ablative fractional CO2 laser resurfacing in Asians. Acta Derm Venereol 2015;95:201-205.
5. Cho SB, Lee SJ, Kang JM, Kim YK, Chung WS, Oh SH. The efficacy and safety of 10,600-nm carbon dioxide fractional laser for acne scars in Asian patients. Dermatol Surg 2009;35:1955-1961.
6. Cho SB, Lee SJ, Kang JM, Kim YK, Oh SH. Treatment of refractory arcuate hyperpigmentation using a fractional photothermolysis system. J Dermatolog Treat 2010;21:107-108.
7. Greaves MW, Sondergaard J, McDonald-Gibson W. Recovery of prostaglandins in human cutaneous inflammation. Br Med J 1971;2:258–260.
8. Grimes PE. Management of hyperpigmentation in darker racial ethnic groups. Semin cutan Med Surg 2009;28:77-85.
9. Kim BW, Lee MH, Chang SE, Yun WJ, Won CH, Lee MW, Choi JH, Moon KC. Clinical efficacy of the dual-pulsed Q-switched neodymium: yttrium-aluminum-garnet laser: Comparison with conservative mode. J Cosmet Laser Ther 2013;15:340-341.
10. Lacz NL, Vafaie J, Kihiczak NI, Schwartz RA. Postinflammatory hyperpigmentation: a common but troubling condition. Int J Dermatol 2004;43:362-365.
11. Lee HS, Kim IH. Salicylic acid peels for the treatment of acne vulgaris in Asian patients. Dermatol Surg 2003;29:1196-1199.
12. Lee SJ, Choi SY, Park KY. A simple method for predicting postprocedure pigmentation in Asian patients. J Am Acad Dermatol 2013;69:e119-120.
13. Leyden JJ, Shergill B, Micali G, Downie J, Wallo W. Natural options for the management of hyperpigmentation. J Eur Acad Dermatol Venereol 2011;25:1140-1145.
14. Park KY, Choi SY, Mun SK, Kim BJ, Kim MN. Combined treatment with 578-/511-nm copper bromide laser and light-emitting diodes for post-laser pigmentation: a report of two cases. Dermatol Ther 2014;27:121-125.
15. Tomita Y, Maeda K, Tagami H. Melanocyte-stimulating properties of arachidonic acid metabolites: possible role in postinflammatory pigmentation. Pigment Cell Res 1992;5:357–361.
16. Yamaguchi Y, Hearing VJ. Physiological factors that regulate skin pigmentation. Biofactors 2009;35:193-199.

Nevocellular nevus

▶ Jin Soo Kang, MD

Introduction

The term benign melanocytic neoplasia refers to a spectrum of benign tumors consisting of nevomelanocytes, which originate from melanocytes, in the epidermis, dermis, or other structures. Benign melanocytic neoplasms include common acquired nevomelanocytic nevi, congenital nevomelanocytic nevi, halo nevi, nevus spilus, Spitz nevi, pigmented spindle cell nevi, blue nevi, and nodal nevi.

Common acquired nevomelanocytic nevi

Common acquired nevomelanocytic nevi, also known as moles, are the most common form of benign melanocytic neoplasms and are subcategorized into junctional, intradermal, and compound nevi according to the location of their nevomelanocytic nests.

Junctional nevi

Acquired junctional nevi are relatively sharply demarcated, homogeneous dark brown to black macules or papules. They range in size from a few millimeters to more than 2.0 cm, however, the vast majority is are less than 1.0 cm in diameter. In addition, most have a round or oval shape and a uniform surface that may occur anywhere on the skin or visible mucosa.

The nevomelanocytes in junctional nevi present histologically with pale-staining, vacuolated or reticulated nuclei, which are arranged in nests in the epidermis. Retraction artifacts separate the nests of nevomelanocytes from the surrounding epidermal cells.

Intradermal nevi

Intradermal nevi are the most common type of common acquired nevomelanocytic nevi. They can present as smooth, dome-shaped papules, but many comprise papillomatous or polypoid, flexural areas. They are usually flesh-colored or may be slightly pigmented. Coarse hairs may protrude from the surface of the nevus.

Compound nevi

Acquired compound nevi are sharply circumscribed, round, or oval pigmented papules. Their color ranges from tan to dark brown. In some cases they have regular, fine stippling. Dark compound nevi often have a more lightly pigmented border. Their profiles and surface features are more variable than those of junctional or intradermal nevi. Some are only slightly elevated and have flat surfaces. Others are dome-shaped or sessile and have either smooth or papilliferous surfaces. They may also feature coarse hairs.

Nevi versus melanomas

Common acquired nevomelanocytic nevi usually develop during childhood and early adulthood below 30 years of age. Thereafter, the rate of nevus development generally declines and nevus regression begins to appear. Thus, the new or growing nevomelanocytic nevus-like pigmented lesion have a higher risk of being diagnosed as a melanoma in older patients than in younger patients.

Nevi exist in a variety of characteristic forms that must be recognized to distinguish them from malignant melanomas. Nevi vary in size, shape, surface characteristics, and color. The important fact to remember is that each individual nevus tends to remain uniform in color and shape. Although various shades of brown and black may be present in a single lesion, the colors are distributed over the surface in a uniform pattern.

Melanomas consist of malignant pigment cells that grow and extend with little constraint through the epidermis and into the dermis. Such unrestricted growth produces a lesion with a haphazard or disorganized appearance, which varies in shape, color, and surface characteristics.

Examination with a hand lens and dermoscope

Careful inspection of suspicious lesions with a powerful hand lens and dermoscope will reveal a number of features that cannot be appreciated with the naked eye. During inspection, it should be determined if there has been any malignant change. Various dermoscopes can be conveniently used for this purpose (Figure 07-1). In addition, clinicians should keep in mind that there have been reports of malignancy in an area where a nevus had been removed. Malignant changes can be detected by dermoscopes. A dermoscope that can be attached to a smart phone has also been developed, such as FotoFinder Handyscope™ (FotoFinder Systems GmbH, Bad Birnbach, Germany).

Tips for treatment

Pigmented nevi are very common in the Asian population, and most South Koreans have more than one nevus. In South Korea, therefore, removal of a pigmented nevus is a common procedure, and various techniques have been developed. Patients with pigmented nevi, whether their skin color is light or dark, want to remove these when they are located on the face. Patients also wish to have minimal scars after treatment, and to be able to carry out normal activities such as washing the face and putting on makeup. Furthermore, patients want the surgery site to look natural. In addition, patients tend to think that the treatment was not successful or was a failure when the lesion is not removed in one treatment session, and/or if it reappears. Therefore, the treatment should leave no scar or only small scars that look

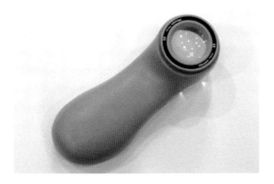
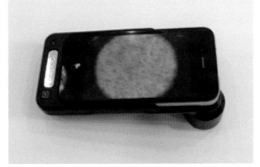

Figure 07-1 Examples of dermoscopes.

natural, and clinicians should explain the possible outcomes to the patients before treatment. In addition, it is recommended that a treatment modality that allows washing of the face and putting on of makeup be chosen, and one that leaves minimal scars and that is not associated with a high rate of recurrence. The carbon dioxide (CO_2) laser is the most frequently used laser for nevus removal. Erbium-doped yttrium aluminum garnet (Er:YAG), long-pulse alexandrite, long-pulse neodymium-doped yttrium aluminum garnet (Nd:YAG), and long-pulse ruby lasers are also used for lesion removal.

▌ Nevus removal using the CO_2 laser

The continuous mode of the CO_2 laser is not safe because in this mode, it is difficult to achieve the right depth of coagulation in the skin, and because this laser mode can cause scars. As such, the continuous mode of the CO_2 laser is rarely used for nevus removal. On the other hand, by using the ultrapulsed and superpulsed (quasi-continuous) modes of the CO_2 laser, the laser/tissue interaction can be controlled more easily, and better outcomes are obtained. To use the CO_2 laser in the proper manner, the spot size and the expected laser-tissue interaction should first be considered. Laser vaporization, a mode between laser excision and coagulation, usually produces good outcomes due to a clean view of the irradiated site and the absence of bleeding (Figure 07-2).

A laser vaporization mode which is closer to the excision mode, i.e., with a smaller spot size, is used when a lesion is located deep in the skin, whereas a laser vaporization mode,

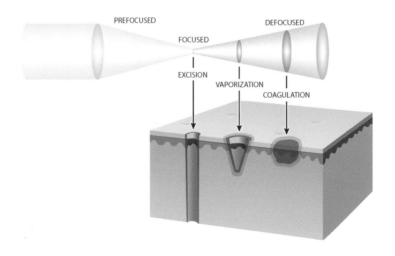

Figure 07-2   Spot size and tissue effect (supplement from Lutronic Corp.).

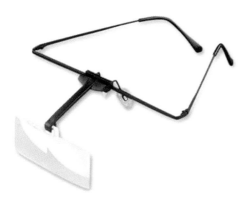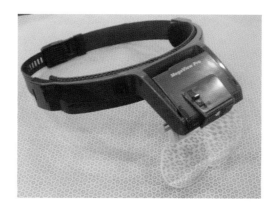

Figure 07-3   A loupe and a magnifier

which is closer to the coagulation mode i.e., with a larger spot size, is used when a lesion is larger and shallow. When these methods are employed, it is important to use a loupe or a magnifier to be able to observe even the minute characteristics of the lesion and the appearance of normal architecture (Figure 07-3).

The relationship between the beam size and the power of the laser should also be considered for proper treatment. The power per unit area, the irradiance or power density, is higher with a smaller beam size at the same laser power, and the laser thus penetrates deeper into the skin. On the other hand, for the same output power as above but with a larger spot size, the power density drops dramatically. There is an inverse square ratio between spot size and power density for the same output power: doubling the spot size cuts the power density by 4, but a spot size 4 times smaller increases the power density 16-fold. A beam with a lower power density will therefore create a more shallow effect in the target tissue. Therefore, the laser beam spot size should be appropriately selected to obtain the desirable power density, which is measured in W/cm^2. The laser vaporization mode causes thermal necrosis in the tissues that immediately underlies the target area (Figure 07-4). With low power densities but long irradiation times, a large area of thermal necrosis occurs, which can lead to major scar formation. A laser beam at a low power density can vaporize only thin layers of tissue and requires a higher number of passes to remove skin of a given thickness. The heat from this is conducted to the underlying tissues causing residual thermal damage, thus inducing thermal necrosis.

A good outcome with less thermal necrosis and minimal scar formation can thus be obtained by using a laser at a higher power density that requires fewer passes to ablate tissue more rapidly thus removing the nevi fast, with minimal residual thermal damage. In addition, to prevent scar development in the normal tisses adjacent to the target tissue, the exposure

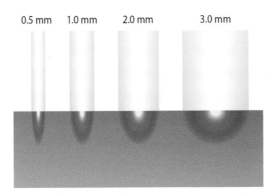

0.5 mm   1.0 mm   2.0 mm   3.0 mm

Figure 07-4 Spot size and tissue effect for the same incident laser power (supplement from Lutronic Corp.).

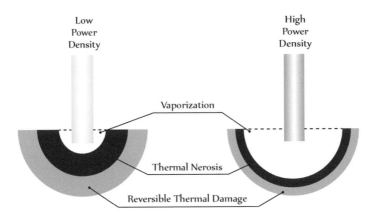

Low Power Density   High Power Density

Vaporization

Thermal Nerosis

Reversible Thermal Damage

Figure 07-5 Thermal effect and power density (supplement from Lutronic Corp.).

time of the laser energy on the target should be limited to within the thermal relaxation time of these tissues (Table 07-1).

Low power densities result in less vaporization of, and greater necrosis around a lesion, thus leaving char. Because the lesion is not neatly removed, the operation field needs to be cleaned off to determine the status of the nevus removal. Scrubbing removes the tissues with thermal necrosis and exposes and removes the underlying area with reversible thermal damage, leading to oozing. Some form of dressing is required to control the oozing, and bigger depressed scars can develop (Figure 07-6).

In contrast, a laser delivering a high power density results in greater vaporization and less thermal necrosis, and clinicians can thus more easily determine if the nevus cells have been

Table 07-1	Thermal Relaxation Time of Some Potential Targets
Target	**Thermal Relaxation Time**
Erythrocyte	2 µm
200 µm hair follicle	40 ms
0.5 µm melanosome	0.25 µs
10 µm nevus cell	0.1 µm
0.1 mm diameter vessel	10 ms
0.4 mm diameter vessel	80 ms
0.8 mm diameter vessel	300 ms

Data from Goldman MP: Cutaneous and Laser Surgery, page 9

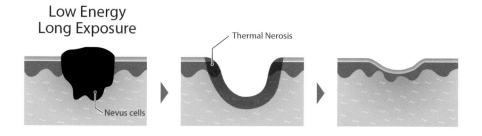

| Figure 07-6 | Thermal damage and scar caused by a laser beam with a low power density and a long exposure time (supplement from Lutronic Corp.).

completely removed. More precise laser treatment can be performed with less scar development when a magnifying lens with higher than 2-3× power is used, because cleaning off charred tissue will not be required, thus eliminating the risk of oozing and the need for dressing (Figure 07-7).

Scar development can be unavoidable if the nevus is large and is located deep in the skin, but the margin of a scar can be managed to an artificial-line appearance or a natural-line appearance (Figure 07-8). An artificial line is very visible whereas a natural line can look natural, as if it were only a pimple mark, because a natural line has an irregular border. A natural appearance is characterized by irregular shaped margins, but an artificial appearance is characterized by straight lines or round shapes, which are more eye-catching (Figure 07-8). A naturally formed line looks like a straight line that is in fact irregular while an artificial line is very straight, thus being very prominent.

To conclude, when a CO_2 laser is used for pigmented-nevus removal, it is recommended that the vaporization mode with a high power density and a short exposure time be used.

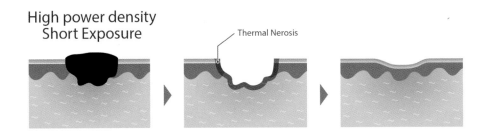

High power density Short Exposure

Thermal Nerosis

Figure 07-7 Thermal damage and scar caused by a laser beam with a high power density and a short exposure time (supplement from Lutronic Corp.).

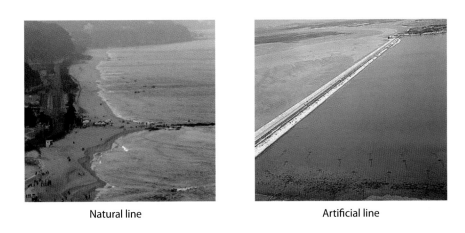

Natural line

Artificial line

Figure 07-8 The appearance of a natural line versus an artificial line in nature.

During surgery, dermatologists should carefully observe the lesion using a magnifying lens, and should limit the irradiation time to within the relaxation time of the surrounding tissues to eliminate the need for scrubbing and to achieve a natural-looking border. It is advised that dressing be avoided. For example, a nevus can be easily removed by quickly passing a 1.4-1.8 W quasi-continuous (superpulsed) laser (frequency: 40-60 Hz; width: 400 µs; on-time: 0.01-0.05/sec; off-time: 0.01-0.05/sec) over the lesion at an appropriate spot size.

Nevus removal using the Er:YAG laser

The Er:YAG laser can ablate tissue precisely but can easily cause bleeding because laser co-agulation is minimal due to the small amount of residual thermal damage left in the tissue. Therefore, the Er:YAG laser should be used very carefully for removing a nevus located in

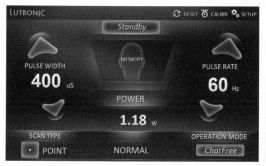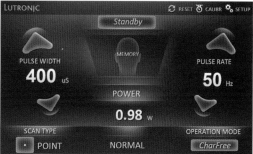

Figure 07-9 Examples of CO_2 laser settings.

the deep dermis, although it can very effectively remove a nevus located in the upper dermis. This drawback has been offset by the recent development of a laser with a dual ablation/co-agulation mode which combines both a CO_2 and long-pulsed Nd:YAG laser in the one system (Figure 07-9).

Important general considerations

- Characteristics of the Asian skin: The Asian skin is prone to scar development because the dermis tends to be thick. Therefore, it is important to use a magnifying lens or loupe to as-certain the precise removal of nevus cells.
- Overtreatment should be avoided. If multiple treatment sessions are necessary, dermatolo-gists should try to reduce the chances of scar development.

Tips for post-treatment care and follow-up

It is recommended that the wounded area be left open after treatment. Some form of dress-ing is required on an oozing wound, but a dressing is not recommended if a laser with a very high power density has been used with quick passes over the lesion.

Applying a 0.3% aluminum solution two to three times a day promotes fast crust for-mation. Patients should be taught that crusts are natural biological dressings under which optimal wound healing occurs. Crusts usually come off spontaneously around seven to ten days after the laser treatment. This process should happen naturally, and crusts should not be pulled off using force or by scrubbing, otherwise reepithelization will be delayed with possible adverse side effects including scar formation or secondary hyperpigmentation.

Important points

- It is important to prevent inflammation after laser treatment of the Asian skin because Asians are very prone to developing tissue inflammation and resultant postinflammatory hyperpigmentation (PIH). Inflammation is almost always followed by PIH in Asians. Therefore, the use of topical antibiotics and dressing in ointment forms should be avoided. Instead, water-based topical antibiotics and dressing are recommended.
- Heavy cleansing is not recommended after crust formation, although light makeup is allowed.

REFERENCES

1. Mitchel P, Goldman. Cutaneous and Cosmetic Laser Surgery. Elsevier; 2006.
2. Randall K, Roenigk, et al. Dermatologic Surgery - Principles and Practice : Second Edition. CRC Press;1996:947-976.
3. Text Book compliation committee of Korean Dermatological Association: Skin Science:Rev.3;418.

Seborrheic keratosis

Jin Soo Kang, MD

Introduction

Seborrheic keratoses are benign tumors that resemble warts and that develop on the faces and/ or trunks of middle-aged men and women. The cause of seborrheic keratoses is unclear, but it is suspected that they originate from keratinocytes whose differentiation process has stopped. Some cases are inherited through an autosomal-dominant inheritance mode and are related with weight gain, exfoliative erythroderma, or an inflammatory skin disease.

Seborrheic keratoses appear with a tan or black color and in papules or disks with clear borders. They are usually very small, rarely larger than 3 cm in diameter. The surfaces resemble a wart. As a lesion develops, the color darkens, and the surface thickens and accumulates oily and scaly crusts. When the crusts are removed, a moist basal layer becomes visible. Seborrheic keratoses develop on seborrheic areas such as the chest and abdominal region, but they also develop on the face, neck, and extremities. They are not observed on the palms and soles. They develop in patients in their 40's and 50's, and there is no difference in the prevalence between men and women. Women usually develop seborrheic keratoses during menopause. There are few subjective symptoms, but patients may feel an itchy sensation.

Tips for diagnosis

A diagnosis can be easily made based on the characteristics of a lesion and its surrounding area. A seborrheic keratosis is either smooth and has tiny, round, and embedded peals, or is rough, dry, cracked, and stuck onto the epidermis. Its color varies from brown to black. The margins of a lesion have a circumscribed border.

Most dermatologists can make an accurate diagnosis by observing the lesion, but biopsy is recommended if the dermatologist cannot be certain. Seborrheic keratoses should be differentially diagnosed from melanomas, which have a smooth surface and are malignant, and from actinic keratoses, which are characterized by squamous erythema with an unclear border and by the development of dark spots on an exposed lesion.

Tips for treatment

Seborrheic keratosis removal using a carbon dioxide (CO_2) laser

The CO_2 laser is used for seborrheic-keratosis removal in a similar way as it is used for the removal of a pigmented nevus where the incident power density is set to give mainly a vaporization mode, but for seborrheic keratosis the laser is set closer to the coagulation mode. In the case of thick lesions, the vaporization mode is used for the removal of most of the lesion and then the coagulation mode is used to irradiate the remaining area. Crusts will then form which function as a biologic dressing. It is important not to scrub off the tissue that is left behind after using the coagulation mode. If left alone, this tissue will form crusts that will come off in 7-14 days, thus minimizing the development of postinflammatory hyperpigmentation (PIH) or post-therapy erythema. If this tissue is scrubbed off, some form of dressing will be required due to the occurrence of oozing, and more severe and long-lasting PIH and erythema can develop. It is possible to misjudge the thickness of a lesion and to leave some parts of it behind. In this case, dermatologists may want to scrub and see the base of the lesion to confirm the thickness. It is recommended, however, to wait for about two months before removing the remaining lesion in the next treatment session rather than cause PIH (Figures 08-1 and 08-2). When the lesion is irradiated in the coagulation mode, crusts will form and will function as a biologic dressing. Full recovery will then be faster because only a small amount of erythema will remain after the crusts come off.

Seborrheic keratosis treated with an erbium-doped yttrium aluminum garnet (Er:YAG) laser

The Er:YAG laser is a good choice for precisely ablating only the epidermal component if the lesion is thin. For a precise view of the treated area, the use of a magnifying lens or loupe is recommended. If the blood vessels of the dermis are damaged by the Er:YAG beam, coagulation is minimal and bleeding will occur, which can be used to determine whether the laser has reached the dermis, and which can be a reference for adequate treatment. Ideally, howev-

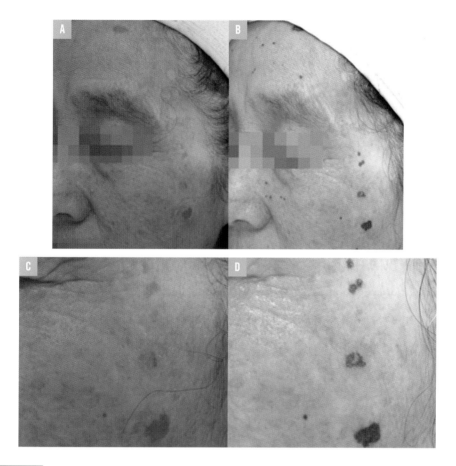

Figure 08-1   **Treatment of seborrheic keratoses using carbon dioxide (CO_2) laser. A.** before treatment. **B.** 8 days after treatment. **C.** Another case before treatment. **D.** 8 days after treatment.

er, the treatment should be stopped before bleeding occurs. When the laser penetrates to the dermis, coagulation will not occur, thus leading to oozing. Therefore, some form of dressing is not necessary when only the epidermis has been ablated, but it becomes necessary when dermal ablation has occurred with oozing. To offset this drawback, a long-pulsed Er:YAG laser set to the coagulation mode, or an Er:YAG laser can be used in combination with a CO_2 laser set to achieve coagulation.

Seborrheic keratosis removal using a combination of Er:YAG and CO_2 lasers

If there is oozing from a surgery site after Er-YAG irradiation, a CO_2 laser in coagulation mode can be used to stop the oozing. This also eliminates the need for any form of surgical dressing (Figure 08-3).

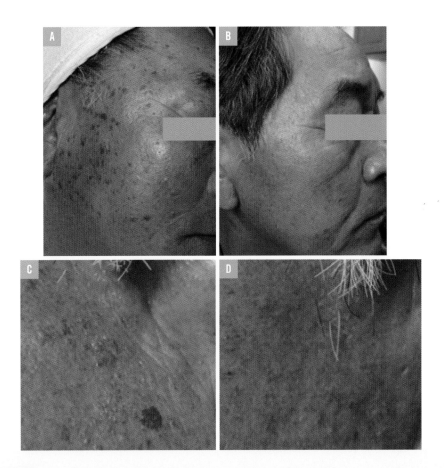

Figure 08-2 **Treatment of seborrheic keratoses using CO$_2$ laser. A.** before treatment. **B.** 15 days after treatment. **C.** Another case before treatment. **D.** 15 days after treatment.

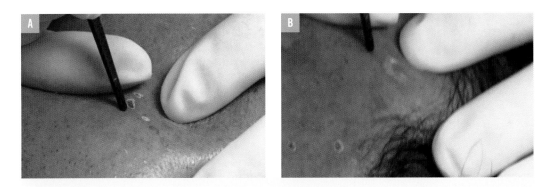

Figure 08-3 **Treatment of seborrheic keratoses using erbium-doped yttrium aluminum garnet (Er:YAG) and CO$_2$ laser. A.** A case treated with Er:YAG laser alone without remarkable lesional oozing. **B.** If there is lesional oozing after Er:YAG treatment, a CO$_2$ laser in coagulation mode can be combined to stop the oozing.

Seborrheic keratosis removal using frequency-doubled Q-switched neodymium-doped yttrium aluminum garnet (Nd:YAG), alexandrite, and ruby lasers

A 532 nm Q-switched frequency-doubled Nd:YAG laser (spot size, 3-4 mm; fluence, 1.0-2.0 J/cm^2) is passed over the lesion once or twice until the lesion is frosted. If the lesion is thick, the laser energy can be increased or another treatment session can be held following healing. A similar approach is used with the ruby and alexandrite lasers.

Seborrheic keratosis removal using long-pulsed lasers

The long-pulsed lasers, including the 755-nm long-pulsed alexandrite laser, 595-nm pulsed dye laser, and 532-nm potassium titanyl phosphate (KTP) laser, deliver pulse widths of microseconds to milliseconds. Although Q-switched lasers are the most widely used devices, long-pulsed lasers also have been effectively used in the treatment of epidermal pigmentary lesions, including freckles, lentigines, and seborrheic keratoses with satisfactory therapeutic outcomes. Additionally, long-pulsed lasers can reportedly reduce the risk of PIH compared to Q-switched lasers. The longer pulse widths of the laser devices treat the target pigments through photothermolysis only, whereas Q-switched lasers, delivering high energy with ultrashort pulses in the nanosecond, produce both photothermal and photomechanical effects on both target pigments and adjacent vascular structures.

When using a 755-nm long-pulsed alexandrite laser, the use of 3-5-msec or a shorter pulse width compared to the 20-, 40-, and 60-msec and laser fluences of 35 to 50 J/cm^2 is generally recommended. When using a 532-nm long-pulsed KTP laser, a pulse duration of 2 msec and a fluence of 9-12 J/cm^2 or a pulse duration of 10-12 msec and a fluence of 15-18 J/cm^2 can be used for the treatment of epidermal pigmented lesions. However, adjustment of treatment parameters should be made according to the individual device and patient/lesion characteristics.

NOTE

- Overtreatment should be avoided in Asian skin due to its high pigment content, and propensity for PIH formation.
- The risk of PIH increases due to severe inflammation, especially if the laser is used at high power densities.

Tips for post-treatment care and follow-up

The risk of PIH can be decreased by applying an alum solution or a water-based moisturizer as post-treatment care because it helps crusts come off easily. If an appropriate sunscreen is regularly and routinely used after the crusts come off, even and normal distribution of skin pigmentation will be achieved.

> **NOTE**
>
> When severe erythema develops or persists for a long time after the crusts come off, the risk of PIH development increases. In this case, post-treatment care using the pulsed dye or copper laser or LED phototherapy is recommended.

REFERENCES

1. Kim YK, Kim DY, Lee SJ, Chung WS, Cho SB. Therapeutic efficacy of long-pulsed 755-nm alexandrite laser for seborrheic keratoses. J Eur Acad Dermatol Venereol 2014;28:1007-1011.
2. Mitchel P, Goldman. Cutaneous and Cosmetic Laser Surgery. Elsevier;2006:1-30.
3. Randall K. Roenigk, et al : Dermatologic Surgery - Principles and Practice : Second Edition. CRC Press;1996:865-879.
4. Text Book compliation committee of Korean Dermatological Association. Skin Science;Rev.3;418.
5. Thomas P, Habif. Clinical Dermatology - A Color Guide to Diagnosis and Therapy : 5th ed. Elsevier;2009:776-781.

09

Café-au-lait macule / Nevus spilus / Becker's nevus / Lentiginosis

▷ Un Cheol Yeo, MD, PhD

Introduction

Brown macules

The skin consists of the external epidermis and the inner dermis. The dermis supports the skin. Its major components are collagen, elastic fibers, and mucopolysaccharides. The epidermis consists of epidermal cells, melanocytes, and immunocytes. Of these, melanocytes protect the skin from ultraviolet rays by producing melanic pigment. The activity of melanocytes varies by ethnicity (e.g., more melanin is produced in Mongoloids and blacks than in whites). The amount of melanic pigment is generally normal, though it varies between skin types.

Brown macules are clearly defined and large or small brown spots on the skin. In a brown macule, the amount of pigment is larger than in normal skin. A brown macule wherein melanin increases mostly in the epidermis can be differentiated from a locus ceruleus wherein melanin increases in the dermis. The typical finding with respect to brown macules is the increased production of melanin due to abnormal melanocytes in the epidermis. In brown macules, it is presumed that an anomaly exists not only under the epidermis but even in the dermis, because though brown macules are believed to be easily cured, they are actually not easily cured via treatment such as treatment with a pigment-specific laser. As such, the pathological phenomenon of brown macules remains unclear. Some researchers refer to the dermis and epidermis with a brown macule as "a garden of abnormal melanocytes."

Types of brown macule

Café-au-lait spot

A café-au-lait spot is a brown macule with a café au lait color. It can occur anywhere in the skin. It is commonly found at birth or in childhood. If untreated, it sometimes becomes larger or thicker. If café-au-lait spots are large and many, chances are that they constitute neurofibromatosis, from which neurofibromas will develop after adolescence.

Nevus spilus

The lesion known as nevus spilus is a macule with a café-au-lait spot-like background. In some cases, if there are nearly no spots or if they have not been formed yet, the macule is first considered to be a café-au-lait spot and is later diagnosed as nevus spilus when the spots are formed.

Becker's nevus

This occurs frequently in the shoulder or chest areas and mostly in adolescence. Unlike other brown macules, almost all forms of Becker's nevus have hair. Some cases of Becker's nevus are first diagnosed as café-au-lait spots when there is no hair, but are later re-diagnosed as being Becker's nevus when hair grows from them. Becker's nevus proliferates in the epidermis as well as in the dermis, often resulting in an uneven dermal surface.

Agminated lentiginosis

This occurs when a large group of small spots, such as freckles, are formed in a small area. If it occurs on the face, it can be confused with nevus of Ota, a type of locus ceruleus. If the color of the agminated lentiginosis is similar to that of a café-au-lait spot, it is nevus spilus. Agminated lentiginosis is a group of agminated lentigines without a brown macule in the background.

Diagnosis tips - café-au-lait spot

How to distinguish a café-au-lait spot

A café-au-lait spot is a darker brown macule than the normal surrounding skin color. Its color varies from slightly darker than the neighboring skin color to very dark. In newborn infants, its diameter is 0.2-4 cm, and it becomes larger in proportion to the skin area as the patient grows. In adults, its diameter is 2-5 cm on average, with the diameter of the smallest spot 0.2 cm and the largest, 20 cm or more. In some cases, the diameter is much greater than 20 cm, and can nearly cover an entire arm.

The lesion may be distinctly or indistinctly demarcated. In some cases, one side of the lesion is distinctly demarcated and the other side is not. The shape of the lesion varies from circular to square or irregular. The lesion sometimes appears as a lump or as separate spots in one area. The interior color of the lesion is commonly uniform café au lait but is sometimes dark brown. The histological finding concerning the café-au-lait spot is an increased melanic pigment in the epidermis without an increase in the number of melanocytes.

When does a café-au-lait spot appear?

Café-au-lait spots are congenital, meaning they occur mostly at birth or immediately after birth. They are commonly left unnoticed for several months if they are light-colored due to their non-exposure to ultraviolet rays because the person stays indoors or because the skin is still reddish. Over time, the number of spots increases and the spots thicken. Café-au-lait spots were reportedly found at birth and before 1 year of age in 43% and 63% of all confirmed cases of neurofibromatosis, respectively.

Does a café-au-lait spot become larger if untreated?

In some cases, the café-au-lait spot grows in number after it is first detected. The number commonly increases in adolescence, although it may also increase in childhood. Even if the number does not increase, the café-au-lait spot becomes larger as the child grows. If a café-au-lait spot that was once observed below the elbow subsequently appears to have expanded to above the elbow, it should be considered that the lesion has grown disproportionately more than the person's age would merit. As the patient becomes an adult, the café-au-lait spot often becomes thicker, although it may become faint.

What is the incidence rate of café-au-lait spots?

The incidence rate was reported to be 12% in non-Caucasian newborns and 0.8% in Caucasian newborns. The incidence rate in normal adults was reported to be 10-20%. Café-au-lait spots are so common that even the author and his second son have café-au-lait spots. Ninety-eight percent of normal adults with café-au-lait spots have three or fewer lesions, and in rare cases, some people have four or more lesions.

Nevus spilus

What is nevus spilus?

Nevus spilus is also called speckled lentiginous nevus. It appears to be a group of spots with café-au-lait spots in the background. It has light brown macules and some scattered darker brown macules. The background is very thick brown so that in some cases, the macules do not stand out well. Some people are first diagnosed as having café-au-lait spots and later re-diagnosed as having nevus spilus when spots form. Nevus spilus may rarely appear at birth, but occurs mostly in infancy. Although black spots sometimes occur together with brown macules, in general, brown macules occur first and then black spots occur later. There was a report that black spots occurred several years or decades later. The black spots may protrude slightly. Generally, the nevus spilus lesion is 1 to 20 cm in diameter, commonly occurs in the abdomen and back, but can also occur in the face, legs, and arms.

Becker's nevus

What is Becker's nevus?

The American dermatologist Becker first gave his name to this disease in 1949. It is a type of brown macule accompanied by hairy brown macules. It appears mostly in adolescence but also at birth or infancy. In many cases, the brown macule appears light-colored but gradually becomes darker. One to 2 years after its onset, it often becomes darker and sometimes becomes slightly lighter when patients reach middle age. Its diameter is generally about 10-20 cm. The lesion border is often irregular yet distinctly demarcated. Hair often grows and thickens over time rather than from the start. Becker's nevus can occur anywhere on the skin. It has been reported that 45% of cases of Becker's nevus occur in the chest and shoulders. It is a common disorder in males, occurring in one out of every 200 men.

Why does the surface of Becker's nevus become uneven?

In many cases of Becker's nevus, in addition to the increase in the brown pigment, the surface becomes slightly uneven over time because of perifolliculitis, which is a form of acne that is due to congestion and clogging of the follicles and thickening of the smooth dermal muscle. Unlike other brown macules, Becker's nevus can be felt with one's eyes closed.

When it is laser-treated at an early stage, its surface becomes uneven over time. Although this uneven surface is sometimes misunderstood as a side effect of laser treatment, the surface of Becker's nevus naturally becomes uneven over time even if untreated. Differential diagnosis is required between serious cases of Becker's nevus and smooth muscle hamartoma.

Does Becker's nevus have much hair from the beginning?

In many cases, hair gradually appears and thickens rather than being obvious from the start. Some people with Becker's nevus do not have hair on the macule at all. Generally, Becker's nevus in men has a great deal of hair, although hair is not found in all cases of Becker's nevus.

The dermatologists can witness patients whose Becker's nevus was originally diagnosed as a café-au-lait spot that appeared in their childhood, but then hair began to grow in the lesion. If the lesion has been treated with laser, then in this case parents or guardians can naturally think that the hair is a side effect of laser treatment. Thus, when there is no hair even if Becker's nevus is suspected, the physician should, before initiating the laser treatment, inform the patient's parents that hair may grow later as part of the disease progression. Other studies reported that about 50% of all cases of Becker's nevus have hair.

What is the possible co-morbidity of Becker's nevus?

There are some reported cases, though rare, that Becker's nevus was accompanied by acne in the lesions, a smaller breast on the affected side, and a musculoskeletal anomaly on the affected side.

When does Becker's nevus occur?

It occurs mostly in adolescence, but can also appear at birth or in infancy.

Agminated lentiginosis

What is agminated lentiginosis?

Agminated lentiginosis is also called agminated lentigines (lentiginosis), partial unilateral lentiginosis (PUL), and unilateral lentigines. Close observation of agminated lentiginosis will reveal that multiple lesions resembling lentigines are clustered together in close proximity to form the agminated lentiginosis. A lentigo is about 2-10 mm in diameter. It can occur anywhere on the skin, and when it occurs at the site where nevus of Ota occurs frequently, it is sometimes confused with nevus of Ota. Agminated lentiginosis mostly appears at birth or in infancy, and studies have shown that it has been found at up to about 15 years of age. It is often distinctly demarcated, and its distribution frequently does not exceed the midline of the body. Its distributional patterns are segmental (limited to an area), dermatomal (along the sensory nerves), curvilinear (in curved lines), and swirled (having a swirl pattern).

What is the difference between café-au-lait spots, agminated lentiginosis, and nevus spilus?

A café-au-lait spot is a macule that appears as a lump rather than a cluster of small lentigines. Agminated lentiginosis is a cluster of small macules such as freckles. An agminated lentiginosis that has café-au-lait-spot-like colors in the background can be considered as a nevus spilus. A lesion that does not have such brown macules in the background but has small clustered lentigines is true agminated lentiginosis.

Can lentiginosis and nevus of Ota be confused?

It is always easy to diagnose these diseases differentially if they are in their typical forms. If they have exceptional features, however, they are commonly confused. Some cases of lentiginosis occur around the eyes and have ocular symptoms. These cases of lentiginosis can be easily confused with nevus of Ota. As lentiginosis is an epidermal disease, and nevus of Ota is a dermal disease, a wrong diagnosis leads to wrong treatment methods and treatment failure. Lentiginosis around the eyes and nevus of Ota require particular precautions. Figure 09-1 shows a case of lentiginosis around the eyes, and because it is accompanied by ocular symptoms, it could be more easily confused with nevus of Ota.

Treatment tips

Laser treatment or surgery?

A brown macule is not easily cured, even with laser treatment. At the beginning of the 1990's, treatment with pigment-specific lasers was heavily commercialized, using such laser

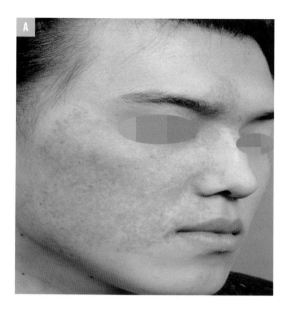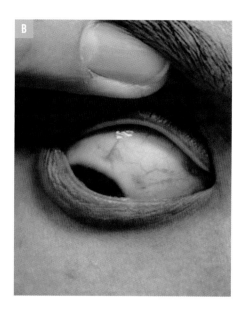

Figure 09-1   A case of agminated lentiginosis confused with nevus of Ota. (**A**) Multiple lentigines on the right side of the face, primarily in a V1-3 distribution. (**B**) Discrete area of brown pigmentation on right medial bulbar conjunctiva. (Kim EH, Kang HY. Eur J Dermatol. 2006)

systems as the high-powered argon (especially the 514.5 nm band), potassium titanyl phosphate (KTP) 532 (532 nm) or pulsed dye laser (580-590 nm). Because of the specificity of these wavelengths for melanin, laser treatment was frequently performed for brown macules with the expectation that it would be a good treatment option, but the result was often very disappointing. Nearly all the brown macules relapsed after the laser treatment. Since then, whenever a new laser treatment method was introduced, it was actively used to treat brown macules but the results have been generally poor. Thereafter, the development of new treatment methods for pigmented lesions using laser tailed off. However, since 1995, researchers have been attempting to successfully treat brown macules using laser but with different approaches, and they found that repeated treatments were effective and some wavelengths more effective than others.

As the successful and total removal of brown macules still presents a problem, however, patients sometimes ask about the possibility of surgery. Surgical treatments include excision and filling the excised site with a skin graft mobilized from neighboring skin, tissue expansion, and skin grafting using remote autologous skin. For large brown macules, however, no surgical treatment has achieved a better aesthetic outcome than that of laser treatment. Thus, surgical treatment is never recommended in these cases.

Laser treatment of brown macules

Treatment with specific lasers is now widely used for brown macules. Laser treatment of pigmented lesions is currently performed with a Q-switched laser, including the neodymium-doped yttrium aluminum garnet (Nd:YAG), alexandrite, and the ruby lasers. Intense pulsed light (IPL), the carbon dioxide (CO_2) laser, and the erbium:YAG (Er:YAG) laser are also used. Recently, treatments using a fractional laser, long-pulsed Nd:YAG, long-pulsed alexandrite, and the micropulsed 1444 nm AccuSculpt system (Lutronic Corp., South Korea) have been introduced.

Here is an important tip. Once the patient or their parents have identified a physician to treat that particular patient, it is recommended that the patient receive treatment using the laser which that physician routinely uses. In other words, the identification of the treating clinician should precede the laser selection, and the laser selection should rest with the physician. Treatment of brown macules is very sensitive and requires minute adjustments to the parameters, and a physician can thus achieve treatment success only when he or she uses the laser that he or she has been using every day for several years. For example, the author has 3 Nd:YAG laser systems, the minute adjustment methods of each of which differ.

Standard treatment methods

Brown macules are treated with lasers using a general approach. However, it is important to note that not all treatments are the same, and all patients are individuals. Inappropriate treatments, even though repeated, cannot produce successful outcomes. Appropriate treatments are as follows.

First, the lesion should be seen to have disappeared when the crust falls off after the laser treatment. If the lesion does not disappear even temporarily, repeated treatment is of no use. Appropriate whitening should follow the treatment so that the lesion may disappear after the crust falls off. The degree of the lightening of the lesion should be decided based on experience. Too strong whitening is highly likely to cause hypopigmentation, but too weak lightening is likely to leave a brown color without temporary disappearance of the lesion even when the crust falls off after the treatment.

Second, the treatment interval is important. After a good treatment, the lesion will temporarily disappear, and within about two months, the brown color will generally reappear. When the brown color reappears, retreatment should be initiated immediately. Delayed treatment will result in a poor outcome. If only the treatment effect is considered, a treatment interval of shorter than two months may seem better, but it is highly likely to cause a scar. For skin restoration with the treatment of brown macules, a two-month interval with a total of three

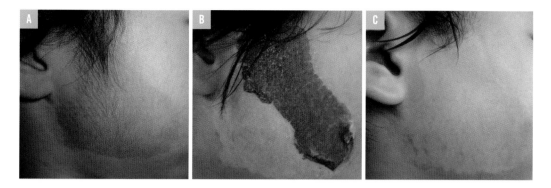

Figure 09-2   **An example of a propely treated cafe-au-lait macule. A.** The pre-treatment lesion on the Rt. mandibu-lar area. **B.** Some of the crust fell off and some did not. In the curst off area, there is erythema but no cafe-au-lait macule. **C.** When the erythema has gone completely, it is clearly seen that cafe-au-lait macule is removed temporarily, and the color of the treated lesion is brighter than the surrounding skin. The hypopigmentation is temporary and the brown macule recurs.

to four treatment sessions is appropriate. Figure 09-2 shows an example of a well-treated lesion. Figure 09-2A shows the pre-treatment lesion, and Figure 09-2B shows that some of the crust had fallen off and some did not. In Figure 09-2C, where the crust has completely fallen off, the brown macules have completely disappeared, though only temporarily.

Importance of early treatment

The importance of early treatment of brown macules cannot be overemphasized. Figure 09-2A shows that the brown macules in the abdomen, chest, and arms of a child have been nearly completely cured, whereas the treatment outcome of the brown macules in the arms of an adult is poor (Figure 09-3B). Brown macules are more easily cured in children than in adults. The author recommends that the treatment be started as early as two or three months after birth. The treatment outcomes during the neonatal period and at 1 year old differ. The earlier the treatment is, the better the outcome will be.

Individual differences in treatment response

The responses to and the effects of laser treatment greatly vary between individuals. It is, however, difficult to identify who will be well cured. Only after several treatment sessions are performed will it be possible to identify who will be well cured and who will not be. It was reported that generally, certain lesions are easily curable and others, not. The author believes that individual differences and the age at which the treatment is performed are the

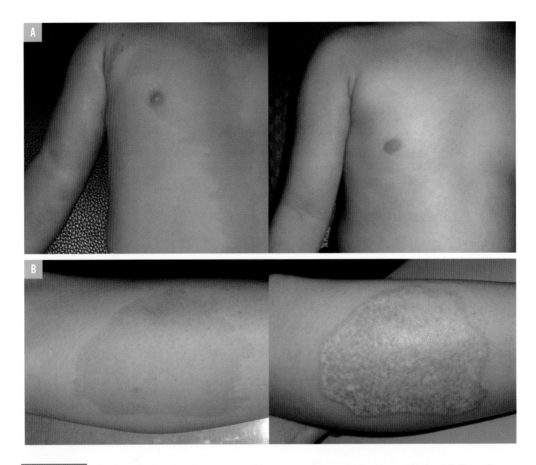

Figure 09-3 **The importance of early treatment of brown macules cannot be overemphasized. A.** It can be seen that the brown macules in the abdomen, chest, and arms of a child have been nearly completely cured, when it is treated in the early stage. **B.** the treatment outcome of the brown macules in the arms of an adult is poor. With repeated treatment the lesion shows peripheral hyperpigmentation, uneven coloration with spots of both hyper- and hypopigmentation.

most important factors. That is, the earlier the treatment is, the better the lesion cure will be.

Before treatment initiation, patients are most curious about how many treatment sessions are required for brown macules to disappear; if the brown macules will completely disappear and if not, how much will the color decrease in intensity; and if side effects will occur. These are called the prognosis. In the case of brown macules, however, a prognosis cannot always be made before treatment. That is, before treatment, it is impossible to identify who will be well cured and who will not be. Although there are several prognostic factors, the prognosis can be predicted only after several treatment sessions, as individual differences can significantly influence the outcome very strongly. The adult patient shown in Figure 09-4 has a large café-au-lait spot in his face. In this patient, the café-au-lait spot was cured after only

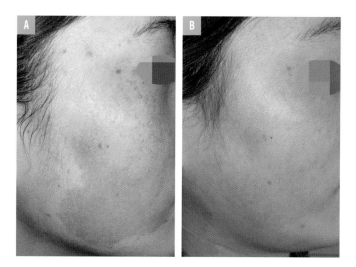

Figure 09-4   **The adult patient has a large café-au-lait spot on her face. A.** is before treatment. **B.** 18 months after 2nd treatment (1.4 J/cm², 532 nm, VRM). The lesion shows nearly complete remission and no recurrence.

two treatment sessions, which is unlike the general treatment progress of other large café-au-lait spots. It is quite clear that, in this patient, it was impossible to predict if the lesion would be well cured in such a short period.

Darkening of the demarcation line after the treatment of brown macules

In some cases, the demarcation area of brown macules darkens. This pigmentation normally disappears within three to six months. This phenomenon is commonly considered attributed to the failure to treat the demarcation area of brown macules. In most cases, however, even if the entire lesion has been treated it is attributed to the particularly high production of pigments in the demarcation area in the course of the wound healing process after the crust falls off, although there may be cases when the demarcation area has not actually been treated because it was faint. When melanocytes in the lesion die due to laser treatment, the brown macules attempt to restore the lesion. One way by which the lesion is restored is when melanocytes and associated pigments migrate back up into the lesion through the follicles. First, the pigments gather around the treatment site to form black spots around the follicles; then some time later, melanocytes and associated pigments migrate up through the follicles, and are consequently deposited in the entire treatment site.

Another way by which the brown macules restore the treatment site is when melanocytes migrate from the demarcation area, darkening the treatment site. At this time in some patients, if melanocytes in the demarcation area produce a large amount of pigments before

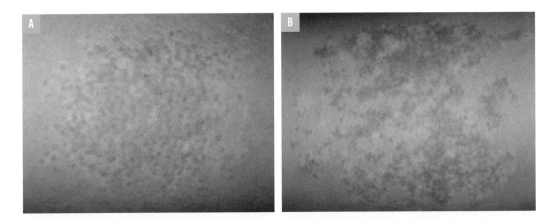

Figure 09-5 **Irregular dyspigmentation after laser treatment. A.** After laser treatment, café au lait macule showed irregular dyspigmentation showing spots of slightly white color, spots of original color and areas of lightened color. **B.** After a few more treatment, it became more irregular showing depigmented, darkened areas in addition to lightened spots.

they migrate, the demarcation area blackens. The pigmentation of the demarcation area sometimes does not disappear even after two years, as described in this article. When the Q-switched laser is used again on the pigmentation of the demarcation area, the pigmentation of the demarcation area normally reoccurs. Treatment using IPL often makes the pigmentation of the demarcation area faint.

Mottled skin due to treatment of brown macules

Care must be taken when treating brown macules in areas other than the face such as the arms, legs, and trunk of adult patients. In these cases, the treatment may worsen the mottling, as shown in Figure 09-5. Mottling means parts of the lesions become faint and others darken, resulting in irregular colors. In this case, further treatment may make all parts of the lesion more faint, but the patient may be not satisfied with the lightening of the entire lesion, and being generally stressed out during the treatment course, may consider continuous treatment a burden.

This type of mottling occurs after treatment is continued, even though slightly abnormal signs were observed after the initial treatment rather than after the entire lesion became mottled after the initial treatment. The abnormal signs include a case wherein parts of the lesion became darker than the hypopigmented macule or the original brown macule. Thus, if slightly abnormal signs are observed after the initial treatment, the treatment should be discontinued and then the mottling will generally improve within six to 12 months.

Café-au-lait spots

Early treatment of café-au-lait spots

As mentioned above, a café-au-lait spot appears mostly at birth or within a few months after birth. As it would last a lifetime without treatment, early treatment is desirable. Early treatment of café-au-lait spots has many obstacles, though. First, the treatment procedure is painful, even for adults. Babies often cry during the treatment procedure because of fear of the environment of the hospital, or because of anger due to their immobilization (due to the laser treatment), or about not being able to move at their own will even if they do not feel pain too much. Second, although a dressing should be applied and babies' wounds should be managed well, infants are often uncooperative during the wound management after the treatment procedure, whereas adults comply well with the instructions. Third, for small lesions, laser treatment can be performed in a short time by holding babies even if they cry. For large lesions, however, this is impossible. In this case, sedative anesthesia is unavoidable. For babies aged 1 year or older, sedative anesthesia is considered, and for babies 1 year or younger, an anesthetic agent is applied to the skin before the treatment.

Given these obstacles, is early treatment still required?   First, many parents have their babies receive early treatment because they want to remove a café-au-lait spot before their child experiences adaptive difficulties in society, that is, before their child's feelings get hurt by negative comments from their peers. Second, the earlier the treatment is, the better the outcome will be.

Is there any test before the treatment of a café-au-lait spot?

Generally, tests are performed before treating any pigment disorder for the following reasons, but on the other hand, there are also several reasons for not doing the tests. Whether or not to perform tests solely depends on the physician's viewpoint. First, a test is performed before treatment to decide whether or not to perform the treatment, because it is uncertain if the lesion will be cured. As everyone knows, a round of tests is not sufficient to remove the lesion. As a relapse on the treated site is common, repeated tests on the same site are normally required. In addition, repeated tests on the same site with two-month intervals take a long time. Thus, it may be better to start the treatment of the entire lesion if no particular problems occur.

Second, physicians may want to first perform a test in parts of the lesion to determine the optimum strength of the laser treatment and the suitable type of laser treatment, and then apply the results of the test to the next treatment. The author performed a test on several spots in the first treatment, and then used the strength that could have a good outcome for the next entire treatment. If a physician is highly experienced in laser treatment, he or she is more likely to decide on the therapeutic parameters based on the instantaneous response to the treatment at the time of the treatment rather than wait until the crust falls off after the laser treatment or two months after the treatment.

Third, after being briefed on the treatment, the patient may sometimes say that he or she does not know how much pain and discomfort he or she would experience during the treatment, and if he or she could manage the treatment site well. In such a case, the author explains the treatment by showing the patient pictures of changes over time after the treatment, and recommends a treatment for the entire lesion. If a patient dislikes treatment of his or her entire lesion, a test of parts of the lesion is performed. Given the safety of this procedure, the test must be performed on a site that is not easily exposed.

There are several reasons why the author dislikes test treatment. First, in some cases, partial treatment makes the color of the untreated parts different from that of the treated parts, and repeated treatments thereafter fail to dispel this difference in color. Second, due to partial treatment, if normal melanocytes (i.e., melanocytes of the nevus) around the partially treated lesions participate in the regeneration of the partially treated lesion, the possibility of relapse of the brown macule is high. Even when an entire lesion is treated, the melanocytes that migrate from the follicles or the surrounding skin become abnormal melanocytes, and form a café-au-lait spot. If abnormal melanocytes participate in the regeneration process, it would be difficult to expect a good outcome. Third, in some cases, even when the test treatment is successful, the treatment of the entire lesion may be unsuccessful. In addition, there may be opposite cases. That is, a test may not reflect the prognosis of the entire treatment.

How is the prognosis of a café-au-lait spot after the treatment?

Although there are various types of café-au-lait spots, the author expects the lesions to become significantly faint in about 50% of the patients who receive treatment and to become very much less faint in the other 50%. It is impossible to expect complete disappearance of a café-au-lait spot in adults, however aggravation is rare with good management after treatment.

What types of café-au-lait spots are well cured?

Levy et al. reported in 1999 that treatment outcomes would be good if the skin color is light, the demarcation is irregular, the lesion consists of multiple pieces, the lesion is small, the color of the lesion is distinct from that of the surrounding skin, and the patient is young. From the author's experience, the most important factor is individual differences. That is, even if all other conditions are good, the outcomes will be poor in some patients; and on the contrary, even if the outcome was expected to be poor, it would be good in some patients. The second most important factor is the age at which the treatment is performed. The younger the patient is, the easier it would be to cure the lesion. Third, a lesion on the face is easiest to treat, and the farther the lesion is from the face, the more difficult it is to treat. That is, a lesion on the face of a child is easy to cure and a lesion on the arm of an adult is the most difficult to cure.

Is there any case wherein the color of the lesion darkened after the treatment?

Dr. Grevelink reported in Archives of Dermatology in 1995 that a café-au-lait spot disappeared or became faint or darker after one session of laser treatment, and that if a lesion only temporarily darkens after treatment, it will later return to its original color. From the author's experience, there were cases wherein the lesion darkened after treatment due to wrong management after the treatment (e.g., the crust separated prematurely while the patient was playing around; the blister was peeled off by mistake; or the treated site was heavily exposed to solar ultraviolet rays while on a trip after the treatment). In these cases, after extensive whitening treatments, most of the lesions recovered their previous dark brown color within two to six months.

The author often experienced cases, however, wherein café-au-lait spots were partially tested at other hospitals much earlier and were later presented for checkup to the author for the first time, at which the partially tested area of the lesion had become darker than the untested area of the lesion. That is, in the author's view, after laser treatment, though a café-au-lait spot may darken temporarily, it may also darken semi-permanently.

When does an entire lesion become white after treatment?

When the crust falls off after the treatment, although the brown color has already disappeared, erythema will be seen. When this erythema disappears, the treated site often looks whiter than the surrounding normal skin color. In this case, the patient initially thinks the treatment was successful; but several months later, he or she worries that the whiter area would be permanently white. In fact, the author considers the outcome good if the lesion is merely lighter-brown than the surrounding normal skin. In this case, the color of the lesion will become normal after one to two years, and the lesion will be cured. The author has never seen a case wherein the lesion was semi-permanently hypopigmented for two years or more.

Judgment on the perfect cure of a café-au-lait spot

In an article published in 1997 in Aesthetic Plastic Surgery, Shimbashi et al. adjudged a lesion perfectly cured when no relapse occurred for six months after the completion of the treatment. In an article published in 1999 in the Journal of Cutaneous Laser Therapy, Levy et al. adjudged a lesion as perfectly cured when no abnormal findings were observed for 12 months after the completion of the treatment. The author deems a lesion perfectly cured when no relapse occurs for 12 months after the completion of the treatment, as he had the experience of a patient who had a relapse one month after the patient was found to have been perfectly cured 11 months after the completion of his treatment. In fact, however, when no relapse occurs for six months after the treatment, the chance of a relapse thereafter is low.

Nevus spilus

What type of laser is used to treat nevus spilus?

Nevus spilus is also treated with laser, as are other brown macules. Generally, spots in the middle are better cured, and the brown macules in the background show a prognosis similar to that of other brown macules. Generally, the Q-switched laser that is used for pigment disorders is used for this disorder. The Q-switched lasers include the ruby, alexandrite, and Nd:YAG lasers. In a comparative study by Polder et al., the results of the treatment with the ruby and Nd: YAG laser for pigment disorder were similar.

Is it possible to treat only the dark spots in nevus spilus?

Normally, the dark spots that are superimposed on the light brown macules in the background are better cured than the light brown macules in the background. If the brown background color is light, only the dark spots are treated; and if the brown background color is dark, the entire lesion is treated.

Becker's nevus

Becker's nevus may be with or without hypertrichosis. Besides, there have been cases wherein Becker's nevus had no hair at first but later became hairy. If a lesion is suspected as Becker's nevus but without hair, the physician should explain to the patient that hair may grow during the course of the treatment as part of the natural progression of the lesion. Otherwise, the patient or his/her parents would consider the hair growing in the course of the treatment as a side effect of the laser treatment. In addition, the physician should explain to the patient that Becker's nevus may well develop a bumpy surface as part of its natural progression. Otherwise, the patient would think that some form of scar has appeared due to laser treatment.

In the treatment of Becker's nevus, a laser for brown macules and a laser for hair removal are used in combination. Regarding the time point at which a laser should be used for hair removal, contrary opinions exist. When laser hair removal is performed from the initial phase, it is better to treat the reservoir of melanocytes in the hair bulge, a cause of the relapse of brown macules. Thus, it is known as good to treat the reservoir of melanocytes early to perform treatment using a laser for hair removal. Physicians who advocate that brown macules should be treated first and then the hair on them should be removed claim that the epidermal side effects can be prevented if the laser hair removal is performed after the color of the brown macules becomes light, because strong laser hair removal may cause epidermal burn injury and consequently, a scar. It is recommended that treatment be performed and a different approach be applied to each case after examining the response to the treatment of brown macules and the degree of the brown color of the skin, by considering both opinions.

Agminated lentiginosis

Laser treatment of agminated lentiginosis is similar to that of a café-au-lait spot. In agminated lentiginosis, however, the lesion is not entirely brown but contains parts of normal skin. Thus, for agminated lentiginosis, treatment is mostly performed on each small lentigo. Thus, it takes longer to treat agminated lentiginosis than a similar-sized café-au-lait spot.

Tips for post-treatment care and follow-up

What drugs are prescribed after the treatment?

After the treatment of brown macules, oral drugs are normally not prescribed. Drugs are prescribed, however, though rarely, in the following cases. First, drugs are prescribed when patients have pain after the treatment because a large area was treated. If the pain causes discomfort, an analgesic can be prescribed; or if it is not prescribed, the patient could take an over-the-counter analgesic. Second, drugs can be prescribed when the lesions become itchy during the healing process of the wound several days after the treatment. This itch does not adversely affect the prognosis, and would not necessarily reoccur in the next treatment. The problem is that scratching an itchy spot can adversely affect good wound healing. An itchy lesion should be protected with a gauze, or the patient can get a prescription for an antihistamine or take an over-the-counter antihistamine.

Is protection using a gauze or other form of dressing after the treatment good?

- Generally, covering the treated site provides protection, and is thus helpful. A non-adhesive form of dressing, such as Mepilex or Mediform, or gauze dressing can be bought from a drug store and applied to the treated site. (Caution: Adhesive hydrocolloid dressings, such as DuoDERM®, should be avoided. If it is used, the crust may also be removed along with the adhesive dressing).
- When replacing the dressing, care should be taken not to knock or pull off the crust. If the crust looks as if it is about to be pulled off together with the dressing, a wet pack should be first applied to the crust before the dressing is removed.
- If a child is bothered by the dressing and thus keeps touching it, it would be good to cover the lesion only while the child is sleeping.

How can vesicles that have occurred after the treatment be managed?

- As vesicles are signs of good treatment, patients do not need to worry about them. If they are well managed, a good treatment outcome can be expected.
- If vesicles occur, the patient can puncture them at home using a needle (the needle should first be heated in a flame and then rinsed in water before use). Then the vesicles should be pressed using a gauze bought from a drug store, after which another clean gauze should be applied to the wound.

- If vesicles reoccur, the previous step can be repeated.
- In addition to draining vesicles after puncturing them using a needle, a wet pack is good for vesicles.

How should a wet pack be applied?

- Saline water bought from a drug store should first be chilled in a refrigerator A disinfected gauze soaked in the saline water should be placed on the treated site.
- The fully soaked gauze should be left on the treated site; and once it dries it should be replaced with a new gauze that was again soaked in saline water.
- If a wet pack is applied to vesicles two to three times (15-20 min per session) a day, they will be alleviated. In addition, the itch and inflammation will improve. A gauze that is not easily removable can be soaked in water so that it can be easily removed.

  *When is a wet pack is required? : When a vesicle appears or when the gauze cannot easily be removed.

How long should protection against ultraviolet rays be provided after the treatment?

After the crust falls off, some form of protective compound to screen out ultraviolet (UV) A and B rays (UVA+UVB sunblock) with a minimum SPF of 30 should be applied routinely before going outdoors. The first month after the treatment is the most important, and the second month is the next most important. As a matter of course, however, anyone who has been treated for brown macules, should be advised to use UVA/B sunscreens routinely as part of their daily skin care regimen.

REFERENCES

1. Becker SW. Concurrent melanosis and hypertrichosis in distribution of nevus unius lateris. Arch Dermatol Syph 1949, 60:155–160.
2. Grossman MC, Anderson RR, Farinelli W, Flotte TJ, Grevelink JM. Treatment of cafe au lait macules with lasers. A clinicopathologic correlation. Arch Dermatol 1995;131:1416-1420.
3. Kim EH, Kang HY. Partial unilateral lentiginosis with ocular involvement. Eur J Dermatol 2006;16:582-583.
4. Levy JL, Mordon S, Pizzi-Anselme M. Treatment of individual café au lait macules with the Q-switched Nd:YAG: a clinicopathologic correlation. J Cutan Laser Ther 1999;1:217-223.
5. Polder KD, Landau JM, Vergilis-Kalner IJ, Goldberg LH, Friedman PM, Bruce S. Laser eradication of pigmented lesions: a review. Dermatol Surg 2011;37:572-595.
6. Shimbashi T, Kamide R, Hashimoto T. Long-term follow-up in treatment of solar lentigo and café-au-lait macules with Q-switched ruby laser. Aesthetic Plast Surg 1997;21:445-448.

10

Tattoos

10-1 Artistic tattoo

Introduction and history

Where did the word 'tattoo' come from? When in doubt, turn to the dictionary. According to the Oxford English Dictionary, the etymology of the word 'tattoo' is as follows: "In 18th c. tattaow, tattow. From Polynesian tatau. In Tahitian, tatu." The first mention of the word 'tatau' in the English language was in a journal written in 1769 by Joseph Banks, Captain James Cook's naturalist, while he was travelling with Cook in the South Seas on *HMS Endeavour*. Banks wrote of the 'tatau'; "I shall now mention the way they mark themselves indelibly ...". The word 'tatau' was subsequently introduced as a 'loan word' into English, and Anglicized into 'tattoo' to match the phonological criteria of the English language. Eighteenth century sailors on later voyages therefore both introduced the word and reintroduced the concept of tattooing as body art to Europe and North America. It was said to be a good way of enabling identification of seafarers should they be found drowned, and it evolved from that into the more decorative forms of tattoo which persist amongst mariners (and many landlubbers) to the present day.

Around Cook's time and even now, specific tattoos had a meaning for seamen. For example, an anchor, such as that seen on the arm of the cartoon character 'Popeye the Sailor Man', is believed to show that a sailor had crossed the Atlantic Ocean, a tattoo of a square-rigged sailing ship under full sail indicated that the wearer had sailed 'around the Horn' (Cape Horn), and crossing the equator was marked with the tattoo of a turtle, complete with shell.

Tattooing is by no means such a comparatively recent phenomenon. Marking of the body with some form of pigmented material either rubbed into wounds (scarification) or injected under the skin with sharp implements predates the 18th century by tens of millennia. Tattooing in

Japan is thought to go back some ten thousand years and more to the Paleolithic era. In Europe, the history of tattooing dates back to the Neolithic or 'new stone age' times, and some of the most famous tattooed warriors or peoples of over two millennia ago were the northern British Picts (from the Latin, '*picti*', painted people') described by Julius Caesar in 54 BC in Book V of his *Gallic Wars*. The Picts were marked (or scarified) with woad, a dark blue dye of plant origin, although copper may also have been used.

Enforced tattooing

Around the same time, in Ancient Rome the word for tattoo was 'stigma', and these were marks which were branded or tattooed into the skin of slaves and convicted criminals (to mark them as such) and conscripted legionnaires (so they could be recognized as deserters should they try to desert). The same prejudice against tattoos was true in Ancient Greece, where anyone with a tattoo was marked as not being Greek, i.e., 'not civilized' and therefore a barbarian. The modern meaning of the word stigma owes its provenance to Ancient Greece and Rome, namely; "a mark of disgrace associated with a particular circumstance, quality, or person."

Other more modern forced identification tattoos are seen such as the 'D' for 'deserter' in the British army up till around the late 1800's. Criminals in civilian life during this era could also be marked with tattoos, where 'D' indicated 'drunkard', 'V' was a vagabond, and 'F' was a 'fray maker', or common brawler. More recently, the identification number tattooed on the inner forearm of Jews in the Nazi concentration camps in World War II is a chilling example of a forced tattoo.

Group tattoos, good and bad

Apart from the forced tattoos just mentioned, very few of these ancient versions of tattooing were for pure decoration, but were an essential part of rites of passage, were believed to imbue magical or protective properties, or denoted belonging to some particular tribe, family or group. Many of the tattoo markings had religious significance in pre-Christian civilizations. A different and more practical reason is presently seen among top notch elite fighting groups (the UK SAS, for example) who will often get a tattoo of their blood group somewhere on their body.

Another use of tattoos was, and still is, to show 'belonging' to some organization, usually with negative connotations, such as gang members exemplified by the very famous example of the members of the Japanese underworld organization, the yakuza. These gentlemen (and

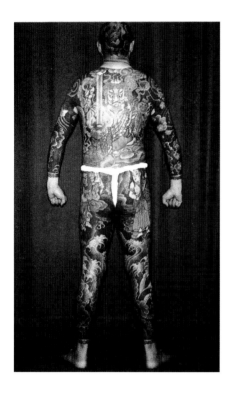

Figure 10-1-1   Example of a Japanese full 'suit of color', usually associated with members of the Japanese yakuza.

some ladies) proudly acquire and wear their 'suit of colors', but only display their '*irezumi*' (Japanese, meaning 'insertion of ink') when they are with fellow *yakuza*. For this reason, Japanese full suits of color end at the neck, wrists and ankles, so that wearing a business suit with a collar and tie can disguise the fact that the wearer is tattooed at all. Figure 10-1-1 shows an example of such a complete 'suit' of tattoos, all of which have some significance in the Japanese Buddhist or Shinto faiths. Many true disciples will have their heads shaved and get their scalp tattooed, and then grow their hair back to hide the tattoo.

The Korean equivalent to the Japanese yakuza, the *Kkangpae* (literally 'thug' in Korean), are also associated with tattoos, but not to anywhere near the same extent as with the Japanese yakuza. (whom, incidentally, the *Kkangpae* hate, and vice versa). The three main groups have identification tattoos, namely a pattern of seven stars on their chest (*Chil Sun Pa*, 'Seven Stars Mob); the Korean Hanja character for 'Son' (where the 'o' is as in 'song', the *Hwan-Song-Sung-Pa*, origin unclear, but believed founded by a gentleman whose family name was Son); and two dragons twined around each other on the upper arm (*Ssang-Yong-Pa*, origin unknown, and now believed to be extinct).

The decorative tattoo

As for the purely decorative tattoo, in more recent history a short-lived vogue for tattoos was started amongst the upper class in the UK in 1862, when the Prince of Wales (later King Edward VII) had the Jerusalem Cross tattooed on his arm, but this practice died out. Currently, however, with premier league footballers (e.g., David Beckham), other top athletes, male and female top singing stars and other performing artists as role models, there has been a huge upsurge in interest in personal decorative body tattoos amongst younger and not-so-young fans and followers, and it has become a burgeoning business. Apart from wishing to emulate the wearer's role model, the reasons for getting a tattoo are many and various, including showing undying affection to the significant other in the recipient's life, undying love for a relative, usually one's mother, or an simple desire to be a little 'different' which may on occasion be somewhat alcohol-fuelled. Figure 10-1-2 illustrates two very differently tattooed shoulders, the main illustration being that of an athlete and the smaller inset being that from a female media star. The philosophy behind the two examples could not be more different. The athlete's tattoo is clearly spiritualistic with a strong native design, whereas it appears as if the

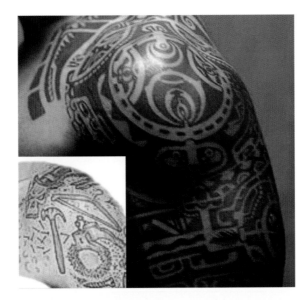

Figure 10-1-2 **Different concepts behind acquiring a tattoo illustrated.** In the main image, the shoulder of an athlete is depicted with a very symbolic tribal-type tattoo. In the inset, the shoulder of a media starlette is shown for comparison. There is no clear linked symbolism, simply a random collection of mundane objects. The athlete has probably had his tattoo designed to help develop inner strength, whereas the starlette's tattoo has no clear purpose, other than potentially to attract attention.

other tattoo artist has just filled spaces with random everyday objects, although one wonders why the handcuffs are so prominent.

Sadly, significant others do not always last for ever, role models may fall out of favor, the tattoo may become an obstacle to getting a job, and simple regret can occur for ever having had a tattoo, especially when the effect of the alcohol wears off. In all these cases, the wearer wants the tattoo removed, and tattoo removal is also becoming a burgeoning business.

The tattoo which is not for ever

For those who only want to try out a tattoo on their own, or for amusement at fairs and other such public events, tattoo transfers or decals are available which are easily applied to the surface of the skin but which can be removed very quickly with liberal applications of soap and water, or left to fade naturally over some days, depending on the quality of the transfer. Special tattoo transfer paper is now available whereby you can design your own tattoo on your computer and print it out on an inkjet printer.

Another form of removable tattoo without any needling is achieved with the use of the active ingredient of the henna plant, which is also based on traditional uses in South Asia where it was (and is) known as 'Mehndi' before it became popular as an artistic expression in the West. Authentic henna 'tattoos' are restricted in color to a range of shades of reds and browns to a near-black, take some time to darken completely after application, and can last for a month or more before they fade naturally. These decorations can be as small or as large as the wearer wants or decreed by the creative limitations of the artist (Figure 10-1-3). However, care must be taken that so-called 'black henna' is not being applied. This compound is very fast-staining, unlike true henna, but is in fact potentially extremely harmful due to the active ingredient para-phenylenediamine (PPD) which causes blistering, eruptions and long term allergic reactions. Even true henna powder has been restricted for sale by the US FDA for hair coloring only, and is regarded as an 'adulterant'.

Infinitink™

For those more adventurous but not yet quite ready for the traditional artistic tattoo approach, a new form of tattoo ink has become available in some countries for traditional needled tattoos. It offers the relative permanence of normal tattoo inks, but if the wearer has a change of heart (or of significant other), these tattoos are designed to be removed easily and completely with a single laser treatment. The tattoo ink, with the trade name of 'Infinitink™', stemmed from the work of a group of clinicians and scientists, prominent amongst whom was Profes-

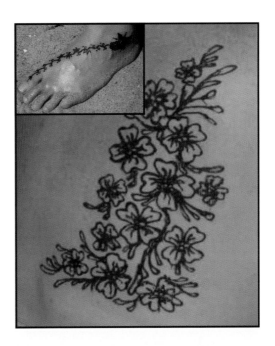

Figure 10-1-3   Temporary henna tattoo designs illustrated, covering the entire back (main image) or the foot (inset) of the wearer. The sand in the background of the foot suggests a holiday tattoo, however, the tattoo looks suspiciously black, so it may have been inked in with 'black henna' with the potential for allergic or subsequent inflammatory reaction. It may not be as temporary as hoped.

sor R. Rox Anderson. The group founded a company called 'Freedom2' in the late 1990's, and the first iteration of the ink received widespread media acclaim, including TIME magazine which named Freedom2 ink the "2007 Invention of the Year" in fashion. The final iteration is available as Infinitink, manufactured via a proprietary process by Freedom2 Inc., and is the first and only tattoo material to be designed by clinicians and bioscientists to undergo clinical and safety testing. The group wanted to develop a method of allowing the easy laser removal of tattoos, based on bioremovable dyes encapsulated in microscopic laser-labile plastic nanobeads, which would remain in the tissue without provoking any foreign body reaction, but would rupture easily with a single laser application, allowing the dye particles to escape and be removed naturally. Infinitink is currently available in only red and black, but has received acclaim from tattoo artists, and their human canvases, in a growing number of countries (Figure 10-1-4).

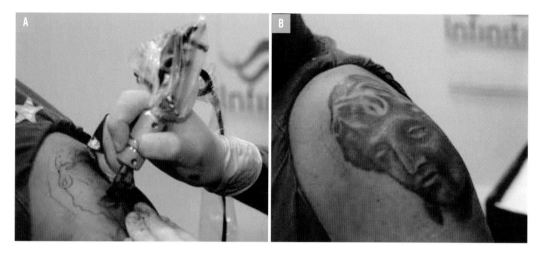

Figure 10-1-4   **An Infinitink™ tattoo in the process of tattooing (A), and the finished article (B).** If the wearer is happy with this image, then it is as permanent as conventional tattoos. However, if the image is not what the wearer really wanted at any time it may be cleared with one single laser treatment.

The tattoo process

Before looking at how decorative tattoos can be removed, it is important to understand the process of the placement of the image. Tattooing involves placing pigment into the upper dermis underneath the epidermis. This is most usually managed by professional tattoo artists with a specially designed motor-driven tattooing machine, whereby ink-laden needles are repeatedly pushed to a certain distance into the skin. Alternatively, a traditional tattoo master might use a bundle of hand-held needles: many Japanese tattooists still use this method. Each artists mixes his or her own colors from a variety of pigments. Amateur tattoos can be placed with a variety of sharp objects, including conventional sewing needles, fine hobby knives and ballpoint pens, the latter having a convenient supply of ink. The major difference between the amateur and professional tattoo is the distribution, depth and type of pigment. The profession tattoo artist will place all pigment at similar depths and densities to achieve the desired effect, and will ideally use a range of the appropriate health regulatory authority approved pigments. The amateur tattoo on the other hand varies widely in depth and density, and the material used as the pigment, such as India ink, ashes, soot, graphite (from pencils) and ballpoint pen ink. All of these contain impurities, however, and can cause a range of adverse side effects.

When they are first needled into the skin by a tattoo artist or an amateur, pigment particles

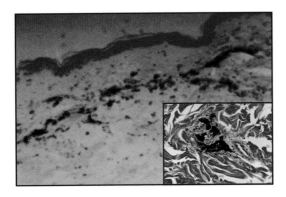

Figure 10-1-5   **(Main image):** Typical histopathological findings of densely clustered tattoo pigment particles in the upper dermal layer. Note the uniformity of the depth of the particles. **(Inset):** higher magnification of a clump of tattoo pigment particles, isolated from the dermal extracellular matrix by a clearly visible fibrotic layer with different optical characteristics from the rest of the extracellular matrix.

can be found from the epidermis down to the required depth in the dermis, with the majority of the pigment located at the target depth. The particles in the epidermis are removed through the crusting process, as are the more superficial particles in the dermis. Some of the smaller particles at the target depth are phagocytosed as part of the wound healing and foreign body reaction. Most of the larger particles however, while still recognized as foreign bodies, are isolated by the body from the surrounding dermal matrix by incorporation and encapsulation in a layer of denser fibrotic tissue surrounded by fibroblasts (Figure 10-1-5), where the particles remain in a stable state and can collectively be seen through the epidermis as the tattoo. Over decades, however, this fibrotic layer tends to migrate deeper into the dermis, accounting for the faded appearance and loss of detail in older tattoos. This fading is not due to deterioration of the pigment particles, but is caused by simple optical physics.

Visible 'white' light enters the skin as an admixture of photons having the wavelengths of the 'colors of the rainbow'. When these photons encounter red pigment in the skin, all the other wavelengths are absorbed by the pigment and only the photons in the red part of the spectrum are reflected back though the skin which are perceived by the human eye as 'red'. The skin is an extremely complex mixture of different-sized biological elements with a large variety of optical characteristics, and thus diffuses or scatters incident light in direct proportion to depth. The deeper the layer of the skin between the red pigment and the surface of the skin, the more that layer absorbs or scatters the incident light, the less light actually reaches the pigment and the less it is reflected back through the skin to the eye of the observer. Thus, although the pigment actually remains the same color, the color seems to become more faint the deeper the pigment is located in the skin. Black tattoo pigment can thus be placed by the master artist to achieve an entire range of colors from black through to a faint blue-gray. As an example of this in a nevus, the variety of color which typifies a Nevus of Ohta lesion all originate from the same black pigment, namely melanin. From a practical viewpoint, this also means that the clinician removing a tattoo should bear in mind that he or she may not need to remove the deepest-located tattoo pigment, as the intervening upper layers of the extracellular matrix which have been cleared of pigment will be more fibrous in any event because of mild scar formation, and thus act as a natural biological optical neutral density filter between the eye of the observer and the pigment.

Artistic tattoo removal

The histological appearance of the pigment particles comprising a tattoo gives a strong clue as to the method of removal of the tattoo. The ink or pigment remains a foreign body, and is alien to the natural composition of the skin. By removing the fibrotic encapsulation which has surrounded tattoo pigments, they are once again exposed as alien substances and trigger the foreign body reaction, resulting in their natural excretion from the body by the kidneys and liver via phagocytosis and the lymphatic system. The methods to achieve this have evolved with time. Abrasion of the skin over the tattoo exposed the pigment so that it could be removed, but for even smaller tattoos this resulted in a deep wound which could not heal by primary intention and almost always left a visible scar with some degree of hypertrophy with or without hyper- or hypopigmentation. In addition to mechanical dermabrasion, salabrasion was popular amongst seafarers who always had a plentiful supply of salt available. Excision of the tattoo followed by a skin graft was also used, again with potential for textural changes and scarring at both the site of the tattoo and the donor site for the skin. Other methods were tried involving creating inflammation in the tissue containing the tattoo pigments with the aim of speeding their expulsion: these included injection of a variety of substances including wine, lime and even pigeon excrement.

In the 1970's, continuous wave lasers, such as the argon at its main lines of 488 nm and 514.5 nm, emerged as a potential method with Professor Leon Goldman of the University of Cincinnati as one of the pioneers, and it was found that matching the wavelength of the laser to the absorption spectrum of the tattoo pigment gave better results. However the unavoidable photothermal damage to the tissue overlying the tattoo particles, due to conducted heat from the long irradiation times, still gave rise to the potential for scarring. The pulsed ruby laser was next found useful for more superficial tattoos, and at pulse widths of 1 millisecond or less, could achieve selective photothermolysis of certain pigments. However, the advent of the nanosecond pulse domain Q-switched laser finally gave clinicians a much finer tool for tattoo removal, and the Q-switched laser was first reported for this application by Taylor and colleagues in 1990.

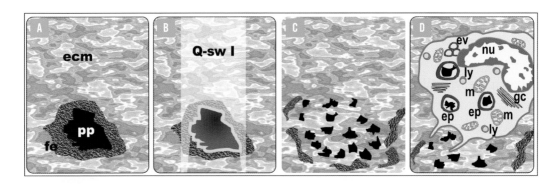

Figure 10-1-6   **The process of tattoo pigment disruption with Q-switched Nd:YAG laser energy. A.** Schematic showing a tattoo pigment particle (pp) encapsulated in a dense fibrotic layer of tissue (FE) in the middle of a normal extracellular matrix (ecm). **B.** The nanosecond domain Q-switched beam (Q-sw I) is transmitted through the ecm and fe, but is preferentially absorbed in the tattoo pigment, heating it up almost instantaneously and explosively. **C.** The tattoo pigment particle disintegrates into small fragments, and the photoacoustic shock wave generated by the explosive reaction shatters the fibrotic protective capsule, exposing the tattoo particles once more as foreign bodies to the ecm and the organism. **D.** Recruited by the foreign body reaction, a macrophage is attracted to the tattoo pigment (chemoattraction): It engulfs and internalizes the pigment in vesicles (ep). The cellular components are as follows: nu, nucleus; ep, engulfed pigment in vesicles; m, mitochondrion, which drives the phagocytosis process through adenosine triphosphate (ATP) production; ly, lysosome, the macrophage enzyme factory which synthesizes the enzymes required to internalize and excrete the pigment; gc, Golgi complex; ev, empty vesicles which have already passed on their pigment for excretion through the lymphatic system.

When targeting tattoo pigments with laser energy in the ns pulsewidth domain, the Q-switched laser beam achieves tremendously high peak powers and generates power densities at the absorbing pigments in the MW/cm² or even GW/cm² regions. For example, a 5 ns Q-switched Nd:YAG laser at a dose of 6 J and a spot size of 7 mm in diameter generates a power density of over 3 GW/cm². At these irradiances, a nonlinear almost athermal dissociative reaction occurs and the target pigments violently disintegrate, resulting in destruction of their protective fibrotic capsule through the generation of a short-acting photoacoustic and photo-osmotic shock wave, but leaving surrounding and overlying normal tissue undamaged. The tattoo particles are once again recognized as alien substances, and naturally removed. This process is illustrated schematically in Figure 10-1-6. The Nd:YAG wavelength of 1064 nm is somewhat absorbed in melanin, but is extremely preferentially absorbed in dark-colored tattoo pigment particles which makes it an ideal wavelength for the Q-switched treatment of tattoos, even in darker skin types.

The length of the treatment period and number of sessions required for successful laser tattoo removal varies from patient to patient, or even for different tattoos on the same patient, and depends on the interaction of a number of factors such as patient age and skin type, scarring propensity, the location, color and extent of the tattoo and the depths and density of the pigments. For those clinicians starting out on Nd:YAG Q-switched laser tattoo removal, especially for patients in the Asian skin phenotype for whom the formation of hyperpigmentation secondary to damage or inflammation is a major problem, the use of a recently published predictive scale, the Kirby-Desai Scale, is recommended. Drs Kirby and Desai evolved their scale based on 6 parameters to which numerical values are assigned: namely skin type, tattoo location, color, pigment density, scarring or tissue change in the tattoo site, and attempt to overlay or disguise the tattoo with another pigment. The scores from each parameter are summed to give a combined value based on which the number of sessions can be calculated which will be required to remove the tattoo successfully. The accuracy and sensitivity of the scale have been well-verified.

In addition to taking the Kirby-Desai scale into consideration for calculation of the number of sessions required, the optimum parameters for the Q-switched 1064 nm Nd:YAG laser treatment of tattoos have evolved from clinician experience and reported papers in the peer-reviewed literature. Tattoo treatment at a 5-7 ns pulse width with 5-8 J pulse energy and a 5-7 mm spot size in general produces excellent results in black and dark-colored tattoos. Treatment will need to be repeated as required at 6-8-week intervals, to allow complete removal of the pigment liberated by each treatment and repair to the tissue damage induced locally by the photoacoustic shock. Complete clearance may not be achieved, which is usually associated with the constituent materials of the pigment, but in general excellent results can be obtained with the Q-switched Nd:YAG laser in black or dark-colored tattoos with patience on the part of both the clinician and the patient. Figure 10-1-7 shows what can be achieved in a uniformly pigmented dark-colored tattoo in 7 treatment sessions (SPECTRA Q-switched Nd:YAG system, Lutronic Corporation, Goyang, South Korea: 1064 nm, 5-7 ns, 4 mm spot diameter, 6-8 J/cm^2). The 1064 nm beam is very compatible with black, very dark blue and red pigments, but different wavelength options are required for effective removal of other tattoo colors. For example, frequency-doubling a Q-switched 1064 nm Nd:YAG beam will deliver visible green at 532 nm, ideal for the lighter red pigments which do not absorb 1064 nm so well. Solid dye handpieces are available for some Q-switched Nd:YAG systems to convert the Q-switched 532 nm beam into appropriate yellow and red wavelengths, suitable for yellow, sky-blue and red pigments and green and dark yellow pigments, respectively. Figure 10-1-8 shows excellent clearance of the darker regions of a multi-colored tattoo after only 2 sessions with the 1064 nm Q-switched beam (SPECTRA, Lutronic Corporation, Goyang, South Korea: 1064 nm, 5-7 ns, 3-4 mm spot size, 4-8 J/cm^2). However, although they have faded somewhat, smaller regions of the red and green pigments remain which could be successfully cleared with the yellow and red dye dye handpieces, respectively.

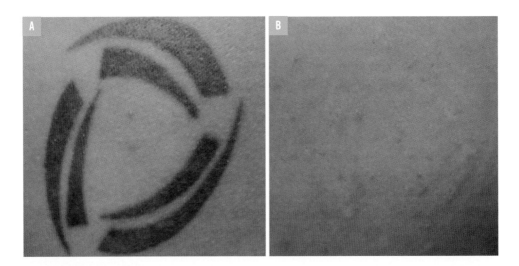

Figure 10-1-7 **Tattoo removed with the Q-switched 1064 nm Nd:YAG laser. A.** Baseline findings in a professionally-applied monochromatic tattoo. **B.** The excellent result achieved after 7 treatment sessions (see text for treatment parameters). Some very faint residual pigment can be seen, with very mild textural changes. Clinical photography courtesy of J Kevin Duplechain MD FACS, Los Angeles, USA.

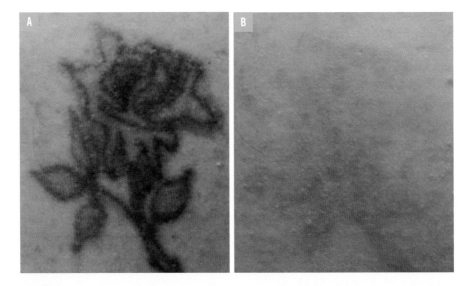

Figure 10-1-8 **Multicolored artistic tattoo removal with Q-switched Nd:YAG laser treatment. A.** Baseline findings showing a dark pigment-outlined tattoo of a rose with green and red for the leaves, petals and shading. **B.** Findings after only 2 treatment sessions (See text for treatment parameters). The dark pigment has been successfully cleared, and the red and green areas have significantly faded following the 1064 nm treatment. The remaining red pigment could be further cleared using the 585 nm yellow dye handpiece driven by the Q-switched 532 nm green beam, and the green pigment could be selectively attacked with the 650 nm red dye handpiece, also driven by the 532 nm beam. Clinical photography courtesy of J Kevin Duplechain MD FACS, Los Angeles, USA

Side effects and complications

According to Kirby and colleagues, approximately 50% of all patients undergoing laser tattoo removal will have some degree of pigmentary or configurational change in the area previously occupied by their tattoo. These changes may resolve over 6-12 months, but may also remain permanently. Purely pigmentary changes are mostly related to the patient's skin type, with Fitzpatrick types IV – VI at risk of changes irrespective of the laser wavelength used due to their propensity to PIH. If PIH occurs, a regimen of bleaching agents such as hydroquinone and daily application of UVA/B sunscreens at a minimum SPF of 30 may help resolve or at least alleviate the problem. Low level light therapy (LLLT) with an LED system delivering 830 nm in the near infrared can be very beneficial in controlling PIH, as can the Q-switched Nd:YAG laser used in low fluence 'laser toning' (see the appropriate section in this book for a description).

As for unwanted textural and configurational changes, taking a careful patient history will reveal if the patient has a tendency towards hypertrophic or keloid formation, in which case he or she must be warned about this increased risk of scarring as part of the pretreatment in-formed consent process. In all patients, if blistering or crusting occurs at the treatment area, the patient must be instructed not to remove this under any circumstances before it falls off naturally, which can take up to two weeks. Early picking at, or other accidental dislodgement of, crusts dramatically increases the chance of scarring and pigmentary changes, and can pro-long wound healing.

Tattoo pigments are alien substances, some more alien than others, and some are even toxic. Through its powerful selective photothermolytic action, the Q-switched laser releases these particles back into the organism which had originally isolated them through encapsula-tion (cf Figure 6 above), where they may produce allergic or other reactions. Oral antihista-mines and anti-inflammatory steroids have been used to treat allergic reactions to tattoo ink, and LED phototherapy at 830 nm will also prove beneficial. In the case of some particular pigments, a photoallergic reaction might occur over the site of the target pigment which will present as pruritis and erythema, with the potential for inflamed nodules, papules, or granulo-mas. Strict solar protection is required in these cases, with intralesional steroid injections. In extreme cases, excision may be necessary.

Very rarely, some pigments will change color following exposure to the laser, resulting in the phenomenon of paradoxical tattoo darkening. If this occurs, the patient should return after 8 weeks, when the darkened pigments can be treated as if they were normal tattoo par-ticles. The potential of this phenomenon should be included in the pretreatment consultation, together with its resolution.

The most serious, but fortunately not so common, side effect is death from some form of hepatitis (B or C) or even HIV. Tattooing involves needles repetitively piercing the skin and drawing blood. One understands that reputable tattoo artists will thoroughly clean and assiduously sterilize their needles between clients, but it is the less reputable tattoo parlors which put their clients at risk through sloppy needle care and imperfect cleaning. In a large population study by the American Association for the Study of Liver Diseases, there was a significant association between having one or more tattoos and having hepatitis C virus (HCV). The results showed that patients with HCV were three times more likely to have a tattoo. Thus, although the study did not conclusively prove causality, it did strongly suggest a link between tattoos and hepatitis infections.

Finally, a note on laser safety during tattoo removal. Protective eyewear appropriate for the wavelength being used is essential. Please remember that eyewear which protects at 1,064 nm might not offer enough protection at 532 nm. In addition, here is an intraoperative precaution for the surgeon to consider. The explosive reaction associated with nanosecond Q-switched photothermolysis can produce the ejection of a fine laser plume from the point of impact consisting of particulate matter, which might include blood and blood-borne pathogens if the laser bean targets a vessel. The use of a dedicated smoke evacuator is therefore recommended during tattoo removal procedures, and face masks for surgical personnel.

REFERENCES

1. Anderson RR, Parrish JA. Selective photothermolysis: precise microsurgery by selective absorption of pulsed radiation. Science 1983;220:524-527.
2. Bini EJ, Dhalla S, Tenner T, Aytaman A, et al. Strong Association Between Tattoos and Hepatitis C Virus Infection: A Multicenter Study of 3,871 Patients. 58th Annual Meeting of the American Association for the Study of Liver Diseases. Boston. November 2-6, 2007.
3. Ellis J. Tatau and Malu: Vital Signs in Contemporary Samoan Literature. PMLA 2006;121:687–701.
4. Goldman L. Effects of new laser systems on the skin. Arch Dermatol 1973;108:385-390.
5. Kirby W, Desai A, Desai T, Kartono F, Geeta P. The Kirby-Desai Scale: A Proposed Scale to Assess Tattoo-removal Treatments. J Clin Aesthet Dermatol 2009;2:32-37.
6. Kirby W, Koriakos A, Desai A, Desai T. Undesired Pigmentary Alterations Associated with Q-Switched Laser Tattoo Removal. Skin and Aging. August 2010. Please visit http://www.drtattoff.com/images/articles/Undesired-Pigmentary-Alterations-Associated-with-Q-Switched-Laser-Tattoo-Removal-Skin-and-Aging-Aug-2010.pdf
7. Ohshiro T. Laser Treatment for Nevi. Tokyo: JMLL; 1981.
8. O'Brian. P. Joseph Banks: A Life. London: Collins Harvill Press; 1987.
9. Taylor CR, Gange RW, Dover JS, Flotte TJ, Gonzalez E, Michaud N, Anderson RR. Treatment of tattoos by Q-switched ruby laser. A dose-response study. Arch Dermatol 1990;126:893-899.

FURTHER READING

1. Gilbert S. The Tattoo History Sourcebook. New York: powerHouse Books;2000.
2. Wysong P. Tattoo Removal Comes Of Age - An Expert Interview With Dr. William Kirby and Dr. Rady Rahban. Medscape;2011. http://www.medscape.com/viewarticle/747828. (Please note that the reader will have to register with Medscape to view this article, but registration is free)

10-2 Traumatic tattoo

Definition

Traumatic tattoos arise from the percutaneous implantation of foreign materials such as asphalt, gravel, dirt, glass, and metal. This is the most common type of tattoo seen in patients. Explosive traumatic tattoos may also form, particularly in male patients, when gunpowder granules from homemade bombs, dynamite, firearms, or fireworks enter the skin. Most traumatic tattoos result from the lack of proper wound management right after acquiring an injury. Therefore, traumatic tattoos should be treated with immediate removal of the foreign body particles whenever possible.

Tips for diagnosis

The diagnosis of a traumatic tattoo is related to the patient's clinical history because most patients with traumatic tattoos visit a clinic long after wound healing. Figure 10-2-1 shows a typical case of a traumatic tattoo. This male patient in his early 20s visited the clinic due to pigments persisting for more than six months. The patient did not properly treat the wounds on his left cheek that were the result of a motorcycle accident. As shown in Figure 10-2-1, traumatic tattoos often accompany some form of visible scar formation, which implies that the trauma was severe enough to allow the percutaneous implantation of a foreign material into the deep dermis. The first step in the diagnosis of traumatic tattoos is to make a differential diagnosis from post-inflammatory hyperpigmentation (PIH), which commonly lasts for a long time after injuries in darker skin types such as the Asian skin. Traumatic tattoos are thus often mistaken for PIH and can accompany PIH in Asian skin. The most important differential diagnosis point is that had PIH spontaneously disappears with time, which is not true for traumatic tattoos (i.e., the pigmentation in the lesion tends to persist). The patient in Fig 10-2-1. complained about pigmentation that had lasted for over six months after the injury that he incurred, and was not likely to have PIH. When it is difficult to make a diagnosis from the clinical features, "i scope" (MORITEX Co., Tokyo, Japan; Figure 10-2-2) can be helpful. In Figure 10-2-3, the dermis is examined using "i scope" in a dimmer mode, where the light reflection is switched off. Blue-black tattoo particles are observed in the deep dermis, parallel to the pattern of the scarring.

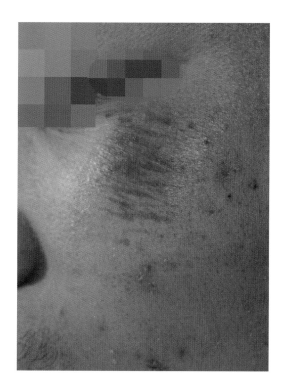

Figure 10-2-1 Typical clinical feature of A traumatic tattoo

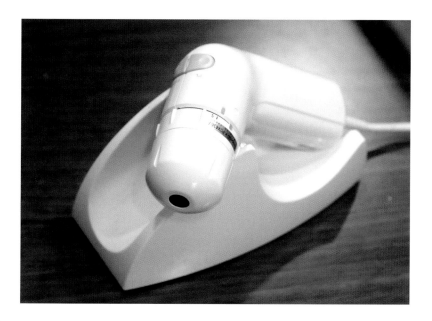

Figure 10-2-2 i scope (MORITEX Co. Tokyo, Japan)

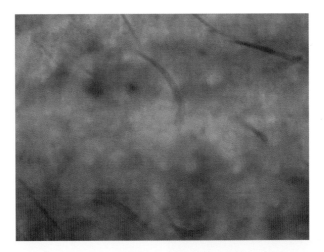

Figure 10-2-3 Lesion in the patient from Figure 10-2-1 viewed in the dimmer mode with light reflection switched off. Blue-black tattoo particles are observed in the deep dermis, parallel to the wound scarring.

Tips for treatment

There are various modalities that are available for removing traumatic tattoos. Some of these, however, have a limited ability to reach particles deeper in the dermis. Cryosurgery, phenol, electrosurgery, and dermabrasion carry a risk of scarring and inadequate tattoo removal. Surgical and microsurgical excisions carry a risk of scarring and cosmetic disfigurement and may be difficult to perform when the individual particles are spread throughout the dermis at varying depths.

Laser-assisted traumatic tattoo removal (Q-switched ruby, Q-switched Nd:YAG) may have a lower risk of scarring and potentially greater success in treating persistent or older tattoos. The Q-switched laser with a nanosecond-pulse width clears tattoo particles through the following mechanisms: (1) immediate vaporization of the particles; (2) transepidermal elimination of the particles during the recovery from the epidermal injuries; and (3) lymphatic clearing of the remaining particles in the dermis through phagocytosis. The majority of the pigments in the tattoo particles disappear immediately after Q-switched laser irradiation while the pigments in nevus of Ota and ABNOM take two to three months to clear after irradiation. A lower-fluence laser could treat traumatic tattoos better compared to the treatments of other dermal pigmented lesions, such as nevus of Ota. Usually, most tattoo particles are densely located in the upper dermis whereas the target pigment chromophores in nevus of Ota are dispersed in the deep dermis. Therefore, laser irradiation not only results in the photothermolysis of the tattoo pigments but can also nonspecifically injure the adjacent epidermis or dermal structures. Therefore, it is very important to use a Q-switched laser with a proper fluence for the treatment of traumatic tattoos. The best practice to determine the amount and depth of the tattoo particles in the dermis is through skin biopsy before the laser treatment. If skin biopsy is not available, it is recommended that a low fluence be used on the dense and superficial pigmentations, and in the second and subsequent sessions, at an interval of 6-8 weeks, a relatively high fluence is used on the dispersed pigment particles. Laser treatments should be done only until the tattoo pigments are whitened, and it is not recommended that irradiation be continued until purpura develops. For the natural appearance of the lesions after laser treatment, the surrounding normal skin can be irradiated along with the lesions. Based on this author's experience, this results in more cosmetically acceptable outcomes, although there can be small changes in the skin texture after the treatment.

Generally, all three types of Q-switched lasers (ruby, alexandrite, and Nd:YAG) can be used for tattoo removal. In Asian skin, however, the Nd:YAG laser is reported to be more effective for tattoo lightening compared to the ruby laser, although both lasers are effective for tattoo removal, the Nd:YAG laser is associated with fewer complications probably because the 1064 nm wavelength is less absorbed by the epidermal melanin.

Figure 10-2-4 shows the case of a male patient in his early 20s who had a traumatic tattoo from a motorcycle accident six months earlier. The patient received one treatment using a 1064 nm Q-switched Nd:YAG laser (3-4 mm spot size; 4.0 J/cm^2 fluence; SPECTRA, Lutronic Co., Goyang, South Korea). Two months after the treatment, most of the tattoo par-

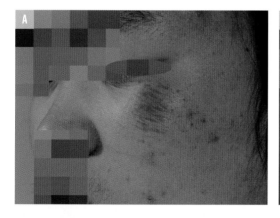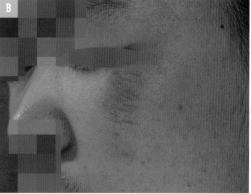

Figure 10-2-4   **Traumatic tattoo in a male (early 20s) after falling off a motorcycle. A.** Before treatment : multiple linear depressed scars after abrasion, with tattoo pigments. **B.** After treatment : 2 months after 1 treatment (Most tattoo particles are removed after treatment with the Q-switched Nd:YAG laser (3-4 mm of spot size, fluence of 4.0 J/cm² fluence).

ticles had disappeared (Figure 10-2-4B). Clinicians should keep in mind that traumatic and general tattoos can be effectively treated with a relatively low fluence compared to the treatment of other dermal melanocytic disorders.

Tips for post-treatment care and follow up

It is not uncommon for traumatic tattoos, compared to other tattoos, to accompany scar development and even, in some cases, foreign-body reactions. When a foreign-body reaction is accompanied by a traumatic tattoo, the inflammation can last for a long time after laser irradiation. This author has experienced a long wound healing period in a patient after treating a "pencil-point tattoo" with a Q-switched laser. Because an unexpected reaction could occur, traumatic tattoos require more cautious wound care compared to other tattoos. Depressed or hypertrophic scars often accompany traumatic tattoos, and it is important to treat these scars. Fractional laser treatment can be helpful for scar revision. Based on this author's experience, the parallel use of a fractional laser in addition to the Q-switched laser can also help the clearance of traumatic tattoos through the wound healing-mediated transepidermal elimination that follows the laser treatment.

REFERENCES

1. El Sayed F, Ammoury A, Dhaybi R. Treatment of fireworks tattoos with the Q-switched ruby laser. Dermatol Surg 2005;31:706–708.
2. Fusade T, Toubel G, Grognard C, Mazer JM. Treatment of gunpowder traumatic tattoo by Q-switched Nd:YAG laser: an unusual adverse effect. Dermatol Surg 2000;26:1057–1059.
3. Lin T, Jia G, Rong H, Li J, Zhou Z. Comparison of a single treatment with Q-switched ruby laser and Q-switched Nd:YAG laser in removing black-blue Chinese tattoos. J Cos Laser Ther 2009;11:236–239.
4. Susan M, Sweeney SM. Tattoo: a review of tattoo practices and potential treatment options for removal. Current Opinion in Pediatrics 2006;18:391–395.

Skin rejuvenation for aged skin

SECTION

02

C / O / N / T / E / N / T / S

01

General concept of multilayer skin rejuvenation approach

▶ Seung Ha Park, MD, PhD, MBA

Aging phenomenon

The aging phenomenon, which is most remarkable on the face, involves systemic phenomena such as changes in tissues including subcutaneous fat, muscles, bone tissue, and changes in metabolism, hormones, and the mental status. The aging phenomenon is attributed to (a) a genetically programmed aging process called the 'program theory'; (b) cellular and organ damage caused by 'wear and tear of tissues' (c) damage to DNA caused by waste products and free radicals due to a harmful environment; and (d) a decreased hormone level and a change in neuro-endocrines.

The facial aging phenomenon includes photoaging and wrinkle deepening on the skin; drooping due to loosening of the retaining ligamenture in the face; sagging and dimpling due to lipodystrophy; and changes in facial muscles and bones. These lead to the facial aging phenomenon, such as forehead wrinkles, crow's feet, nasolabial folds, perioral wrinkles, jowls, and eyebrow and eyelid ptosis. As part of the aging phenomenon of the skin, the epidermis becomes thin due to atrophic change; the epidermal cells become smaller and are distributed irregularly; the stratum corneum becomes thicker; and melanin pigments increase. These epidermal changes are more extensive in photoaging caused by sunlight. In the dermal aging, components of the skin become thinner; the skin appendages including the sebaceous glands undergo atrophy; ground substances decrease; the collagen fiber layer becomes thinner; and elastosis occurs wherein degenerated elastic fibers are irregularly arranged.

Rejuvenation and anti-aging

Although rejuvenation and anti-aging may be confused, they are distinct from each other. Anti-aging involves prevention of the aging process, and rejuvenation is the process of reversion of the already aged status to a juvenile status. As such, anti-aging involves mainly medical and conservative treatments, whereas the rejuvenation approach involves surgical and active treatments. Facial and total rejuvenation includes skin care and rejuvenation; face lifting; anti-aging agents that prevent and treat the aging phenomenon; diet and exercise; non-smoking and abstinence from drinking; a change in lifestyle; psychological and mental therapy; and social support.

Rejuvenation methods

Rejuvenation methods include invasive operations (e.g., face lifting) and less invasive operations (endoscopic lifting, aging blepharoplasty, or lipoplasty). Blepharoplasty and lipoplasty are commonly performed in middle-age patients. Non-surgical methods include laser resurfacing, which is a less invasive treatment. Fractional laser treatment is a minimally invasive form of laser treatment. Non-operative and non-invasive rejuvenation methods involve fillers, botulinum toxin, medical skin care, and anti-aging medicine, which do not require social downtime. Near-infrared light-emitting diode (LED) phototherapy is attracting attention, especially as an adjunctive modality.

"No pain, no gain" applies to rejuvenation methods. Thus, non-operative and non-invasive methods are much less effective than operative and invasive methods. A non-invasive or less invasive method that can reduce the patient's discomfort and increase the rejuvenation effect should be developed. Table 01-1 summarizes both invasive and noninvasive approaches.

Table 01-1   **Rejuvenation methods**

Operative, invasive	Face lifting
Operative , less invasive	Endoscopic operation Blepharoplasty Lipoplasty
Non-operative, invavise	Resurfacing laser
Non-operative, non-invasive	Non-ablative laser Medical skin care Filler material Botulinum toxin Anti-aging medicine

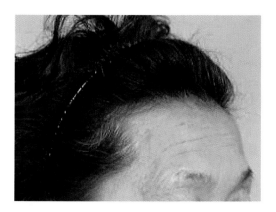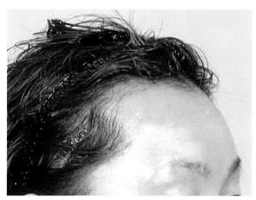

Figure 01-1 Endoscopic forehead lifting, a less invasive method achieved remarkable rejuvenation effect in the upper face.

Face lifting

Face lifting is the most invasive and aggressive surgical rejuvenation method, and most effectively improves deep facial wrinkles and soft tissue drooping and sagging. According to the surgical dissection level, face lifting can be classified into subcutaneous lifting, superficial musculoaponeurotic system (SMAS) lifting, composite lifting, and subperiosteal lifting. Endoscopic lifting is a less invasive lifting method and can be effective mainly for the upper and mid-face. Blepharoplasty, which is a treatment for aging-related eyelid ptosis, is the most commonly performed form of plastic surgery in middle-age people. Liposuction can be effective for tissue drooping or jowls on the face.

Lipoplasty

Atrophy of subcutaneous and soft tissue due to aging requires volume replacement. Fat injection is a procedure wherein the fat harvested in liposuction from the lower abdomen or thigh, in which fat accumulation is high, is injected into the desired area using a syringe to correct deep wrinkles or sunken areas. To achieve a good outcome with fat injection, the fat should be injected evenly into multi-layers and tissues whose vascular circulation is good, using a fine tip with a small diameter. The disadvantage of fat injection is the high absorption of the injected fat. Within 6 months after the injection, about 50% of the injected fat is absorbed and the remainder would remain for life. To prevent the absorption of the injected fat, over-correction in the first procedure or a fat booster injection several months later can be used.

Filler

Fat injection is performed in the cheek, temple, lips, or forehead, where volume replacement is required. When a small volume must be replaced, the injection can be performed easily using a filler. No filler lasts for life and is safe. Currently, the hyaluronic acid filler is widely and safely used, though it is absorbed highly after its injection, and thus results in a decreased volume. Hyaluronic acid is made of non-animal stabilized hyaluronic acid using genetic engineering, and thus has no risk of bovine spongiform encephalopathy, unlike bovine-derived collagen. It is safe and has no side effects, so a hypersensitivity skin test is not required. Injection of a large volume in a single site may have side effects and thus, only a small amount should be injected into an appropriate area.

Botulinum toxin

Botulinum toxin is a substance produced by *Clostridium botulinum* bacteria. Among botulinum toxins, type A is the most powerful. Botulinum toxin blocks muscle contraction by inhibiting the secretion of acetylcholine at the neuromuscular ending. It effectively improves dynamic facial wrinkles such as crow's feet, as well as glabella wrinkles, by blocking facial expression muscles. Although botulinum toxin can easily and effectively improve dynamic facial wrinkles via injection, the effect of the injection lasts for only 6 months or less. This relatively short effect duration is due to the formation of a new nerve ending in the muscle duet or acetylcholine exocytosis. Thus, repeated treatment every 6 months is required. Injection into the forehead may result in side effects such as eyebrow ptosis, and eyelid ptosis and injection into the perioral area may cause side effects such as an unnatural mouth expression. Thus, the injection should be carefully performed only in appropriate areas. For facial lipoplasty, liposuction and fat injection can be performed using a syringe. Syringe rejuvenation is a process of achieving a rejuvenation effect using a syringe, and includes fat injection, lipoplasty, botulinum toxin, and filler injection.

Anti-aging therapy

Anti-aging therapy mostly involves medical treatment, wherein anti-oxidant vitamin C and E are administered to reduce free radicals. As people age, growth hormones, melatonin, and dehydroepiandrosterone (DHEA) decrease; and particularly in women, estrogen decreases after menopause. The level of growth hormones reaches its peak at 16 years of age and then decreases gradually to only 20% of the peak at 60 years of age. Growth hormones are required in the growth period as well as for the metabolism of the body. It is known that exercise increases growth hormones. In postmenopausal women, subcutaneous fat and the skin tone decrease due to the decreased estrogen level. Estrogen replacement can produce a skin rejuvenation effect. There is a concern, however, that the administration of estrogen in post-menopausal women may increase the probability of the development of breast cancer, though there is no scientific evidence of such. Regular tests for breast cancer may be helpful, though. It is recommended that anti-aging therapy be individualized depending on the level of hormones, vitamins, and metabolites in each patient, as assessed with the relevant tests.

Medical skin care

In elderly people, aging spots and fine wrinkles form in the skin. Skin care can make the skin fair and improve wrinkles in aging skin. For skin care, bleachers, exfoliants, soothers, and sunblock creams are mainly used. Moisturizers, nutrition creams, the anti-oxidants vitamins C and E, and facial cleansers are also used. Whitening agents inhibit the formation of melanin pigment in melanocytes. The most commonly used whitening agents are hydroquinone and kojic acid. For exofoliants, peeling creams, retinoic acid, and α-hydroxy acids (AHA) are commonly used, and the effect and irritability of the peeling cream varies according to the concentration. Peeling creams remove the keratin layer, promote epidermal renewal, and regenerate atrophic epidermal cells. They also peel off aging spots by removing melanin pigments, and rejuvenate the skin by improving fine wrinkles. These exofoliants are effective only for the epidermis but not for the dermis. Thus, if the use of an exofoliant is stopped, the effect would disappear after about 6 weeks. Whitening and peeling creams are highly irritable to the skin and thus may cause irritation such as redness and itching. Concomitant use of hydrocortisone, an anti-inflammatory soother agent, may alleviate the symptoms.

Laser rejuvenation

Resurfacing laser and non-invasive laser

The carbon dioxide (CO_2) laser and erbium: yttrium aluminium garnet (Er:YAG) laser may have good rejuvenating effects such as increased skin tightness and elasticity, and removal of aging spots. These treatment methods require a long wound healing time, however, because they peel the skin extensively from the surface to parts of the dermis. When wound healing is delayed or not accomplished, serious sequela such as hypertrophic scars or dyschromia may be left. After laser ablation, erythema may last for a long time. In Asians, laser ablation may

Table 01-2	Rejuvenation lasers
Ablative laser; resurfacing laser	CO_2; invasive, powerful Er:YAG; less invasive
Non-ablative laser	Diode; infrared laser IPL
Non-ablative fractional laser	Er:glass fractional
Ablative fractional laser	CO_2 fractional Er:YAG fractional
Other	RF LED Photodynamic therapy Fractional RF
Combination	Laser + RF

CO_2, carbon dioxide; Er:YAG, erbium: yttrium aluminium garnet; IPL, intense pulsed light; RF, radiofrequency, LED, light-emitting diode.

cause postinflammatory hyperpigmentation (PIH) , which leads to considerable discomfort in social life. Lower-power infrared laser, diode, or LED phototherapy do not have the disadvantages of laser ablation but can tighten the skin. Although they do not cause such side effects as erythema or PIH, physicians or patients do not use them widely because of their less noticeable weak effect. Intense pulsed light (IPL) polychromatic light energy with a broadspectrum waveband (450-1,200 nm) that is effective for melanin pigments and telangiectasia in aging skin but cannot increase skin elasticity.

▌Fractional laser

This is as safe as the infrared laser, and causes no discomfort in the patient's daily life. It is also almost as effective as laser ablation. Although laser ablation removes the full thickness of the epidermis and thus causes problems, the nonablative fractional laser delivers heat to the deep dermis without damaging the epidermis and thus, can induce skin tightening. With the nonablative fractional laser, a micro-columnar central pore may be formed. The micro-columnar central pore is a kill zone, a central necrosis caused by irreversible change due to thermal damage. The edge of the kill zone forms a coagulation zone wherein such reversible change due to a weaker thermal effect such as degeneration of proteins occurs. The kill zone in the center and the coagulation zone form a micro-thermal zone (MTZ). Treatment with the nonablative fractional laser results in erythema and edema that last for only about a day; and on the next day of the treatment, allows the patient to lead a normal life. It also causes no downtime in the patient's social life (i.e., the patient can already wash her face or wear make-up). Besides, after the treatment, PIH does not occur, except in patients whose skin is sensitive; and even if PIH occurs, it would be very slight. Although the nonablative fractional laser cannot remove epidermal lesions, it lightens pigmented lesions and improves slightly hypertrophic or atrophic scars as well as hypopigmented scars. Besides, it improves wrinkles and acne scars with its skin tightening effect, though only slightly. Thus, 3-5 sessions at intervals of 3-4 weeks are required. The nonablative fractional laser is advantageous in that it does not peel off the skin and is more effective than the low-power infrared laser. It is, however, less effective than the ablative laser approach. To optimize the benefits of the fractional approach, an ablative fractional technique that uses the CO_2 laser and Er:YAG laser has been developed. The ablative fractional laser has the features of both the fractional laser and the ablative laser but with minimal downtime. The CO_2 fractional lasers achieve partial ablation through vaporization of water in tissue. With the ablative fractional laser, the tissue is ablated in the form of a micro-ablative column (MAC), and the surrounding tissues tighten due to the thermal effect.

Other treatments and combination treatments

Radiofrequency treatment, which uses radiofrequency energy and has a fractional function, has been developed to preserve the epidermis and promote dermal regeneration to prevent the disadvantage of resurfacing treatment and to increase skin elasticity. Radiofrequency treatment can be used in combination with laser treatment.

Summary

For facial rejuvenation, clear understanding of the aging phenomenon is necessary. For total rejuvenation, all possible options such as laser skin rejuvenation, face lifting, and volume replacement should be combined to achieve a better outcome.

REFERENCES

1. Babak A, et al. Master techniques in facial rejuvenation. Saunders 2007:263.
2. Calvin MJ, Aamsey A. The Aging Face, a systematic approach. Saunders 2002.
3. Glogau RG. Physiologic and structural changes associated with aging skin. Dermatol Clin 1997;15:555-559.
4. Goldman MP, et al. Cutaneous Laser Surgery, Mosby. 2nd ed, 1999.
5. Goldman MP, Marchell N, Fitzpatrick RE. laser skin resurfacing of the face with a combined CO_2/Er:YAG laser. Dermatol Surg 2000;26:102-104.
6. Hamra S. Composite Rhytidectomy. Plast Reconstr Surg 1992;90:1-13.
7. Hohenleutner R, Hohenleutner S, Bäumler W, Landthaler M. Fast and effective skin ablation with an Er:YAG laser: determination of ablation rates and thermal damage zones. Laser Surg Med 1997;21:13.

8. Isee NG. Endoscopic facial rejuvenation: endoforehead, the functional lift. Aesthetic Plast Surg 1994;18:21-29.

9. Park SH. Laser dermatologic plastic surgery, Ch 10, Laser rejuvenation, 2nd Ed. Seoul: Koonja Pub Co.; 2014. p.366-386.

10. Patrick LT, Alexis MV. The MACS-Lift. short scar rhytidectomy. Quality medical publishing;2004.

11. Walsh JT, Deutsch TF. Er:YAG laser ablation of tissue: measurement of ablation rates. Laser Surg Med 1989;9:327.

12. Zering CL. Cutaneous laser resurfacing with the erbium:YG laser and the char-free carbon dioxide laser: a clinical comparison of 100 patients. Int L Aesthetic Reconst Surg 1997;5:29.

Fine lines & deep wrinkles (skin laxity)

▶ Won Serk Kim, MD, PhD

Introduction

Skin wrinkles are the most important and common symptoms of the aging skin. The distribution and movement of facial muscles play an important role in the formation of wrinkles. People who always frown tend to develop deep, thick wrinkles in the brow, whereas those who smile a lot tend to develop lots of wrinkles at the lateral aspect of the eye, so-called crow's feet. Genetic factors are also believed to be involved in the formation of wrinkles. For example, wrinkle patterns vary across human races. Koreans tend to have thicker wrinkles than Caucasians. In Koreans, thick wrinkles are remarkable mostly in the brow and around the eyes and lips, whereas in Caucasians, many fine wrinkles rather than thick ones develop in the brow and cheek. There are differences even between Koreans of the same age. The causes of fine wrinkles, deep wrinkles, and decreased skin elasticity, all of which are important clinical symptoms of aged skin, include a decrease in extracellular matrix proteins in the dermis. It is well known that the amount of collagen in the dermis decreases by 1% each year in adults. Particularly, in photoaged skin that had been exposed to ultraviolet rays for a long time, the amount of collagen decreases more than in skin aged due to intrinsic factors. In addition, wrinkles are intensified by the effect of gravity on age-damaged soft tissues, particularly in the superficial musculoaponeurotic system, and by repeated contraction and relaxation of facial muscles of expression.

Tips for diagnosis

Wrinkles are generally classified depending on their pathogenesis and severity. By pathogenesis, they can be grouped into four types. First, fine wrinkles such as those under the eyes appear due to thinning of the epidermis and the dermis due to a decrease in collagen and elastic fibers after prolonged exposure to ultraviolet rays through the action of the degenerative enzymes, matrix metalloproteinases I and II. Second, wrinkles such as crow's feet, frown lines, and forehead wrinkles are caused by dents in the epidermis or dermis formed by repeated contraction and relaxation of the muscles of expression. Third, accordion pleat wrinkles are caused by atrophy of the epidermis, dermis, and adipose layer, and the consequential loss of elasticity and the formation of excessive skin, as exemplified by sagging cheeks. Finally, nasolabial folds are caused by skin folding due to repeated contraction and relaxation of muscles and consequential sagging of the skin, subcutaneous fat, and muscles due to gravity.

Tips for treatment

Treatment procedures for aged skin can be grouped into invasive and non-invasive ones. Invasive treatment procedures, the most common of which is carbon dioxide (CO_2) or erbium: yttrium aluminium garnet (Er:YAG) ablative laser treatment, treat pigmentary and structural changes related to photoaging by ablating off the epidermal layer and depositing heat in the dermis, so-called residual thermal damage. The epidermis is stimulated to regenerate, and the collagen in the dermis is rearranged through the remodeling process following photothermal damage and induction of the wound healing process, including neocollagenesis. Although results can be excellent, downtime can be prolonged with the potential for severe side effects including hyper- or hypopigmentation and scar formation.

With the introduction of procedures that are less invasive and cause less damage to the skin, however, both physicians and patients can feel less burdened by the procedure, and the procedures can now be performed safely with much less downtime. For skin rejuvenation, such non-invasive methods included so-called nonablative skin rejuvenation using systems such as the 1064 or 1320 nm neodymium:yttrium aluminium garnet (Nd:YAG) laser, 1440 or 1450 nm diode laser, 1540 or 1550 nm erbium:glass laser, and intense pulsed light (IPL). Although they caused less side-effects, these nonablative approaches had disadvantages, however, in that multiple treatment sessions were required and the treatment effects were delayed and not dramatic compare to those of the invasive procedures.

Devices that combine radiofrequency (RF) with laser or IPL and infrared thermal energy that directly act on the dermis are also used as non-invasive rejuvenation methods. Those approaches are not influenced by the skin color, can promote the regeneration of collagen without damaging the epidermis, and patients who have received this kind of treatment can immediately feel greater 'skin tightening' due to the initial contraction of collagen. Although patients feel satisfied immediately after the treatment mostly due to the skin shrinkage effect, this effect is temporary. An important point is that heat-induced rearrangement of collagen gradually occurs over several weeks or months, after which lax skin can recover its tightness through the remodeling process.

Full-thickness ablation using the laser

The biggest advantage of skin ablation using a laser is that in the ideal situation the skin can be removed up to the desired depth, complications can be minimized via skin restoration through regeneration and contraction of the dermal collagen fibers, and maximum correction of aged skin can be achieved. The CO_2 laser used first for this approach, emits mid infrared light at a wavelength of 10600 nm. Although it cannot perform pigment-selective destruction, it acts through absorption of tissue water, as water is the major chromophore for the 10600 nm wavelength. In the early days of this technique, the continuous wave (CW) CO_2 laser was widely used. Although results could be excellent, CW CO_2 full face ablation induced serious side effects such as prolonged erythema and scar formation. CW was thus gradually replaced by pulsed, superpulsed, and ultrapulsed lasers. Since the mid-1990s, skin ablation using the ultrapulsed CO_2 laser has been widely used as the gold-standard treatment for wrinkles, acne scars, and surgical or wound scars. Skin irradiation with the CO_2 laser that emits a short pulse wave with high energy (thermal relaxation time <700 μsec and pulse duration: 250 μsec – 1 msec) results in necrosis of the epidermis and thermocoagulative changes in the papillary and upper reticular epidermis, as assessed histologically, and reversible contraction of highly heat-sensitive dermal collagen. A histological examination may show that new collagen has formed in the dermis some 4 weeks after the laser treatment, and remodeling of this collagen can continue for up to one year or more, leading to such clinical outcomes as the disappearance and improvement of wrinkles, and restoration of a youthful-looking skin.

Numerous clinical studies have shown that laser ablation using a CO_2 laser could improve the skin tone and wrinkles by 50% or more in a single session. Full-thickness ablation using a CO_2 laser, however, could take 1 week or more to for reepithelialization, and at least 1 month or more before the patient could return to their social or working life, causing serious disruption to their normal activities of daily living. Besides, full-thickness ablation using a CO_2 laser may cause complications such as infection, swelling, redness, or dyspigmentation due to damage of the entire epidermal layer and partial damage in the dermal layer.

The Er:YAG laser, a next-generation laser that addressed the disadvantages of the CO_2 laser, emits a wavelength of 2940 nm, the absorption of which in water is more than one order of magnitude better than that of the CO_2 laser. Thus, the 2,940 nm wavelength acts very superficially, with clean epidermal ablation and residual thermal damage in the dermis limited to 1-3 μm per J/cm^2, dramatically better that of the CO_2 laser. Because of the Er:YAG short pulse width of 250-300 μsec, it has a shorter thermal diffusion time and causes less damage to neighboring tissue. Thus, the exact depth to be ablated can be adjusted with the Er:YAG laser because if the dermoepidermal junction is exposed after 4-5 passes with the laser, pin-point bleeding occurs and the laser irradiation can be stopped. Comparisons in numerous studies of the treatment effects and side effects of the CO_2 laser and the Er:YAG laser have shown that the mean recovery time with the CO_2 laser was 10-14 days and with the Er:YAG laser, 5-10 days; the morbidity and incidence of complications were lower with the Er:YAG laser; and the Er:YAG laser was more suitable for skin regeneration in Asians. The same studies showed, however, that for the treatment of severely photoaged skin or deep wrinkles, the Er:YAG laser had a weaker treatment effect both clinically and histologically due to less delivered thermal damage to the dermal matrix, and provided a poor view of the surgical area due to poor hemostasis during the surgery.

To address these disadvantages, the long-pulsed and dual-mode Er:YAG lasers for abla-tion and coagulation were developed and are widely used in ablation for aesthetic purposes and for photodamaged skin, hypertrophic scars, seborrheic keratosis, and pigmented nevi. There was also a system which combined both the CO_2 and Er:YAG wavelengths in one system, which was reported to have excellent effects. Nevertheless, full-thickness ablation is associated with the risk of post-treatment scarring or infection. Thus, the ablation should be performed several months after discontinuing the administration of retinoic acid; and before the procedure, prevention of infectious diseases such as herpes simplex is suggested. In ad-dition, care must be taken in treating areas such as the neck or hands that have few skin ap-pendages, because wound recovery is slow and formation of scars is common in these areas, and patients must be highly compliant in their wound care regimen.

Regeneration using the non-ablative and ablative fractional lasers

The CO_2 laser and the Er:YAG laser, though highly effective in the treatment of facial wrin-kles and acne scars, have disadvantages in that they require a long healing time and have risks of various side effects, as mentioned already. The conception of fractional photother-molysis (FP), which was introduced in 2003, presented a new paradigm for skin regeneration treatment. FP is a principle wherein the laser beam is 'fractionated' into many microbeams, creating a series of deep microscopic thermal zones (MTZs) to depths varying from around 700 μm to 1300 μm with a diameter of 400 μm or less to induce the migration of uninjured cells in the neighboring region thus swiftly achieving regeneration of the skin. FP is advantageous in that it can reduce the healing time by regenerating the epidermal and dermal layers while maintaining the barrier function of the skin, and can minimize complications. FP was first utilized with an erbium-doped fiber (Er:glass) laser operating at a wavelength of 1550 nm. The Er:glass laser is a non-ablative fractional laser (NAFL) that is typically capable of forming 2000 MTZs per 1 cm^2 (15-20% of the entire skin area in one treatment session) without involving any of the biological pigment chromophores, thereby stimulating fibroblasts and epidermal stem cells. Since then, various types of NAFL systems with various wavelengths, pulse energies, and injury patterns have been developed following the NAFL principle. Since 2007, ablative fractional lasers (AFLs) were developed based on the CO_2 or Er:YAG lasers to deal with more severe skin aging than the NAFL systems were capable of.

Thus, currently available fractional lasers can be grouped into the NAFL and AFL systems. The 1550 nm or 1540 Er:glass laser, the most representative NAFL system, can activate a healing process that consists of shrinkage of the treated site for one week after the treatment, relaxation of the treated site thereafter and followed some 4-6 weeks later by tightening of the treated site through the remodeling phase of the wound healing process. The NAFL approach is therefore used to repair wrinkles, treat enlarged pores, and deal with age-related skin sequelae such as skin laxity. NAFL was known to improve fine, moderate or wrinkles by up to 80% without complications with 2-3 sessions of treatment at an interval of 2 weeks. Despite its advantage of a short healing time, though, it is less effective for deep wrinkles, even if it is performed repeatedly. Thus, the patients are sometimes not fully satisfied when NAFL is performed as monotherapy. NAFL treatment can also be used to improve various skin conditions such as freckles, dyspigmentation, stria distensae, and disseminated superficial porokeratosis and scars.

As already mentioned, in 2007, the AFL technique was developed to combine the benefits of full-thickness ablation with the fractional approach. The AFL creates macroablative columns (MACs) in the epidermis and dermis, so unlike the NAFL, the epidermis as also ablated. Immunohistochemistry of AFL-treated skin has shown that, after treatment using the fractional CO_2 laser, the healing process continued for 3 months or longer due to the thermal injury-mediated wound healing process from the epidermal stratum corneum right through deep into the dermis. This prolonged healing process was thus expected to more significantly improve wrinkles and skin texture than with the NAFL. In fact, a comparative clinical study wherein a test was performed with a split-face design showed that one treatment session with a CO_2 AFL improved facial wrinkles by 75%, whereas one session with a 1550 nm Er:glass NAFL improved facial wrinkles by only 25%. In addition, CO_2 AFL is known to remarkably improve age-related skin lesions with only 1-2 sessions of treatment, unlike the NAFL, which requires multiple sessions. After AFL treatment, exudates normally appear in the treated site for 1-2 days, and thus some degree of wound management of the treated site is necessary. The regeneration starts within 2 days, however, and patients can go back to their normal life within 5-10 days. In addition to the CO_2 AFL systems, Er:YAG based AFL systems are now also available. Comparative studies with split-face designs showed that the CO_2 AFL system more significantly improved the skin texture and wrinkles than the fractionated Er:YAG laser, because of the more superficial action of the Er:YAG wavelength and the small amount of residual thermal damage. The number of indications for the fractional laser is expected to expand, as numerous centers are currently conducting studies on this approach.

Regeneration using nonablative laser skin rejuvenation

Truly nonablative laser skin rejuvenation (NAR), which is non-fractionated, allows patients to return to their normal life immediately after the treatment, and was developed in the mid 1990's to counteract the long down time and severe side effects of full-face ablative laser rejuvenation. NAR achieves its effect by delivering thermal energy to the dermal matrix collagen under an aggressively cooled epidermis, thereby leaving the epidermis intact. NAR systems include the 1320 nm Nd:YAG laser, the 1450 nm diode laser, and the 585 and 595 nm pulsed dye lasers, etc, all of which are equipped with an epidermal cooling device and though not actually a laser, IPL is also used in nonablative skin rejuvenation. Generally, treatments are performed at intervals of 3-4 weeks, and patients can go back to their normal daily life immediately after the treatment. The treatment effect of NAR and IPL systems remains however controversial, with patient dissatisfaction often reported. Slight swelling may occur and, though rarely, redness, blisters, and pigmentation at the treated site. No serious complications have been reported, but results are considerably less robust those achieved with the NAFL and AFL approaches.

Skin rejuvenation with other approaches

Laser ablation using the interstitial lipolysis laser is now being tried for regeneration of aging skin. The lipolysis laser delivers micropulsed laser energy to the deep dermis and subdermal fat layer through an optical fiber either via a microcannula with a 1 mm diameter that is placed under the incision line, or using the bare fiber through a microincision, and the laser is fired while the fiber is moved back and forth in a radial, fan-like motion. The effect of the laser is achieved by combining photoacoustic and photothermal energy. In addition to the photoacoustic effect that induces degeneration of adipocytes, the photothermal effect is achieved when laser light is absorbed in the connective tissues such as collagen fibers after it

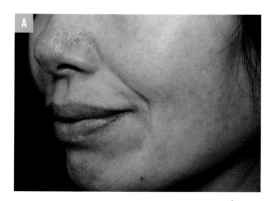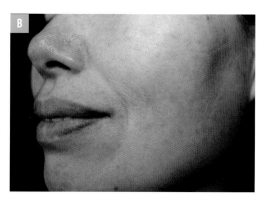

Figure 02-1   **Effect of 1444 nm pulsed neodymium:yttrium aluminium garnet interstitial fiberoptic-delivered laser treatment on the nasolabial fold. A.** Before treatment. **B.** 3 months after one treatment session.

is first absorbed in the fat layer using water and fat as the chromophores and then delivered to the dermis. The thermal energy converted from the laser energy in the subcutaneous fat layer reaches sufficient temperatures to achieve liquefaction of adipocytes, and tightening and retraction of dermal tissue are induced when the temperatures in the deep dermis might reach around 50°C. Thus, high collagen regeneration in the dermis can be achieved without damage to the epidermis. The most recent of these laser lipolysis systems is a 1444 nm Nd:YAG laser, which was developed in South Korea (AccuSculpt; Lutronic Corp, Goyang, South Korea). This interesting system has been reported to increase skin elasticity via collagen contraction by maximizing both water and fat absorption in the subdermal fat layer and creating a milder photothermal effect in the dermal collagen (Figure 02-1).

RF energy has also attracted attention for skin rejuvenation and treatment of skin laxity in recent years. When RF energy is applied via a surface electrode, however, high power cannot be used because of epidermal burns, so to achieve adequate dermal thermal effects, some form of skin cooling is essential and multiple treatments are usually required. To overcome this, fractional RF has been developed. When the RF energy is fractionated over multiple needle electrodes, and furthermore the needles are insulated apart from the very tip, then RF energy is selectively delivered to a preset depth in the dermis with no electrothermal damage to the epidermis, and no need for skin cooling. A novel system which combines microneedling fractional RF (MFR) with superficial fractional RF (SFR) has been recently developed (INFINI; Lutronic Corp.). It is therefore now possible to deliver powerful electrothermal damage to the dermis while minimizing the damage to the epidermis, and to perform skin rejuvenation by inducing the formation of collagen in the photoaged dermis (Figure 02-2). In the very near future, MFR will be able to be delivered in combination with superficial

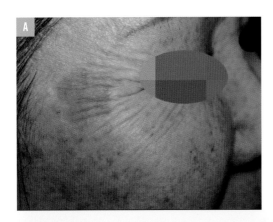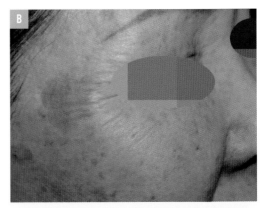

Figure 02-2 **Effect of microneedling fractional radiofrequency (MFR) on periorbital wrinkles. A.** Before treatment. **B.** 3 months after three treatment sessions.

fractional RF delivering controlled energy only to the epidermis and very superficial dermis, with the one system, thereby delivering true three-dimensional skin tightening.

REFERENCES

1. Alexiades-Armenakas MR, Dover JS, Arndt KA. The spectrum of laser skin resurfacing : Nonablative, fractional, and ablative laser resurfacing. J Am Acad Dermatol 2008;58:719-737.

2. Brightman LA, Brauer JA, Anolik R, Weiss E, Karen J, Chapas A, Hale E, Bernstein L, Geronemus RG. Ablative and fractional ablative lasers. Dermatol Clin 2009;27:479-489.

3. Doherty SD, Doherty CB, Markus JS, Markus RF. A paradigm for facial skin rejuvenation. Facial Surg 2009;27:479-489.

4. Goldberg DJ, Rogachefsky AS, Silapunt S. Non-ablative laser treatment of facial rhytides. A comparison of 1450 nm diode laser treatment with dynamic cooling as opposed to treatment with dynamic cooling alone. Lasers Surg Med 2002; 30:79–81.

5. Goldberg DJ, Samady JA. Intense pulsed light and Nd:YAG laser non-ablative treatment of facial rhytides. Lasers Surg Med 2001;28:141–144.

6. Holcomb JD, et al. 1444 nm Nd:YAG lipolysis laser assisted facial contouring – A new paradigm for facial sculpting and rejuvenation. Abstract presented at American Society for Laser Medicine and Surgery Conference, 2010, Phoenix, AZ.

7. Jih MH, Goldberg LH, Kimyai-Asadi A. Fractional photothermolysis for photoaging of hands. Dermatol Surg 2008:34:73–78.

8. Tannous Z. Fractional resurfacing. Clin Dermatol 2007;25:480-486.

9. Tark KC, Jung JE, Song SY. Superior lipolytic effect of the 1,444 nm Nd:YAG laser : comparison with the 1,064 nm Nd:YAG laser. Lasers Surg Med 2009;41:721-727.

10. Tierney EP, Kouba DJ, Hanke CW. Review of fractional photothermolysis : treatment indications and efficacy. Dermatol Surg 2009;35:1445-1461.

11. Trelles MA. Short and long-term follow-up of nonablative 1320 nm Nd:YAG laser facial rejuvenation. Dermatol Surg 2001;27:781–782.

Enlarged pores

▶ Kee Yang Chung, MD, PhD & Sung Bin Cho, MD, PhD

Introduction

'Enlarged or dilated pores' applies to the visible topographic feature at the skin surface corresponding to enlarged openings of pilosebaceous follicles. These visible funnel-shaped pores are physiologically present in all individuals but recently, many patients complain of these pores as a cosmetic problem and seek treatment. Various factors such as sex, genetic predisposition, aging, chronic ultraviolet exposure, comedogenic xenobiotics, acne, and seborrhea are known to be responsible for enlarged pores.

Tips for diagnosis

Skin pores appear as empty funnel-shaped structures or as cornified cylindrical plugs, corresponding to comedones. Visible empty funnel-shaped pores are physiologically present in all individuals. Horny impacted pores are normally seen in the facial skin, especially on the nose and cheeks, but the appearance of pores differs among individuals. Oily skin results from large quantities of sebum produced by the sebaceous glands, filling the follicular reservoir and leaking onto the body surface. On the face, greasy skin is shiny and may be accompanied by enlarged pores, follicular plugs, sebaceous filaments and comedones.

In Caucasians, some investigators have regarded enlarged pores as a phenomenon of photoaging. While it is true that enlarged pores are one manifestation of photoaging, many Asian patients with enlarged pores are young and do not necessarily show other photoaging-associated symptoms such as sallow skin tone, dilated pore structure, crepe-paper-like inelasticity of the eyelids and rhytides. Instead, many patients with enlarged pores seem to complain of greasy or oily skin compared with other patients with normal pore size. The appearance of skin oiliness results from the presence of an excess of sebum secreted by the sebaceous glands onto the skin surface.

Tips for treatment

Previous reports regarded enlarged pores as a phenomenon of photoaging and treated them using methods such as intense pulsed light, retinoic acid cream, oral isotretinoin, isotretinoin iontophoresis and glycolic acid peeling. Some reports mentioned the pore size reduction effect while focusing on the acne scar treatment.

Recently, 1064 nm neodymium-doped yttrium aluminum garnet (Nd:YAG) laser treatment showed effect in reducing pore size (Figure 03-1). Until now the 1064 nm Nd:YAG laser has been widely used to remove tattoos, unwanted hair and dermal pigment. However, both Q-switched (QS) Nd:YAG (QSNY) and long-pulsed (LP) Nd:YAG have been shown to induce dermal collagen formation in the mid to upper dermis which explains their effect

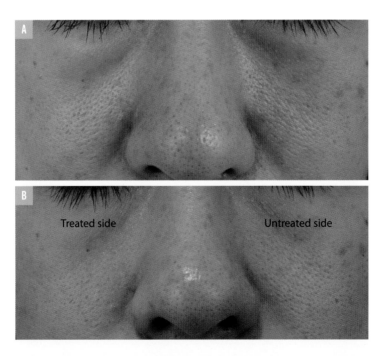

Treated side   Untreated side

Figure 03-1 Effect of quasi long-pulsed 1064 nm Nd:YAG laser treatment on enlarged facial pores. **A.** Before treatment, **B.** 3 months after five sessions of treatment (3.0 J/cm^2, 300 μs pulse width, 7 mm spot size, three laser passes).

on wrinkles and possibly on the reduction of pore size. In several studies, both QS Nd:YAG and LP Nd:YAG showed effectiveness in reducing the size of enlarged facial pores but the optimal mode and parameters are still under debate. For treatment using a collimated beam, the handpiece of the laser is held approximately 2 cm away from the skin and passes over the skin are made in a painting motion until the clinical end-point is reached. The clinical end-point is moderate erythema and/or mild petechiae over the treatment area. Multiple treatments at an interval of 2 to 3 weeks are required.

Systems based on the principle of fractional photothermolysis (FPS) are also used to treat enlarged pores. The nonablative FPS creates hundreds to thousands of microthermal treatment zones (MTZs) and coagulated columns which are surrounded by untreated tissue under an intact epidermis. Because the epidermal architecture is more or less intact, the epidermis is rapidly repaired. Ablative FPSs, on the other hand, create microablative columns (MACs) including the epidermis. Once again the ablated column is surrounded by residual thermal damage (coagulated zone) and beyond that, normal epidermal and dermal tissue. Because the ablative damage is fractionated, the surrounding normal tissue helps the MACs to heal rapidly, and reepithelization occurs in 2-4 days. By rearrangement and stimulation of collagen production, the FPS approach may improve the texture of the treated area. Fractional 1545 and 1550 nm erbium glass (Er:glass) lasers representing the nonabalative FPS, and fractional carbon dioxide (CO_2) and Er:YAG lasers representing ablative FPS, have shown efficacy to improve enlarged facial pores. However, multiple treatments are required especially with the nonablative FPS approach.

A fractional radiofrequency (RF) device using penetrating microneedles also has been effectively used for treating enlarged facial pores. The penetration depth of the microneedles can be precisely controlled to effectively deliver RF energy into the dermal tissue as well as to prevent unwanted excessive thermal injury in the epidermis. The RF-induced electrothermal tissue reaction usually results in generating water-drop or cocoon-shaped coagulation around the tip of electrode in the dermis, whereas ablative FPS makes a conical zone of photothermal coagulation presenting the widest injury in the epidermis and narrower in the dermis. Until recently, several types of fractional RF devices have been used which can be subdivided by monopolar or bipolar, the number of microneedle electrodes, such as 5 to 49 microneedles in a disposable tip, and insulated or non-insulated electrodes.

An *in vivo* micropig study reported that the characteristics of RF-skin interaction were dependent on a variety of factors, including the depth of the microneedles, tissue impedance and permittivity of the skin layers, RF exposure times, and level of power When the treatment settings of RF exposure time and power level are apprpriately set, a bipolar RF device using insulated microneedles can produce a larger zone of electrothermal coagulation in the deeper reticular dermis or subcutaneous layer compared with the epidermis and papillary dermis. However, the concentration of electrothermal tissue reaction is higher in the papillary dermis and lower in the reticular dermis or subcutaneous layer. Additionally, histometric values of RF-induced coagulated column, including height, width, and calculated volume, are usually significantly affected by the RF exposure times. However, the level or power setting of the RF current reportedly affects the degree of tissue coagulation rather than to histometric values, i.e., the quality of the coagulation rather than the volume. Previous investigations demonstrated that RF-treated skin comprised regenerated collagen and elastic fibers. Additionally, the compact rearrangements of thick collagen fibers after RF treatment in both the upper and lower dermis have been suggested as one of the major contributing factors for improving enlarged pores.

Enlarged pores can be treated with several sessions of fractional microneedle RF treatment at 3-6 weeks intervals. The use of topical anesthetic cream prior to the RF treatment is usually recommended. The device settings for treating enlarged pores include microneedle depths of 1.0 to 2.0 mm and single or multiple passes depending on the skin-RF response. The power level and exposure time should be set according to the characteristics of each individual patient. Factional microneedling RF treatment for enlarged pores is generally well tolerated without remarkable side effects, except for transient post-treatment minimal oozing, crusting, and scaling, these, and erythema, improve spontaneously in 3-5 days. However, caution should be exercised when treating enlarged facial pores in patients with melasma, especially in the periorbital area.

- The concept of beauty in Asian women is different from that in Caucasians. In Asians, there is a high demand for rejuvenation treatments that can reduce pore size and/or have a "whitening effect" on skin color. The Nd:YAG 1064 nm laser and fractional lasers can be used as effective treatments to improve the appearance of enlarged pores in Asian patients (Table 03-1).

Table 03-1 **Summary of combination laser treatment options for enlarged pores.**

	Modality	Laser parameter
1064 nm Nd:YAG laser	Q-switched Nd:YAG	2.5-6 J/cm^2
	Long-pulsed Nd: YAG	3-15 J/cm^2
Fractional photothermolysis system	Ablative carbon dioxide laser	70 mJ, 150 spots/cm^2
	Nonablative erbium glass laser	20-28 mJ, 400-900 spots/cm^2

Tips for post-treatment care and follow-up

For Nd:YAG laser treatment, topical anesthetic cream is not mandatory. However, cooling during and after laser treatment is recommended. Side effects observed have mainly been pain during treatment, post-treatment erythema, petechiae and edema, all of which resolve within a week after treatment.

For the fractional laser approach, both ablative and nonablative, a topical anesthetic cream should be applied prior to the laser treatment due to pain during treatment. Side effects are mild pain during treatment, mild post-treatment erythema, and edema, all of which resolve within a few days with the nonablative systems and around a week or so with the ablative systems. Other possible adverse events include hyperpigmentation, hypopigmentation, crusting, itching, and scarring.

- Side effects of Nd:YAG treatment for enlarged facial pores are very subtle so that patients do not experience any limitations in their normal activities.
- Fractional photothermolysis systems may have side effects such as prolonged erythema and hyperpigmentation in dark-skinned Asians.

REFERENCES

1. Cho SB, Lee JH, Choi MJ, Lee KY, Oh SH. Efficacy of the Fractional Photothermolysis System with Dynamic Operating Mode on Acne Scars and Enlarged Facial Pores. Dermatol Surg 2009;35:108-114.
2. Cho SI, Chung BY, Choi MG, Baek JH, Cho HJ, Park CW, Lee CH, Kim HO. Evaluation of the clinical efficacy of fractional radiofrequency microneedle treatment in acne scars and large facial pores. Dermatol Surg 2012;38:1017-1024.
3. Jung JY, Lee JH, Ryu DJ, Lee SJ, Bang D, Cho SB. Lower-Fluence, Higher-Density versus Higher-Fluence, Lower-Density Treatment with a 10,600-nm Carbon Dioxide Fractional Laser System: A Split-Face, Evaluator-Blinded Study. Dermatol Surg 2010;36:2022-2029.
4. Kim JE, Lee HW, Kim JK, Moon SH, Ko JY, Lee MW, Chang SE. Objective evaluation of the clinical efficacy of fractional radiofrequency treatment for acne scars and enlarged pores in Asian skin. Dermatol Surg 2014;40:988-995.
5. Lee CN, Kim YJ, Lee HS, Kim HS. Effects of Q-switched and long-pulsed 1064nm Nd:YAG laser on enlarged facial pores. Photodermatol, Photoimmunol & Photomed 2009;25:328-330.
6. Roh M, Han M, Kim D, Chung KY. Sebum output as a factor contributing to the size of facial pores. Brit J Dermatol 2006;155:890-894.
7. Roh MR, Chung HJ, Chung KY. Effects of various parameters of the 1064nm Nd:YAG laser for the treatment of enlarged facial pores. J Dermatol Treat 2009;20:223-228.
8. Wattanakrai P, Rojhirunsakool S, Pootongkam S. Split-Face Comparison of Long-Pulse-Duration Neodymium-Doped Yttrium Aluminum Garnet (Nd:YAG) 1,064-nm Laser Alone and Combination Long-Pulse and Q-switched Nd:YAG 1,064-nm Laser with Carbon Photoenhancer Lotion for the Treatment of Enlarged Pores in Asian Women. Dermatol Surg 2010;36:1672-1680.
9. Zheng Z, Goo B, Kim DY, Kang JS, Cho SB. Histometric analysis of skin-radiofrequency interaction using a fractionated microneedle delivery system. Dermatol Surg 2014;40:134-141.

04

Resurfacing laser

▶ Seung Ha Park, MD, PhD, MBA

Skin peeling

Ablation involves removal of a thin layer of the skin, and the ablation procedure involves removal of the surface of the skin for treatment. The skin consists of the epidermis and the dermis. The cells in the epidermal basal cell layers move regularly toward the keratin layers, and thereby constantly renew the epidermis. The epithelial cells are found in the epidermis and in some parts of the appendages of the dermis. They also exist in the secretary ducts of the sweat and sebaceous glands. In addition, epithelial cells surround hair follicles.

The existence of epithelial cells is essential for the epithelization of the skin. Since skin wounds heal well in the epidermis where there are epithelial cells and in the upper papillary dermis where there are many dermal appendages, the skin in these regions heals normally even after ablation of a thin layer of the skin. Thus, ablation is normally compared to onions because as with onions, layer after layer can be peeled off.

Laser resurfacing

In 1989, the possibility of performing ablation of the skin using carbon dioxide (CO_2) laser with a continuous wave (CW) was suggested. As CW lasers can cause increased thermal skin damage, however, superpulsed and ultrapulsed lasers were developed to avoid the severe side effects associated with CW lasers. This development led to the use of high-power lasers for ablation of the skin. In the mid-1990s, laser ablation became widely used owing to its treatment effect for skin lesions and its good rejuvenation effect.

In the early 2000s, the erbium: yttrium aluminium garnet (Er:YAG) laser started to be used for ablation. Because the penetration of the light emitted from the Er:YAG laser was more shallow than that from the CO_2 laser, the Er:YAG laser did not lead to the severe erythema, associated with deep ablation. Thus, the Er:YAG laser is now widely used for laser ablation.

The biggest advantage of laser ablation is that it makes it easy to control the depth of penetration, unlike other ablation procedures. For chemical peeling, it is not possible to know the depth of the ablation until the crust falls off, and mechanical ablation involves hemorrhage, whereas laser ablation does not involve so much bleeding and thus makes it possible to know the exact depth of the ablation. With laser resurfacing, it is easy to control the depth of the ablation, and thus, the upper dermis can be ablated safely and deep ablation can be performed effectively without such side effects as formation of hypertrophic scars. Ablation using a high-power laser can vaporize only the tissues in the intended site, without destroying the normal tissues. Unlike dermabrasion, laser resurfacing does not involve bleeding, and thus, the scar can be tidy. As laser resurfacing caogulates capillary vessels, lymphatic glands, and nerve endings that are less than 0.5 mm in diameter, bleeding and effusion are low and post-treatment pain is slight, which increases patient comfort. Unlike with chemical peeling, laser ablation forms less of a crust. Thus, the patient can wash her face immediately after the treatment, and wound treatment is convenient. With laser resurfacing, ablation can be done up to the desired depth because the depth of the penetration can be easily controlled. Besides, ablation-related sequela can be avoided. Laser resurfacing can be safely performed even on eyelids and the neck, where the skin is thin. It is more effective for wrinkles and scars as it tightens the skin and increases the elasticity of the skin due to its thermal effect.

CO$_2$ laser

The CO_2 laser emits energy at with a wavelength of 10600 nm and with a depth of penetration of 0.1 mm or less because of its target in tissue. The energy emitted by the CO_2 laser has been used for ablation because it has a strong affinity to water and can destroy skin tissues non-selectively regardless of the presence of hemoglobin and melanin. The early CO_2 laser emitted in continuous wave (CW), which caused serious thermal damage in the target tissue. To overcome this problem, superpulsed and ultrapulsed modes were developed instead of the CW mode. The Silktouch laser that was developed only at the initial stage was not a pulsed laser, but could achieve the effect of the pulsed lasers by rapidly scanning a small 0.2 mm laser beam over the tissue. A CO_2 laser that could deliver high peak powers in a short pulse width was developed to minimize thermal damage to tissues and maximize vaporization. The Ultrapulse CO_2 laser has an irradiation time (600 μsec) that is shorter than the thermal relaxation time (TRT) of the skin (960 μsec), and a maximum output of 100 W. Besides, its output density is 405 J/cm^2 or more, which is higher than that required for vaporization of tissues. The energy per pulse (diameter: 2.5 mm) of the light from the CO_2 laser is 250-500 mJ.

Er:YAG laser

The Er:YAG laser emits at a wavelength of 2940 nm, with a depth of penetration of 0.02 mm or less. Its affinity to water is 10 times higher than that of the CO_2 laser (coefficient of water absorption: CO_2 laser, 790 μm-1 and Er:YAG laser, 13000 μm-1). A high-power CO_2 laser can achieve a depth of ablation of 50-200 μm at one irradiation, and a depth of residual thermal damage of 80-150 μm. As the depth of ablation is shallow with Er:YAG laser, several irradiations are required to ablate tissue to the same depth as with the CO_2 laser. As the Er:YAG laser causes less thermal damage, however, deep ablation is impossible because of the lack of hemostasis in the ablated site. The Er:YAG laser offers the advantage that the wound healing time is short, since the depth of the thermal damage (30-50 μm) is much lower than that with the CO_2 laser. Although the Er:YAG laser has such advantages as little thermal damage and fast wound healing, it is not very effective in improving wrinkles as it cannot tighten the skin and increase elasticity as much as with the CO_2 laser. If the irradiation time is increased with the Er:YAG laser, an effect similar to that with CO_2 laser can be achieved. The dual-mode Er:YAG (Contour, Sciton Corp., USA, Action II, Lutronic Corp., South Korea) laser has two types of irradiation time: 250-350 μsec (shorter) and 40-1000 msec (longer). With the dual-mode Er:YAG laser, it is possible to use a combination of the ablation and coagulation modes for ablation with good hemostasis (Table 04-1).

| Table 04-1 | Experimental comparison of the CO_2 laser and the Er:YAG laser (from Dr. Kang DH and Dr. Park SH) |

Resurfacing method	Vaporization depth (μm)	Thermal necrosis (μm)	Resurfacing depth (μm)	Grenz zone (μm)	Microfibril density (No./μm^2)
Ablative mode Er:YAG 60 μm	21	34	55	209	16.6
Dual mode Er:YAG 25 μm	35	45	80	208	15.9
Ultrapulse CO_2 250 mJ	53	74	127	358	17.4
Ultrapulse CO_2^+ Ablative Er:YAG	48	58	106	299	15.9

(Normal microfibril density; 5.6/μm^2)

Laser resurfacing indications/contraindications

The purposes of laser ablation can be classified into removal of skin lesions (vaporization or ablation) and increase in the contraction or elasticity of the skin. Depending on the situation, these two purposes are sought at the same time. Skin lesions limited to the epidermis can be easily ablated with a laser. Typical lesions that can be removed easily by a laser include freckles, senile lentigines, seborrheic keratoses, and epidermal nevus. Laser ablation of scars to tighten the skin can also flatten uneven skin surfaces by increasing skin elasticity. Laser ablation is highly effective for depressed scars such as traumatic scars, hypertrophic scars, surgical scars, acne scars, and smallpox scars. Laser resurfacing is not effective for wounds that have not normally healed. It is contraindicated for large and deep scars such as burn scars, and for atrophic skin due to the long-term use of vitamin A. Hyperpigmentation is common after laser ablation especially in darker Asian skin types. Laser ablation should not be performed on patients who are sensitive to skin care, which is required to treat such pigmentation. A face with melasma or a dark skin color is more subject to pigmentation. Patients who are sensitive to hydroquinone or retinoic acid, which are used for pretreatment before laser ablation, should avoid laser ablation. Besides, patients who have non-realistic expectations about laser ablation, or who have mental disorders or a drug addiction problem should avoid laser ablation. Tables 04-2 and 04-3 summarize the indications for and contraindica-

Table 04-2   Indications for and contraindications to laser resurfacing

Indications	Contraindications
Epidermal lesions:	Deep and wide scars
Senile keratosis	Burn scars
Seborrheic keratosis	Melasma (risk of temporary worsening)
Freckles	Sunlight-sensitive skin
Lentigines	Skin sensitivity to whitening agents and exfoliating agents
Epidermal nevus	Unrealistic patient expectations
Milia	Mental patients
Syringoma	Drug addicts
Xanthelasma	
Rhinophyma	
Precancerous lesions in the skin;	
Actinic keratosis	
Keratoacanthoma	
Bowen's disease	
Pagetoid disease	
Skin aging	
Wrinkles	
Traumatic scars	
Acne scars	
Smallpox scars	

Table 04-3	Open dressing and occlusive dressing	
	Open dressing	**Occlusive dressing**
Treatment material	Antibiotic ointment, Vaseline, ophthalmic ointment, physiological saline, diluted vinegar	Colloid, semi-permeable membrane. Duoderm, Flexzan, Askina, Lasersite
Advantage	The patient can immediately wash his/her face, no accumulation of sebaceous glands, the wound is visible, and inflammation can be detected easily	Less pain, and no discomfort related to the dressing Less pigmentation Mild scarring The patient can immediately go out.
Disadvantage	Discomfort related to the dressing Pain, dryness, and tightening sensation More severe pigmentation than before The patient does not want to show scar	Accumulation of sebaceous glands and acne may worsen. Detection of infection may be delayed.

tions to laser resurfacing, and considerations regarding wound dressings.

Laser resurfacing and skin care among Asians

Skin care is important to enhance the effect of ablation and keep the skin tidy after the ablation. Particularly in Asians, hyperpigmentation and postinflammatory hyperpigmentation (PIH) are common, and thus, skin care before and after laser resurfacing is necessary. To prevent pigmentation after laser resurfacing, a bleaching agent (4% hydroquinone or kojic acid) should be used for 6 weeks or more. For a face that has melasma or dark skin, the bleaching agent should be used for 2 months or more. The most representative treatment for pigmentation is the Kligman formula, which consists of hydroquinone (4%), retinoic acid (0.1%), hydrocortisone (1%, or dexamathasone), is a combination of a bleaching agent, an exfoliating agent, and an anti-inflammatory agent. Although there are many types of skin care products, bleaching agents, exfoliating agents, soothers, and sunblock creams are commonly used. Hydroquinone prevents the formation of melanin pigments by inhibiting tyrosine. Retinoic acid peels off keratin, promotes regeneration of the epidermis, promotes blood circulation, and speeds up and evens out healing of wounds after ablation. As 0.1% retinoic acid is highly irritable to the skin, the use of 0.05% or 0.025% retinoic acid is desired. Steroid ointment soothes the irritation from the use of exfoliating agents and bleaching agents, promotes wound healing, and reduces erythema and itching with its sedative action. In addition, steroid ointment has a bleaching effect. Before ablation, a bleaching agent, a low-concentration exfoliating agent, and a soother are normally used for about 4 weeks. For a patient with light skin, they can be used for only 2 weeks; and for a patient with melasma or dark skin, it is desirable that they be used for 6-8 weeks. When a bleaching or exfoliating agent is used, a sunblock must be used concomitantly, as the bleaching or exfoliating agent may cause further pigmentation due to irritation. During the skin care regimen for pre-treatment prior to ablation, the patient can wear makeup as usual. Some patients may develop serious erythema or edema due to sensitive skin. Mild erythema and itching are common during the healing process, however, and this should be sufficiently explained to the patient. If the patient feels discomfort that is too severe to withstand, reduction of the concentration or dose of the exfoliating agent may be helpful. In more severe cases, only a bleaching agent should be applied. If the skin is severely irritated by the exfoliating or bleaching agent, skin care with treatment of the pigmentation after the laser resurfacing is required. Patients who cannot withstand skin care should not undergo laser ablation. Some patients have complained that their skin became darker during the pre-treatment. This might have been due to the rise of preexisting melanin pigments that made the skin look darker as exfoliation occurred, although the irritation might have actually caused the skin to produce more melanin pigments. As steady application of the agent for about 1-2 months can make the skin look white gradually, this should be well explained to the patient. Skin care can be started immediately after the wound heals after laser resurfacing. A steroid cream can be used from the start. Patients should apply the steroid cream first after they wash their face. The earlier a sunblock is used, the better the outcome would be. A sunblock may cause a stinging sensation on the skin. A UVA/UVB sunblock with a sun protection factor (SPF) of 25-30 is more appropriate than one with an SPF of 40-50, and should be used in the morning and at night. The timing of use of bleaching and exfoliating agents should vary depending on what the patient can withstand. Normally, the use of a bleaching agent can start 1 week after the wound heals. The use of an exfoliating agent can begin 2 weeks after the wound heals, and the concentration of the exfoliating agent should be low (0.025% retinoic acid).

If the patient cannot withstand a bleaching or exfoliating agent, its use can start a few days later. One month after ablation, skin care is performed as it is before ablation. If no pigmentation occurs even with 1-2 months of use, skin care should be performed for several months more with a lower dose instead of being stopped.

As the skin is dry after ablation, it is desirable that a moisturizer, Vaseline, and a nutrition cream be applied. Wearing makeup is possible only after the wound heals, and it is normally recommended that makeup be worn 2 weeks after ablation. If the color of the facial skin is outstanding due to erythema and pigmentation in the ablated site, normal makeup or special makeup (with Covermark™ or a concealer) can be used. Covering the glaring colors can be more easily achieved by using complementary colors; that is, a green cover can be used for red skin, and a yellow cover for brown skin.

Effects of laser resurfacing

The skin of young people is pink, and thus, they have a good complexion, clean skin, and good elasticity without blemishes. Young skin has thin keratin layers. In young skin, the melanin pigment is evenly distributed, and there is a constant ratio of the number of melanocytes and the number of epithelial cells in the basal cell layer. Epithelial cells undergo normal division and migration, and show periodic regeneration. In the dermal layer, collagen fibers are regularly arranged and elastic fibers, ground substances, and water are adequately distributed.

Aged skin that has been exposed to sunlight for a long time gradually becomes turbid, yellowish, and rough. Besides, in such skin, blemishes increase, elasticity decreases, and wrinkles form. As histological findings show, the cells in young skin are uniform in size, shape, and arrangement. In aged skin, the keratin layers thicken and undergo degeneration (elastosis) and actinic change. The epithelial cells are diverse in shape and size, are arranged irregularly, and are generally atrophic. Melanocytes are arranged irregularly. Melanin pigments increase and are distributed over wide and thick areas, and appear as mottles. In the dermis, thick and rough elastic fibers that have undergone elastosis exist highly irregularly, and the subepidermal Grenz zone is thin. The rete ridge is flat, and collagen fibers and fibroblasts decrease. Besides, among the ground substances, glycosaminoglycan increases. All these combine to decrease the skin elasticity.

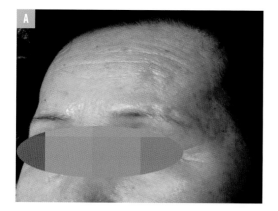 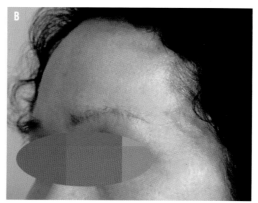

Figure 04-1 **A photograph taken 1 year after surgery on a 72-year-old woman who underwent CO$_2$ laser resurfacing for facial rejuvenation.** Marked improvement of skin wrinkles and an excellent facial lifting effect were experienced. Deep-level laser resurfacing, however, caused discomfort from long-lasting erythema.

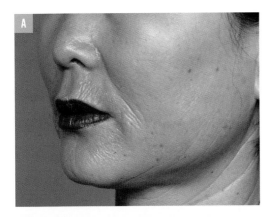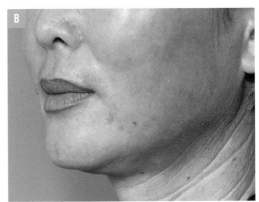

Figure 04-2   Dramatic rejuvenation was achieved with laser resurfacing in prominent perioral wrinkles that could not be improved with a face-lift or other methods.

The regenerated skin after ablation shows no aging phenomenon and has the same features as the skin of young people. The epidermal stratum corneum is thin, the degenerated keratin is removed, the epidermal layer is thick, the shape and size of the epithelial cells are regular, and the epithelial cells are arranged regularly. The melanin pigment decreases and is mostly found in the basal cell layers, and melanocytes are also regularly arranged in the basal cell layers. In the dermis that had been ablated with laser, the characteristic rough and thick elastic fibers that underwent elastosis disappear and are replaced by collagen fibers that are regularly arranged over a thick area. These collagen fibers are short and denser. The glycosaminoglycan in the ground substances decreases, new thin elastic fibers are regenerated, and the number of fibroblasts increases. After laser ablation, the collagen fiber layers of the dermis increase 3 to 6 times, which results in an overall increase in the skin elasticity. Clinical examples can be seen in Figures 04-1 and 04-2. A comparison between the two types of laser used for ablative resurfacing is seen in Table 04-1.

Complications of laser resurfacing

The complications of laser resurfacing include hyperpigmentation, hypopigmentation, depigmenation, hypertrophic scar formation, prolonged erythema, skin contour change, striae formation, infection, acne eruption, and milia formation. Hypertrophic scar formation, depigmentation, and skin contour change, all of which occur due to laser resurfacing that has been performed too deeply, can be avoided by adjusting the resurfacing depth. Erythema and hyperpigmentation are not complications but are resurfacing-related phenomena for which pre- and post-operative skin care is required. This should be sufficiently explained to the patient. In addition, to prevent complications, the appropriate treatment and care should be performed by correctly distinguishing the indications and contraindications of laser resurfacing, as outlined in Table 04-2.

REFERENCES

1. Alster TS, Garg S. Treatment of facial rhytides with a high energy pulsed carbon dioxide laser. Plast Reconstr Surg 1996;8:791.
2. Alster TS. Cutaneous resurfacing with CO_2 and erbium:YAG lasers: preoperative, intraoperative, and postoperative considerations. Plast Reconstr Surg 1999;103:619.
3. Baker TJ, Stuzin JM, Baker TM. Facial Skin Resurfacing. Quality Medical Pub;1998.
4. Collawn SS. Occlusion following laser resurfacing promotes reepithelization and wound healing. Plast Reconstr Surg 2000;105:2180.
5. Fitzpatrick RE, Rostan EF, Marchell N. Collagen tightening induced by carbon dioxide laser versus erbium:YAG laser. Laser Surg Med, 2000;27:395.
6. Fitzpatrick RE, Smith SR, Sriprachya-anunt S. Depth of vaporization and effect of pulse stacking with a high-energy, pulsed carbon dioxide laser. J Am Acad Dermatol 1999;40:615.
7. Fitzpatrick RE. Maximizing benefits and minimizing risk with CO_2 laser resurfacing. Dermatol Clin 2002;20:77.
8. Fulton JE. Complications of laser resurfacing. Dermatol Surg 1997;23:91.
9. Khartri KA, Ross V, Grevelink JM, Magro CM, Anderson RR. Comparison of Erbium and carbon dioxide lasers in resurfacing of facial rhytides. Arch Dermatol 1999;135:391.
10. Kligman AM, Willis I. A new mormaula of depigmenting human skin. Arch Dermatol 1975;111:40.
11. Park SH, Koo SH, Choi EO. Combined laser therapy for difficult dermal pigmentation: resurfacing and selective photothermolysis. Ann Plast Surg 2001;47:31.
12. Park SH. Laser dermatologic plastic surgery, Ch 9, 2nd Ed. Seoul: Koonja Pub Co.;2014:310-364.
13. Rosenberg GJ, Brito MA, Aportella RA, Kapoor S. Long-term histologic effects of the CO_2 laser. Plast Reconstr Surg 1997;104:2239.
14. Ross EV, Sajben FP, Hsia J, Barnette D, Miller CH, McKinly JR. Nonablative skin remodeling:selective dermal heating with a mid-infrared laser and contact cooling combination. Laser Surg Med 2000;26:186.
15. Schwartz RH, Burns AJ, Rohrich RJ, Barton FE Jr, Byrd HS. Long-term assessment of CO_2 facial laser resurfacing: aesthetic results and complications. Plast Reconst Surg 1999;103:592.
16. Seckel BR, Younai S, Wang KK. Skin tightening effects of the ultrapulse CO_2 laser. Plast Reconstr Surg 1998;102:872.
17. Seckel BR. Aesthetic laser surgery. Boston: Little Brown Co.; 1996
18. Stuzin JM, Baker TJ, Baker TM, Kligman AM. Histologic effects of the high energy pulsed CO_2 laser on photoaged facial skin. Plast Reconstr Surg 1996;99:2036.
19. Stuzin JM, Baker TJ. Histologic effects of the high energy pulsed CO_2 laser on photoaged facial skin. Plast Reconstr Surg 1997;99:2036.
20. Wee SY, Koo SH, Park SH, Ahn DS. An experimental study of the histologic changes in laser resurfacing using the ultrapulse CO_2 laser. Kor Soc Plast Reconstr Surg 1997;24:1464.
21. Weinstein C. Erbium laser resurfacing: current concepts. Plast Reconstr Surg 1999;103:602.

Laser-assisted approaches to facial and neck lifting

▷ Jae-Woo Park, MD, PhD

Introduction

Facial rejuvenation is becoming one of the most common procedures in the aesthetic facial surgery field. However, the major classical face lift, in which tissue is dragged laterally and backwards instead of upwards, has not become popular among Asian patients and practitioners. This is because changing the facial shape can change one's identity, and the procedure can leave wide surgical scars that are difficult to hide, involves long recovery times that prevent normal social life, and is expensive. The Asian patient rather wants a procedure which will give a more natural facial shape with minimal change in identity, more upwards lifting than lateralized lifting which is associated with a wider face with bigger mouth, and more exaggerated sharp, small eyes.

Most Asian patients do not have any remarkable configuration problems of the neck that would be addressed by the classical face and neck lift. In other words, the basic concepts of facial and neck lifting in Asians need to be redefined to provide that vertical facial lifting with laser-assisted scar-free neck rejuvenation and lifting. With laser-assisted lipolysis (LAL), applied for facial contouring, localized fat can be removed in the lower face and neck that is dragging the face and its associated tissues downwards. During the process of laser-assisted facial contouring (LAFC), interstitial tightening of the skin can also be accomplished. After LAFC, it is possible to lift the face and neck with minimal scars that are limited to the anterior hairline and anterior auricle. This approach gives the Asian patient a more natural and younger-shaped face. With minimal swelling, the recovery time is very short. The authors propose that this approach will help to popularize facial and neck lifting procedures in Asian subjects.

Laser-assisted lipolysis

The rationale for the use of the laser in LAL is the ability to more easily remove a remarkably large amount of fatty tissue. Interstitial lipolysis achieves selective fat tissue destruction via two mechanisms, namely photoacoustic and photothermal effects. The wavelengths which have been routinely used in LAL are the 980 nm diode laser and the 1064 nm and 1320 nm lines of the neodymium-doped yttrium aluminium garnet (Nd:YAG) laser. More recently, the micropulsed 1444 nm Nd:YAG wavelength has been added to this list, offering significant advantages over the other wavelengths as far as its duality of preferential absorption in fat and water is concerned. During LAL, it is possible to achieve a simultaneous shrinkage of the deeper dermal collagen either directly or indirectly because of thermally mediated denaturation of the collagen fibers in the deeper reticular dermis which occurs alongside laser lipolysis of the subdermal fatty tissue, but without thermal damage in the epidermis. This mild thermal damage in the dermis causes some collagen shrinkage and kick-starts the wound healing process, leading to both collagenesis and elastinogenesis followed by skin tightening and lifting through the remodelling phase of wound healing.

This effect is related to both the laser pulse width, which mediates the photoacoustic and photo-osmotic effects, and also the wavelength, which determines the chromophore targets, namely fat and water. The 1444 nm Nd:YAG laser (AccuSculpt™; Lutronic, Goyang, South Korea) has a pulse width of 100 μs delivering an extremely high peak power via a 600 μm optical fiber. Energy at 1444 nm is much better absorbed in fat and especially water than either the 980 nm, 1064 nm or 1320 nm wavelengths (Figure 05-1). The combination of these factors, namely short pulse, high peak power and high absorption, result in an almost explosive reaction at the fiber tip, but with the resultant heat confined to the tissue immediately adjacent to the tip. For 1444 nm, this means that less energy is required to destroy the same amount of fat compared with the other wavelengths, increasing the safety margin for laser lipolysis, especially in more delicate tissue structures such as the face. In other words, the 1444 nm micropulsed Nd:YAG laser offers a higher performance in fat destruction and tissue tightening but with low collateral damage or side effects such as burns, neurovascular damage and skin necrosis. The lipolysis and tissue tightening effect is dose-dependent. During LAL, fat tissue at the probe tip is swiftly melted simultaneously with the above mentioned photoacoustic/photo-osmotic effect, which collapses adjacent fatty tissue just like a honeycomb (Figure 05-2.). This results in primary tissue shrinkage, perceived as tightening. When the heat from this reaction reaches the deeper dermis, the collagen fibres are mildly coagulated or denatured, and this results in collagen regeneration followed by secondary and

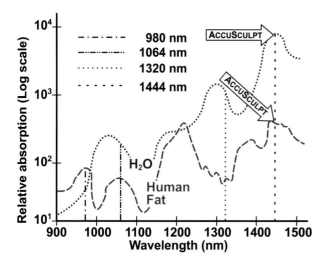

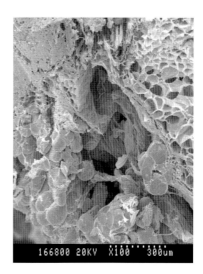

Figure 05-2 After laser-assisted
lipolysis, the peripheral area around
the area of destroyed fat has collapsed,
resembling a honeycomb.

long-lasting tissue tightening through the remodeling process. In an experimental study, the
pulse width- and wavelength-dependent fat destructive effect was compared among the 1444
nm, 1320 nm and 1064 nm lasers. For the same parameters, the crater made by the 1444 nm
beam was 10 times larger than that created with the 1064 nm beam (Figure 05-3).

Laser-assisted face and neck lift with LAL

Plastic surgeons are in general unfamiliar with laser-assisted face & neck lifting based on
LAL. This approach offers correction of lax or drooping skin on the face and neck with, or
even without, actual skin excision. It is ideal for young or middle-aged patients who have
minimal or moderate skin laxity (Figures 05-4, 05-5, 05-6). The lax skin and sagging interstitial tissue can be tightened during LAL based on the photothermal and photoacoustic mechanisms mentioned above. The collagen fibers in the deep reticular dermis are denatured during
the laser treatment followed by regeneration and remodeling. Finally the skin and interstitial
tissue on the face and neck can then be lifted upwards with the conventional surgical approach.

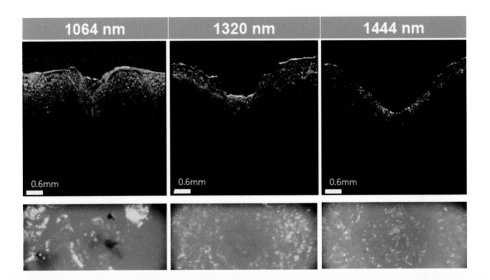

Figure 05-3 In an experimental study, the crater made by the 1444 nm Nd:YAG laser is 10 times bigger than that made by the 1064 nm Nd:YAG laser (Images by using opitical coherence tomograph Countesy of Jong-in. Youn. Ph.D Biomedical Optics Laboratory. Catholic University of Daegu, Korea).

Tips for diagnosis

Before the surgical procedure, the expectations of the patient, especially what surgical result they are looking for, must be carefully assessed. Some patients want to have aggressive face lifting even if it involves heavy edema requiring a long recovery time. On the other hand, most present-day patients want to have a surgical procedure that will have minimal impact on their activities of daily living, either socially or in the workplace. In addition to requiring a desirable surgical result, patients are concerned about maintaining the natural shape of their face with as minimal a change as possible, namely without noticeable scars around the ears, no side effects that will have any severe impact on their ADL, and no change in their identity. For these patients, laser assisted face and neck lifting with LAL is most likely to be the best option.

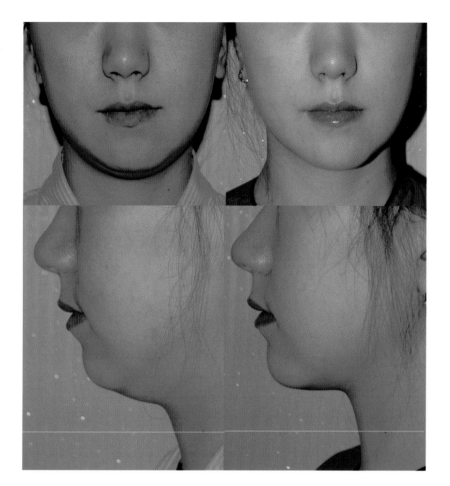

Figure 05-4   A 29 years old woman before (left) and 6 months after (right) laser assisted lipolysis with the 1444 nm Nd:YAG laser.

Tips for treatment

Preoperative assessment & preparation

Preoperatively, the surgeon must assess what kind of surgery the patients are prepared to undergo, i.e., aggressive or minimally invasive. The face and hair must first be cleaned with a gentle cleanser and an antibiotic shampoo. Then the skin laxity must be checked to decide on the extent of skin excision required. Any facial asymmetry and other deformities that the patient may not actually be aware of must be assessed and recorded with precise and repeatable clinical photography and a written report. A dedicated clinical photography system such

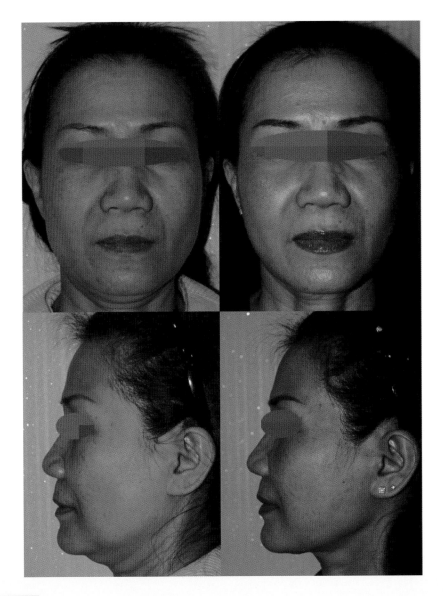

Figure 05-5   A 51 years old woman before (left) and 10 months after two sessions of laser assisted lipolysis with the 1444 nm Nd:YAG laser.

as the Visia™ from Canfield is ideal for this purpose. Almost everyone has facial asymmetry but they are not aware of it. The same applies to mild facial deformity or the actual extent of their lines and wrinkles Because of that, the surgeon must make a thorough assessment, and record the results in detail. After the assessment has been completed, it is a good idea to have the patients sign the pretreatment record.

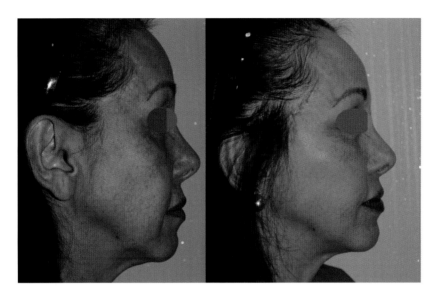

Figure 05-6   A 65 years old woman before (left) and 2 months after (right) surgical midface lift and laser assisted lipolysis with the 1444 nm Nd:YAG laser.

Clinical photography and treatment design

Clinical photography is very important for recording the baseline findings and for perioperative assessment. The pretreatment photography should include the full frontal, oblique, and lateral views in addition to any other required aspects of the patient's face and neck. These photos must be shown on a screen in the operating theater.

The design involves some surface landmarks such as chin tip, lower ear pole, sternocleidomastoid (SCM) muscle, neck wrinkles and lines, tracheal lateral margins, the expected neck line, and so on. After taking all the baseline photographs, the patient is posed in the primary head position. The first line is drawn from the lower ear pole to the tip of the chin The second line is marked to follow the melomental folds (marionette lines). These two sets of lines intersect and divide the lower face into four section. The entry point should be placed in the medial and lower sectors about 1 cm from the drooping tissue and sited so that it is as concealed as possible, but should allow good flexibility for probing with the optical fiber or cannula. With the patient lying down, the most protrusive areas of the cheek are then marked with many circles that let the surgeon know where the tissue is bulging the most. Then the third line is marked to run parallel to the first line, along the lower border of the mandible. The anterior border of the SCM muscle, both tracheal borders and the uppermost neck line should be marked next. Finally the expected cervical angle must be marked, placing it in between the lower mandibular border and the uppermost neck line.

There are some areas to be avoided during LAL. The first is the area just above where the facial artery crosses the mandibular border. If too much suction was performed here, a depressed deformity might develop after liposuction. Any other depressed areas should be marked as areas where suction LAL be avoided. The area to be treated might be divided into power units. The volume of nasolobial prominence, 3×5 cm^2 and 2 cm in thickness, will be the basic unit for the irradiated energy. For this area, the total energy might be 200 J. The total surgical area is divided into basic power units. The total number of the units multiplied by 200 J will be the total energy delivered to the patient. The basic power unit helps to make this procedure easier for the beginner.

Surgical procedure

After completing the design for the procedure, drape the surgical field. The entry points should be covered with surgical tape to prevent maceration and scarring. Local injection anesthesia of the entry points is achieved with 2% lidocaine and 1:100,000 epinephrine solution. The sites are then punctured with an 18 G hypodermic needle and an 18 G blunted cannula is inserted and placed for the tumescent injection. The surgical field for laser lipolysis and lifting is infiltrated with about 5-10 cc of tumescent solution on the nasolabial prominence, 20-30 cc on each cheek, and 50-100 cc on the neck area. After tumescent solution infiltration, wait for 10-15 minutes to allow epinephrine hemostasis to take effect.

LAL of the surgical area is then performed using a multiple layer technique because the tissue thickness has been multiplied with infiltration. The parameters for the face are a frequency of 40 Hz, pulse energy of 150-200 mJ, and 6-8 W power. The nasolabial area is irradiated with a total energy of around 200 J and the other areas are divided into basic units and treated with a total energy of about 200 J per unit. About 50 J total energy should be delivered to the superficial subdermal area. The subcutaneous tissue is divided into 3 layers and is irradiated with a total energy of about 50 J per layer. The appearance of the guide beam through the tissue is helpful for the beginner when performing multiple layered irradiation. When irradiating in the deeper layers, the beam is larger and diffused, becoming smaller and brighter as the more superficial layers are treated. Once the surgeon is familiar with the procedure, the depth of the fiber can be judged by the quality of the sound associated with the photoacoustic effect. When working in the superficial layers, the sound is higher and sharper compared with the deeper and more muffled sound heard when the tip of the fiber is in the deeper layers.

After irradiation, the lysed fat can be removed with a blunted cannula. Some practitioners have said that a 2-3 mm diameter multi-hole cannula is good for lipid removal in LAL. The author, however, uses a 1-1.5 mm single hole cannula, which allows evacuation of the melted fat in multiple layers and gives good control over the manipulation of the cannula to prevent nerve or vascular damage. The volume of fat for evacuation is minimal; 1-2 cc per side for the nasolabial prominence, 3-5 cc per side for lax cheeks, and 5-10 cc per side for the neck and submental area. After LAL, the surgical field should be irrigated with diluted hyaluronidase and triamcinolone solution for thermal quenching and to assist early recovery. The hyaluronidase is the dehydrogenase acting as the bond between n-acetylglucosamine and glucuronic acid in hyaluronic acid that is one of the main structural components of cells and interstitial tissues. This technique breaks down large molecular structures and results in increased tissue permeability for the substance. The hyaluronidase irrigation after LAL might also help to control edema by increasing the absorption of any free oil, tissue fluid and tumescent solution. Triamcinolone is a mid-term lasting adrenal corticosteroid which increases local fluid absorption through the salt/water balance. It also decreases the anti-inflammatory reaction through lowering immune cell activity.

Tips for post-treatment care and follow-up

After irradiation, each of the entry points is taped with a small gauze dressing or a material like Tegaderm™. No other dressing is needed. Compressive bandaging for the face and neck is avoided because the compression around the ears and submental area can cause severe swelling which could prolong the recovery time. The small tape dressings can be removed on the day after treatment and ointment is applied to the entry points without gauze or skin tape. The patient should avoid washing the face until the 2nd postoperative day. From the day after surgery, the use of near infrared LED phototherapy, such as with the HEALITE™ (Lutronic Corp.) is good to reduce pain, swelling, recovery time and to accelerate the disappearance of any bruising. If any patient complains about slight swelling in the treated areas after the 2nd postoperative day, gentle radiofrequency massage might be helpful for them.

The patient should be followed for 2 to 4 weeks after treatment. The laser assisted face and neck lift is not usually associated with any postoperative pigmentation problems after treatment. During the recovery period, fluctuating edema might occur once or twice, but it should not be severe. If this occurs, compressive bandages should not be used on the face and neck, since this might increase the severity of the swelling. The laser-treated area might feel a little hard, especially on the submental area, and this can be softened with intralesional hyaluronidase and triamcinolone injections repeated as required.

The pain after LAL usually lasts for a maximum of 2-3 months, but can be faster depending on the individual patient. Patients are usually able to put up with this pain without any kind of treatment or medication. If somebody complains of severe pain, however, it can be treated with small doses of an analgesic such as acetaminophen (paracetamol) or ibuprofen. It is very rare to need a strong pain killer or tranquilizer but if required, they should be used for the very short term only. LED phototherapy at 830 nm can also be very helpful to alleviate post-LAL pain or discomfort.

For the majority of patients, a single session is required, while some people who have less elastic skin might be need the entire procedure repeated 2-3 times depending on their individual condition.

Side effects

The possible complications of laser-assisted face and neck lifting include bleeding, hematoma formation, burn, infection, scar formation and so on that might happen after any other kind of surgery. The other possible complication that might happen is injury of major neurovascular structures, but if the laser probe has been properly placed in the subcutaneous layer this is very uncommon. The subcutaneous layer is free from any major neurovascular structure. The fiber should be maintained parallel to the skin surface, and not allowed to penetrate into the deeper tissue layers. Major nerve-related complications usually occur due to the mechanical injury during a mechanical liposuction procedure.

Burns are very rare, especially if the probe has not been allowed to remain stationary on the same spot for a long time, such as 5-10 sec. With the recommended to-and fro continuous motion of the fiber and/or cannula in a fan-like pattern, burns do not occur. Paresthesia in the treated area after LAL may last for 2-3 months and is variable in degree from an itching or tingling sensation to mild or even severe pain on touching the affected spot. Paresthesia might be the result of damage to the sensory nerve endings, and probably depends on the dose, or energy, delivered to the treatment unit. It will disappear spontaneously, but sometimes it needs controlled with mild analgesics, tranquilizers or LED phototherapy. A lump might be noticed in the irradiated field, especially under the chin during the healing period which is usually an immature scar or fibrotic tissue. Because these lumps can prevent the desired skin tightening or lifting by its mass effect, they can be controlled with an injection of the diluted and sterilized hyaluronidase and triamcinolone solution.

Midface surgical lift and laser-assisted neck lift with LAL

Nowadays a face lift might be performed with a skin excision and superficial muscular aponeurotic system (SMAS) plication for the mid-face, and LAL for the lower face. After LAL for the lower- and mid-face, the skin incision is made along the anterior hair line with excision of 1-1.5 cm of skin. The skin flap is be elevated subcutaneously up to the malar prominence, nasolabial fold, marionette line, and over the mandibular border. After bleeding control, a cheek SMAS of about 3 cm in width is plicated and fixed to the solid portion of the deep temporal area and under the zygomatic arch with 3-0 vicryl sutures. The orbicularis oculi is split and fixed to the upper lateral deep temporal area. The skin flap is trimmed and sutured without tension. The use of LAL before this procedure can reduce the time for the dissection, bleeding, swelling, and scar formation.

REFERENCES

1. Apfelberg DB, Rosenthal S, Hunstad JP, Achauer B, Fodor PB. Progress report on multicenter study of laserassisted liposuction. Aesthetic Plast Surg 1994;18:259–264.
2. Badin AZ, Moraes LM, Gondek L, Chiaratti MG, Canta L. Laser lipolysis: Flaccidity under control. Aesthetic Plast Surg 2002;26:335-339.
3. Dang YY, Ren QS, Liu HX, Ma JB, Zhang JS. Comparison of histologic, biochemical, and mechanical properties of murine skin treated wth the 1064-nm and 1320-nm Nd: YAG lasers. Exper Dermatol 2005;14:876-882.
4. Goldman A. Submental Nd:YAG laser-assisted liposuction. Laser Surg Med 2006;38:181-184.
5. Ishikawa K, Miyasaka M, Tanaka R, , Tanino R, Mizukami K, Wakaki M. Histologic evaluation of the pulsed Nd: YAG laser for laser lipolysis. Lasers Med Surg 2005;36:43-46.
6. Katz B, McBean J, Cheung JS. The new laser liposuction for men. Dermatol Ther 2007;20:448–451.
7. Kim KH, Geronemus RG. Laser lipolysis using a novel 1,064 nm Nd: YAG laser. Dermatol Surg 2006;32:241-248.
8. Melega J. Liposuction using neodymium:yltrium:aluminium:garnet laser. Plast Reconstr Surg 2003;111:2497.
9. Prado A, Andrades P, Danilla S, Leniz P, Castillo P, Gaete F. A prospective, randomized, double-blind, controlled clinical trial comparing laser-assisted lipoplasty with suctionassisted lipoplasty. Plast Reconstr Surg 2006;118:1032–1045.
10. Tark KC, Jung JE, and Song SY. Superior Lipolytic Effect of the 1,444nm Nd:YAG Laser: Comparison With the 1,064nm Nd:YAG Laser. Lasers in Surgery and Medicine 2009;41:721–727.

Acne

Active acne (Including PDT)

▶ You Chan Kim, MD, PhD

Introduction

Acne vulgaris is an inflammatory disease of the pilosebaceous follicles, peaking in adolescence, and characterized by comedones, papules, pustules, nodules, and often scars.

Pathogenesis of acne includes sebaceous gland hyperplasia with increased sebum secretion, hyperproliferation of the follicular keratinocytes, colonization of the pilosebaceous duct by *Propionibacterium acnes,* and inflammation.

Tips for diagnosis

Acne lesions can be divided into non-inflammatory and inflammatory lesions. Non-inflammatory lesions consist of open comedones (blackheads) and closed comedones (whiteheads). Inflammatory lesions include papules, pustules, and nodules (cysts). Depressed or hypertrophic scarring may follow.

Tips for treatment

Light therapy

Blue light photoinactivates *Propionibacterium acnes* (*P. acnes*) through endogenous photodynamic therapy (PDT), targeting the porphyrins protoporphyrin IX and coproporphyrin III. Red light is less effective at photoactivating porphyrins, especially when they are endogenous and in small quantities, but penetrates more deeply into tissue. Red light may also have anti-inflammatory properties by influencing cytokine release from mast cells, macrophages or other cells.

Light therapies with blue or blue/red light are more likely show benefit than those with yellow, red or green light sources. Red-blue light was more effective that topical 5% benzoyl peroxide cream in the short term. However, light therapy alone may not be enough to treat active acne in some cases and so combination with other therapeutic modalities is usually necessary, although the study by Lee and colleagues on moderate to severe inflammatory acne showed good efficacy for sequential blue and red light-emitting diode (LED) phototherapy on its own.

Photodynamic therapy

Mechanism of PDT

The mechanism of PDT in acne treatment may involve direct thermal injury to the sebaceous glands, destruction of *P. acnes*, manipulation of keratinocyte turnover in the infundibulum, or a combination of any of the above.

Light sources

Noncoherent light sources are better for superficial lesions with large surface areas because they are cheaper to purchase and maintain, and have larger illumination fields.

Route of administration and photosensitizer

Itoh discussed his use of systemic aminolevulinic acid (ALA)-PDT in 96 Asian patients with moderate to severe acne of the face and body. Most (91.6% of patients with facial acne, 92.2% of those with body acne) improved or markedly improved. However, almost all other investigators have used topical PDT. Because of the lack of systemic phototoxicity and ease of use, topical PDT is the favored route of administration. Recently the efficacy and safety of ILI-PDT (PDT with an intralesional injection of ALA) was evaluated in 10 patients with recalcitrant localized acne. ILI-PDT showed a definite statistical superiority in effect after the first and second PDT sessions compared with conventional PDT. In terms of side effects, generalized erythema and exfoliation was not reported after ILI-PDT. ALA and methyl aminolevulinate (MAL) have been widely used and effective in the treatment of acne. Recently indocyanine green (ICG) dye has been tried in the treatment of Asian acne patients. The maximum absorption band of ICG dye ranges from 600-900 nm with the peak in the near infrared, and it can selectively accumulate in sebaceous glands. ICG dye in conjunction with a 805 nm diode laser was effective for acne treatment in 16 Korean subjects and only two cases showed minor side effects.

Wavelength

A photodynamic reaction with blue light irradiation can temporarily eradicate *P. acnes* through its effect on porphyrin-induced apoptosis, particularly coproporphyrin III as already mentioned. Nonetheless, better results may be obtained through the use of broad spectrum light, especially in the more pigmented skin types.

Dosimetry

Both fluence and fluence rate affect the pain of PDT interdependently. In the treatment of acne, a low fluence and fluence rate are recommended.

Contact time

Investigations that used 3-4 h photosensitizer contact time (incubation) were associated with significant patient drop-out due to pain, pustular eruption, exfoliation, edema and erythema. 'Short contact' times of 15-90 min seem to be associated with milder and occasionally less frequent side effects. However, in a recent, randomized, half-facial treatment study for 20 Korean patients with moderate to severe acne, the degree of improvement in inflammatory acne was greater in the long incubation time ALA plus intense pulsed light (IPL) (3 hours) than the short incubation time group (30 min) or the IPL alone group. The investigators suggested that acne vulgaris might be treated more efficiently without complications, even in Asian patients, using PDT with a long incubation time rather than a short incubation time. They suggested that contact times from 30 min to 3 hours should be applied on a patient-by-patient basis.

Number of and interval between treatments

At intervals of one to four weeks, two to four treatments were administered. For adverse events to subside, longer intervals would be required for more aggressive therapy, i.e. higher MAL/ALA concentrations, longer contact times, higher fluencies and fluence rates.

Side effects

Varying degrees of side effects, such as erythema, edema, blistering, pain, acute acneiform eruptions and postinflammatory hyperpigmentation (PIH), have been reported. Wiegell and Wulf compared MAL-PDT and ALA-PDT in patients with acne. In this randomized comparative investigator-blinded split-face study, no statistically significant differences were observed in the pain scores during inflammation. MAL caused as much pain as ALA in diseased skin, but other adverse effects seemed to subside much faster with MAL, which involved a lesser extent reactions in of normal skin.

In 2001, Itoh et al studied the effect of topical PDT in patients with acne. Thirteen Japanese patients with intractable acne were treated with PDT using ALA and polychromatic vis-

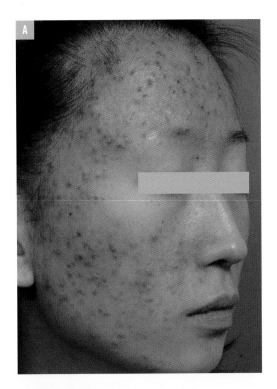
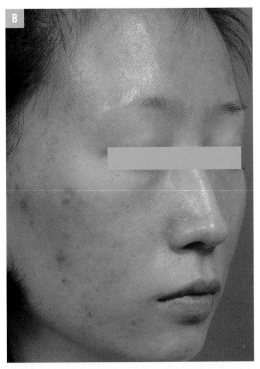

Figure 01-1 (A) Erythematous papules on the face before PDT. (B) Marked improvement after two sessions of PDT using IPL.

ible light. All patients had apparent improvement of facial appearance and reduction of new acne lesions following PDT treatment. A total of 78 Chinese patients with severe facial acne were treated with 1-3 courses of ALA PDT. 22% of patients showed excellent improvement after one-course treatment and another 34% showed excellent improvement after two courses. The rest (44%) required three-course treatment to further reduce the number and size of residual lesions. Adverse effects were minimal. However, MAL-PDT using IPL in 23 Chinese did not lead to significant improvement of moderate inflammatory acne compared with the control group. A proportion of patients could not tolerate the discomfort that was related to PDT despite a short (30 min) MAL incubation time. Recently 180 Chinese patients with moderate to severe facial acne were treated with ALA PDT with different concentrations (5%, 10%, 15%, 20%) of ALA. Increasing the concentration of ALA seems to be beneficial for improving the results, but regarding side effects, a trend towards more serious erythema and PIH was observed with increasing ALA concentration.

In conclusion, several studies have confirmed that PDT is superior to some forms of light alone for the treatment of acne vulgaris. However, the development of PIH is of concern, especially in Asians. Topical MAL or ALA PDT using red noncoherent light sources at low fluence and fluence rates may be suitable for Asian acne patients (Figure 01-1). To avoid PIH, photosensitizers should be sufficiently cleaned off the skin before irradiation. A total of 2-4 treatments at 2-4 week intervals is usually enough to obtain improvement of acne. A contact time from 30 min to 3 hours should be applied considering both the efficacy and side effects of PDT, such as PIH, especially in Asian patients.

Tips for post-treatment care and follow-up

After irradiation, the treated lesions are cooled with an alum solution for 10 minutes. The patient should avoid sun-exposure until the day after treatment. The patient is followed from 2 to 4 weeks after treatment.

REFERENCES

1. Hamilton FL, Car J, Lyons C, Car M, Layton A, Majeed A. Laser and other light therapies for the treatment of acne vulgaris: systemic review. Br J Dermatol 2009;160:1273-1285.
2. Ito Y. Treatment of acne. In: Goldman MP (ed) Photodynamic therapy. Philadelphia: Elsevier Saunders;2005. p.20.
3. Itoh Y, Ninomiya Y, Tajima S, Ishibashi A. Photodynamic therapy of acne vulgaris with topical δ-aminolaevulinic acid and incoherent light in Japanese patients. Br J Dermatol 2001;144:575-579.
4. Kim BJ, Lee HG, Woo SM, Youn JI, Suh DH. Pilot study on photodynamic therapy for acne using indocyanine green and diode laser. J Dermatol 2009;36:17-21.
5. Lee SY, You CE, Park MY. Blue and red light combination LED phototherapy for acne vulgaris in patients with skin phototype IV. Lasers Surg Med 2007;39:180-188.
6. Oh SH, Ryu DJ, Han EC, Lee KH, Lee JH. A comparative study of topical 5-aminolevulinic acid incubation times in photodynamic therapy with intense pulsed light for the treatment of inflammatory acne. Dermatol Surg 2009;35:1918-1926.
7. Papageorgiou P, Katsambas A, Chu A. Phototherapy with blue (415 nm) and red (660 nm) light in the treatment of acne vulgaris. Br J Dermatol 2000;142:973-978.
8. Ryou JH, Lee SJ, Park YM, Kim HO, Kim HS. Acne-photodynamic therapy with intra-lesional injection of 5-aminolevulinic acid. Photodermatol Photoimmunol Photomed 2010;25:57-58.
9. Taylor MN, Gonzalez ML. The practicalities of photodynamic therapy in acne vulgaris. Br J Dermatol 2009;160:1140-1148.
10. Wang XL, Wang HW, Zhang LL, Guo MX, Huang Z. Topical ALA PDT for the treatment of severe acne vulgaris. Photodiagnosis Photodyn Ther 2010;7:33-38.
11. Wiegell SR, Wulf HC. Photodynamic therapy of acne vulgaris using 5-aminolevulinic acid versus methyl aminolevulinate. J Am Acad Dermatol 2006;54:647-651.
12. Yeung CK, Shek SY, Bjerring P, Yu CS, Kono T, Chan HH. A comparative study of intense pulsed light alone and its combination with photodynamic therapy for the treatment of facial acne in Asian skin. Lasers Surg Med 2007;39:1-6.
13. Yin R, Hao F, Deng J, Yang XC, Yan H. Investigation of optimal aminolaevulinic acid concentration applied in topical aminolaevulinic acid-photodynamic therapy for treatment of moderate to severe acne: a pilot study in Chinese subjects. Br J Dermatol 2010;163:1064-1071.

02

Acne related erythema & hyperpigmentation

Jiehoon Kim, MD

Definition

The reactions occurring after acne treatment may vary. These reactions are generally associated with the severity of the acne lesion and the appropriateness of the treatment delivered. Table 02-1 shows post-acne scarring by grade. This chapter discusses the macular change that corresponds to grade 1, the mildest grade of scarring.

It is rare for acne to immediately disappear after various medical and surgical treatments. In most cases, the cure is followed by erythematous or pigmented macules, which are commonly observed in wound healing. Although these macules spontaneously disappear in most cases, they sometimes persist in Asian skin.

Table 02-1 Grades and Examples of Post acne Scarring (reference : Goodman GJ, Baron JA. Post acne scarring: a qualitative global scarring grading system. Dermatol Surg 2006; 32: 1458–1466.)

Grade	Level of disease	Characteristics	Examples of scars
1	Macular disease	Erythematous, hyper- or hypopigmented flat marks visivle to patient or observer irrespective of distance.	Erythematous, hyper- or hypopigmented flat marks
2	Mild disease	Mild atrophy or hypertrophy that may not be obvious at social distances of 50 cm or greater and may be covered adequately by makeup or the normal shadow of shaved beard hair in males or normal body hair if extrafacial.	Mild rollong, small soft papular
3	Moderate disease	Moderate atrophic or hypertrophic scarring that is obvious at social distances of 50 cm or greater and is not covered easily by makeup or the normal shadow of shaved beard hair in males or body hair if extrafacial, but is still able to flattened by manual stretching of the skin.	More significant rolling, shallow "box car," mild to moederate hypertrophic or papular scars
4	Severe disease	Severe atrophic or hypertrophic scarring that is obvious at social distansces of 5 cm or greater and is not covered easily by makeup or the normal shadow of shaved beard hair in males or body hair (if extrafacial) and is not able to be flattened by manual stretching of the skin.	Punched out atrophic (deep "box car"), "ice pick", bridges and tunnels, gross atrophy, dystrophic scars significant hypertrophy or keloid formation

Tips for diagnosis

Erythematous macules

If only the epidermis and superficial dermis are involved, the scars may appear as macules that may be red if inflamed and comparatively early or young scars (under 1 year old) or with altered pigmentation. Figure 02-1A shows the result of a six-week treatment of a patient who presented with acne vulgaris for which medication, extraction, and superficial chemical-peeling treatment (glycolic acid) were performed (Figure 02-1B). As shown, the erythematous macules persisted in the acne lesion.

Hyperpigmented macules

Scar pigmentation may increase in the more olive-skinned patients and represents mostly a post-inflammatory response that will fade in 3-18 months. This requires strict sun protection in patients who do not readily burn and who may not perceive sun avoidance as usually necessary. In Asian skin, however, hyperpigmented macules are the most serious problem occurring after acne treatment. Hyperpigmented macules occur more frequently in Asian skin, despite adequate sun protection, than in Western skin, and usually persist for a long time once they occur (Figure 02-2).

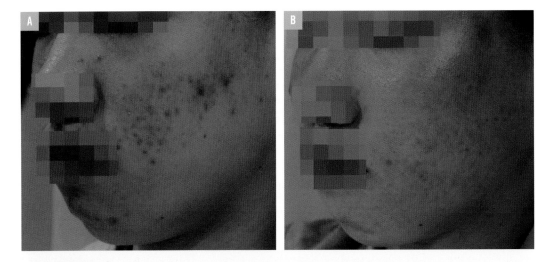

Figure 02-1   **26 years old Korean female with acne vulgaris. A.** Acne vulgaris on the cheek at baseline. **B.** 6 weeks after treatment (combination with medication and superficial chemical peeling). **Note:** Erythematous macules remain on the treated area after treatment.

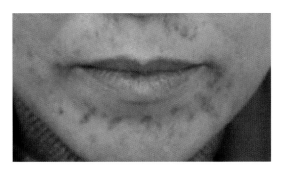

Figure 02-2   **35 years old Korea female with acne vulgaris. Note:** After treatment, post inflammatory hyperpigmentation persisted for a long time.

Hypopigmented macules

Post-acne hypopigmented macules are not commonly found in Asian skin. The white macules seen in the post-acne environment usually represent true scars or post-inflammatory leukoderma.

Tips for treatment

Erythematous macules

Red macular changes are quite well targeted by vascular lasers and light sources such as intense pulsed light (IPL) systems. Theoretically, lasers and light sources may play an important role in the prevention of progression to scarring of inflamed healing acne lesions. In the past, the pulsed dye laser (PDL) was used for the treatment. Recently, however, IPL (Figure 02-3) or low-level light therapy (LLLT; Figure 02-4) is widely used for treatment.

There is an important conisderation that deserves clinicians' attention when performing the aforementioned laser treatments, such as PDL or light treatments like IPL, for post-acne erythematous macules. That is, the irradiation should be performed with a lower fluence for post-acne erythematous macules using PDL or IPL than for vascular lesions such as common telangiectasia.

In some cases, for acne treatment, superficial chemical peeling is performed or comedones are extracted. If LLLT at 633 nm (red light) or 830 nm (infrared light) is performed as a routine procedure after superficial chemical peeling or comedone extraction, pain can be relieved, wound healing can be promoted, and post-acne erythematous macules can be effec-

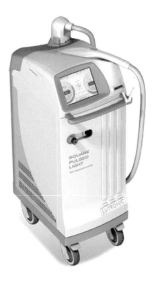

Figure 02-3 Intense Pulsed Light (IPL) system (Solari; Lutronic Corp., Goyang, South Korea)

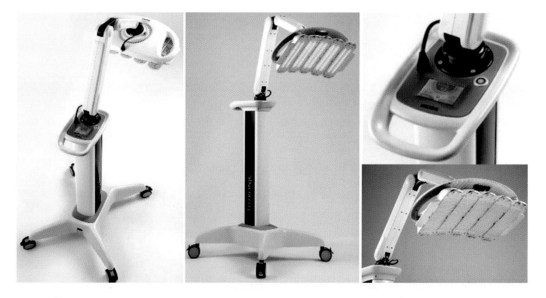

Figure 02-4 LED Low Level Light Therapy (LLLT) system (Healite II; Lutronic Corp.).

tively prevented. These modalities have also been used for moderately atrophic scars as well as hypertrophic scarring.

❚ Hyperpigmented macules

In Asian skin, erythematous and hyperpigmented macules are common. Hyperpigmented macules are associated with post-inflammatory hyperpigmentation. Reparative treatment may not always be required. If treatment is sought, medical therapy may suffice, with topical reparative creams such as retinoic acid, hydroquinone, kojic acid, and azelaic acid used in other examples of post-inflammatory pigmentation. Alternatively or additionally, light skin peels with glycolic acids or Jessner's solution, or variants of retinoic-acid peels, may be utilized.

For the treatment of a resistant case, laser toning (low-fluence 1064-nm Nd:YAG laser treatment; Figure 02-5) could be helpful. Laser toning is a treatment modality that is commonly used for the treatment of melasma in Asian countries such as South Korea. The theoretical principle of the treatment with melasma or PIH via laser toning is based on subcellular selective photothermolysis (Kim IH et al., J Invest Dermatol, 130:2333–2335).

In the past, if post-acne hyperpigmentation occurred, clinicians generally waited until it improved, and treatment was initiated only if no improvement was achieved. As laser toning has almost no risk of adverse events, however, it is advantageous to perform early treatment

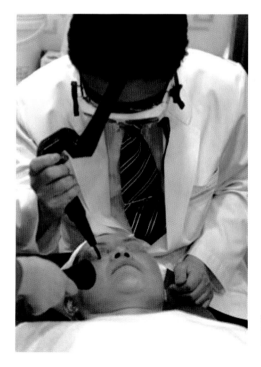

Figure 02-5   Laser toning (low-fluence 1064-nm Nd:YAG laser treatment)

for post-acne hyperpigmentation using laser toning. A Q-switched Nd:YAG laser at 1064 nm (SPECTRA; Lutronic Corp., Goyang, South Korea) was used by this author for the treatment of early-stage post-acne hyperpigmentation, where irradiation with a large spot size and a low fluence of 1.3-1.5 J/cm^2 was performed every one to two weeks, and a satisfactory outcome was achieved.

Hypopigmented macules

Hypopigmented macules have been reported as fairly refractory to treatment. There have been scattered reports of repigmentation after manual or needle dermabrasion (utilizing a tattoo gun without pigment). Some pigment transfer procedures have also been attempted. A particularly difficult type of hypopigmented macular scarring is termed "perifollicular scarring." Perifollicular acne inflammation may produce small hypopigmented macular or papular scars from the destruction and attenuation of the collagen and elastin fibers in the tissues surrounding the hair follicles. This is most common on the trunk and is largely untreatable at present. If they are papular rather than macular, and particularly if facial, such scars may be treated via fine-needle diathermy.

There are a number of techniques that are currently being utilized for the treatment of vitiligo that may also be useful in the treatment of post-acne scarring. Minigrafting holds some promise, but there appears to be little spread of pigment from the grafts into the surrounding skin in patients with scarring. Epidermal suspensions, both cultured and immediate noncultured, may also be somewhat useful.

REFERENCES

1. Alster TS, McMeekin TO. Improvement of facial acne scars by the 585 nm flashlamp-pumped pulsed dye laser. J Am Acad Dermatol 1996;35:79–81.
2. Goodman GJ, Baron JA. Post acne scarring : a qualitative global scarring grading system. Dermatol Surg 2006;32:1458–1466.
3. Goodman GJ, Baron JA. The management of post-acne scarring. Dermatol Surg 2007;33:1175–1188.
4. Kim JH, Kim H, Park HC, Kim IH. Subcellular selective photothermolysis of melanosomes in adult zebrafish skin following 1064-nm Q-switched Nd:YAG laser irradiation. J Invest Dermatol 130:2333–2335.
5. Wang CM, Huang CL, Hu CT, Chan HL. The effect of glycolic acid on the treatment of acne in Asian skin. Dermatol Surg 1997;23:23–29.

03

Acne scars

▶ Won Serk Kim, MD, PhD

Introduction

Acne is a chronic inflammatory disease of the pilosebaceous unit. It presents itself as comedones, papules, pustules, and nodules and sometimes leaves atrophic or hypertrophic scars. Acne conglobata, a severe acne condition, presents with aggregated nodules, large abscesses, and cysts, and as it is a highly inflammatory disease, it commonly leaves scars or keloids even after healing.

Tips for diagnosis

Acne scars can be grouped into four types based on their shape: ice pick, boxcar, rolling, and hypertrophic scars. Of these, the ice pick scar is the most common. It has a deeply dented shape, looking as if the skin had been stabbed with an ice pick. The boxcar shape is also a common type of scar. It has a vertically dented demarcation. It may be shallow or deep and occurs mostly on the cheek. The rolling scar occurs when the dermis has been damaged, and its surface looks like waves. It is not deep but is wide. The hypertrophic scar is an elevated scar with a rough surface. It usually occurs on the back or chest but may also occur on the neck or face. It often occurs at the site where a severe cystic or nodular acne lesion had been. It normally occurs within the boundary of the original lesion and tends to become smaller over time. On the other hand, keloid scars are a different entity, although often confused with hypertrophic scars. Keloid scars grow and extend beyond the borders of the original lesion.

Tips for treatment

There are various treatment methods that are currently available for acne scars, depending on the patient's condition. First, fractional lasers, which are subdivided into nonablative fractional lasers (NAFL) or ablative fractional lasers (AFL) which make thousands of micro-thermal zones (MTZs) or microablative columns (MACs), inducing the regeneration of the dermal matrix collagen. The energy emitted by the fractional laser can affect tissue as deep as 1500 μm for NAFLs and around 2000 μm for AFLs, and can deliver consistent energy to the dermis, inducing neocollagenesis. In the case of the nonablative (NAFL) approach, the epidermis is minimally damaged, whereas in the ablative (AFL) approach, microablative columns (MACs) are created in both the epidermis and dermis Thus, the NAFL is good treatment for milder scarring, and the AFL is better for more severe scarring. Among acne scar types, the treatment outcome of the rolling scar is particularly good with the fractional laser. Recovery time after NAFL is very short, but 3 to 5 treatments are required with 1 month intervals (Figure 03-1). A longer recovery time is required with the AFL approach, but the number of treatment sessions required is much less than NAFL (Figure 03-2). Both NAFL and AFL need considerably shorter downtime than the fully ablative laser technique. The combination of the fractional laser and focal chemical peeling techniques may achieve an even better outcome because focal chemical ablation using high concentration TCA is effective for the treatment of narrow but deeply dented ice pick scars.

Second, the fractionated microneedling radiofrequency (RF) approach can also be used, in which fine needle electrodes are inserted into the skin, and the RF energy delivered from the tip of the needle (in insulated microneedles) stimulates the regeneration of collagen and

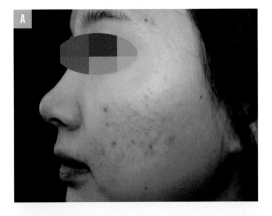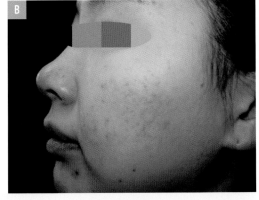

Figure 03-1   Effect of 1550 nm Er:Glass Fractional Laser treatment (nonablative fractional laser) on acne scarring. **A.** Before treatment. **B.** 4 months after three sessions of treatment.

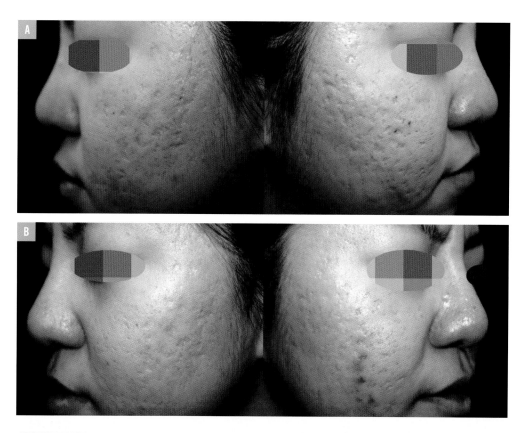

Figure 03-2 Effect of 10600 nm CO$_2$ fractional laser (ablative fractional laser) treatment on acne scars. **A.** Before treatment. **B.** 6 months after two treatment sessions.

elastin in the deep dermis. In some systems, such as the INFINI (Lutronic Corp., Goyang, South Korea) the depth of the needling can be selected so that several layers of electrothermal coagulation in the one treatment session can bring about good three-dimensional shrinkage of the tissue followed by collagen regeneration and remodeling, filling up the scars and toning the skin. Unlike conventional laser procedures, insulated microneedling RF does not cause electrothermal damage to the epidermis and thus allows a shorter recovery time after the treatment.

A third approach is interstitial laser treatment, originally developed for body and facial contouring through laser-assisted lipolysis. One such system is the 1444 nm micropulsed neodymium:yttrium aluminium garnet (Nd:YAG; AccuSculpt; Lutronic Corp) delivered via a 600 μm optical fiber which is inserted into the skin, and the tissue at the fiber tip is irradiated with the high peak power, micropulsed (100 μs) 1444 nm laser energy. As the laser energy directly targets the subdermis, or in the case of acne scars, the dermis, photothermal damage does not occur to the epidermis. For the treatment procedure, a 21 G cannula is inserted via a tunnel created using an 18 G needle, the optical fiber is inserted through the cannula, and then laser energy is delivered interstitially via the fiber. The wavelength of 1444 nm is very well absorbed by water, which constitutes a very high percentage of the dermal matrix, so thermal energy is safely contained in the tissue at the very tip of the fiber. Wide, round rolling scars are depressed due to the dense fibrosis which has formed at the base of the scar, thus tethering or anchoring the scar base and causing the depression. This fibrous tissue is under tension, and by using a subcision (subcutaneous incision) technique with a fan-like motion of the fiber in the dermis at the scar base, the fibrotic tissue is photothermally lysed, releasing the tension and allowing the depressed tissue to assume a more normal depth.

In addition, the neighboring area around the scar can be directly removed via laser. For this, the 2940 nm erbium:yttrium aluminium garnet (Er:YAG) laser (ACTION II; Lutronic Corp.) can be used as it can accurately ablate off a very thin layer of skin due to the vey high absorption in water at this wavelength. This approach can make the demarcation area of the dented scar smooth and can induce neocollagenesis in the dermis, accelerating the improvement of the atrophic tissue. Although Er:YAG treatment has the disadvantage of requiring post-treatment wound management, it can reduce the number of treatment sessions because of the greater treatment outcome of a single session compared with the other procedures.

Immature or young hypertrophic acne scars, which are red and swollen, can be treated using a long-pulsed dye laser (VBeam; Candela Corp., Wayland, MA, USA), which is mostly used for vascular diseases at a wavelength of 595 nm. This approach can reduce the size of a hypertrophic scar. After the treatment, the elevation of the scar is lowered and a reduction occurs in the density of the microvasculature supplying the scar, thus reducing the scar's red tone. There should be three to five treatment sessions with four-week intervals.

In most Asians with Fitzpatrick skin type III-IV, the treatment effect of laser is potentially less than in Caucasian skin, and side effects tend to occur easily. The darker the skin color is, the more melanin there is in the epidermis. Melanin can cause unintended epidermal damage by acting as a chromophore during laser treatment, especially at shorter green/yellow wavelengths, and consequently, blisters, crusts, postinflammatory hyperpigmentation (PIH), and scarring may occur. Due to its shorter downtime and fewer side effects (e.g., PIH) compared with conventional laser resurfacing, the fractional resurfacing laser can be more useful for Asians.

Tips for post-treatment care and follow-up

Before undergoing treatment for acne scars, patients should discontinue taking isotretinoin at least six months prior to the procedure. Photosensitive drugs such as tetracycline should also be discontinued two weeks before the procedure as they will increase the potential for PIH. In addition, it will be beneficial for patients to avoid exposure to ultraviolet radiation and to apply a UVA/B sunblock daily from at least two weeks before the laser treatment, and then daily after the treatment.

REFERENCES

1. Alster TS, McMeekin TO. Improvement of facial acne scars by the 585 nm flashlamp-pumped pulse dye laser. J Am Acad Dermatol 1996;35:79–81.
2. Chapas AM, Brightman L, Sukal S, Hale E, Daniel D, Bernstein LJ, Geronemus RG. Successful treatment of acneiform scarring with CO 2 ablative fractional resurfacing. Lasers Surg Med 2008;40:381–386.
3. Cho SB, Lee JH, Choi MJ, Lee KY, Oh SH. Efficacy of the fractional photothermolysis system with dynamic operating mode on acne scars and enlarged facial pores. Dermatol Surg 2009;35:108–114.
4. Jacob CI, Dover JS, Kaminer MS. Acne scarring: A classification system and review of treatment options. J Am Acad Dermatol 2001;45:109–117.
5. Kang WH, Kim YJ, Pyo WS, Park SJ, Kim JH. Atrophic acne scar scar treatment using triple combination therapy: Dot peeling, subcision and fractional laser. J Cosmet Laser Ther 2009;11:212–215.
6. Rivera AE. Acne scarring: a review and current treatment modalities. J Am Acad Dermatol 2008;59:659–676.
7. Tanzi EL, Alster TS. Comparison of a 1450-nm diode laser and a 1320-nm Nd:YAG laser in the treatment of atrophic facial scars: a prospective clinical and histologic study. Dermatol Surg 2004;30:152–157.
8. Walgrave SE, Ortiz AE, MacFalls HT, Elkeeb L, Truitt AK, Tournas JA, Zelickson BD, Zachary CB. Evaluation of a novel fractional resurfacing device for treatment of acne scarring. Lasers Surg Med 2009;4:122–127.
9. Ward PD, Baker SR. Long-term results of carbon dioxide laser resurfacing of the face. Arch Facial Plast Surg 2008;10:238–245.
10. Weiss ET, Chapas A, Brightman L, Hunzeker C, Hale EK, Karen JK, Bernstein L, Geronemus RG. Successful treatment of atrophic postoperative and traumatic scarring with carbon dioxide ablative fractional resurfacing: Quantitative volumetric scar improvement. Arch Dermatol 2010;146:133–140.

04

Sebum control

◗ Boncheol Leo Goo M.D., B.S.

Introduction

Sebum is a substance that is secreted by the sebaceous glands found in the skin and mucous membranes of mammals. The primary function in human is believed to moisturize, lubricate and protect the outer wall of the human body.

Normally, sebum production is essential for the skin as a protective organ. Sebum is secreted to the stratum corneum to maintain an effective barrier with other proteins and lipids. The composition and the rate of sebum production vary among individual and body parts. In certain disease conditions, abnormal sebum secretion acts pathogenetically. Acne is a representative disease entity with both increased and altered patterns of secretion, while the complete relationship is not well clarified.

When a physiologic condition disturbs normal life, it can be considered a pre-disease condition or illness, which needs medical or procedural intervention.

Tips for the diagnosis

Conventionally, there is no definition or objective value that indicates sebum excess. It gains significance only when the patient argues that it causes some disturbance in his or her normal life. Frequently the patients complain of a greasy, oily and seborrheic skin condition, which is uncomfortable and requires frequent washing and correcitive makeup. Often this descriptive condition correlates with other pathogenetic skin conditions and needs to be diagnosed carefully. A clinically important example is adult-type acne, showing regional variation in the face with different seborrheic or oily conditions, in a 'complex' skin type.

Subjective complaints from the patients have some characteristics in history taking. The patients complain of a 'too fast' oily change after washing, or uneven greasiness in certain facial lesions. This change often accompanies pustules, comedones or acneiform eruption even though the severity is often just subclinical.

Measurement with a Sebumeter™ or comparable devices is only way to quantify the sebum secretion objectively. However, seasonal, environmental or hormonal variations often make biased data, which is can be considered as just additional information or as experimental data. To arrive at a diagnosis and for making a treatment plan, clinical assessment takes more significance.

> Sebum production in dark or Asian skin type is considered to be higher than lighter or Caucasian skin types. Although the 'oily skin' typing is mostly subjective, the demand to decrease sebum is higher in the population with a dark or Asian skin type.

Tips for the treatment

If the patient is unable to take well-known medicine like retinoids, long-lasting and effective treatments with energy-based delivery devices are often recommended. The goal of treatment is to suppress the sebaceous gland activity, not to eradicate the glands themselves. Parameters can be adjusted according to the regional variance even in the individual face, to deliver the proper amount of energy for each sites with different activity or composition of the sebaceous glands.

Photodynamic therapy (PDT) is an effective way of treating acne vulgaris, Usually to control seborrhea, a shorter incubation time or lower intensity of the activating light source is recommended to adjust parameters. The protocol using 633 nm-LED for sebum excess control is as follows:

1. Removal of excessive scales with a skin scrubber or modified Jessner's solution application according to the patient's skin condition. In the summer season or humid conditions, just removing the greasiness with a cleanser is usually enough.
2. Incubation with 5-aminolevulinic acid (5-ALA) for 20 minutes under clear plastic wrap occlusion. Application can be skipped if the lesions are not seborrheic.
3. Swabbing off any 5-ALA remaining on the surface with sterile water-soaked gauze or a sponge is very important to avoid complications like tanning or superficial burning.
4. Activate by irradiating with a 633 nm LED device (e.g. Healite II; Lutronic Corp., Goy-

ang, South Korea, Intensity 4, 60 J (65 mW/cm^2 for 15 min 23 sec)).

5. Clean off any photosensitizer once again, without using soap.

6. Apply mineral UVA/B sunscreens and repeat at 2-week intervals. Treatment can be repeated 3 or 4 times, adjusted according to the skin response.

7. Skin barrier repairing moisturizer should be applied when the air is dry.

A microneedle fractional radiofrequency (MFR) device has recently been introduced which offers a flexible range of biopolar RF energy delivery into the dermis. Because the needle depth is adjustable and available to be close to the sebaceous gland level, the device was thought to be effective in delivering controlled heat damage to the sebaceous glands. Lee et al reported a significant decrease in the sebum level and sebum excretion rate by 30-60% and 70-80% after a single treatment with MFR on the face of Korean subjects, lasting for 8 weeks. Interestingly, the physician's global improvement scores (GIS) for acne severity and acne lesion count also improved with maximum efficacy at week 2, but the efficacy had not lasted in most patients by week 8. This illustrates that sebum control should be done differently from acne treatment, even with the same device.

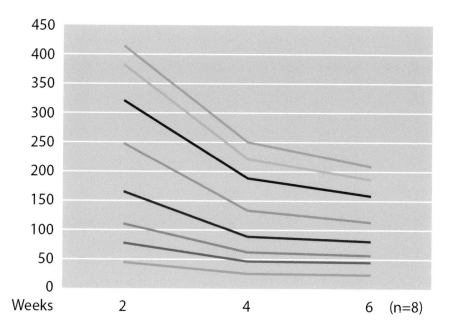

Measured and Analyzed with Sebumeter MPA580 by Courage+Khazaka GmbH Germany.

Figure 04-1　Sebum production change by INFINI™ treatment by time, after single treatment session.

Additional benefits associated with MFR treatment could be a reduction in pore sizes in the skin. Though the size of pores in the skin is affected by many factors including skin laxity and photoaging, sebum secretion is significantly related with regional pore size in the face. The suggested protocol for MFR treatment using MFR (INFINI™, Lutronic Corp.) is as below.

1. Wash the face and apply topical anesthtics (EMLA™ or equivalent) for 30 to 45 minutes. Topical retinoid can be applied as an adjuvant treatment in severe cases, nevertheless systemic retinoid pretreatment is not recommended.

2. Swab off the anesthetic cream, because when the surface dries unevenly the conductance can be different lesion by lesion. Repeat treatments are recommended to reduce the sebum gradually, and to give MFR treatment to each cosmetic unit, when treating the whole face.

3. Apply MFR on the first pass to the cheek area with level 7 (17.5 W), 120-300 ms, depth at 2 mm, and for the second pass on the forehead and nose with level 6 (15 W), 100 ms, depth at 1 mm.

4. Swab any spotty bleeding with hydrogen peroxide-soaked gauze if necessary.

5. Cool the surface with an ice pack for 10 to 15 minutes

6. Skin barrier repairing moisturizer should be applied when the air is dry.

7. Repeat sessions in 4 to 6 weeks according to the skin response.

Seborrhea in dark or Asian skin type can be effectively controlled by several modalities. Usually many sessions are necessary. Compared with acne or other suppurative disease treatment, the treatment parameters should be lowered to decrease the risk of postinflammatory hyperpigmentation. Afterward skin barrier restoring is the state of the art, to prevent dryness and cracking, especially from environmental influences.

Tip for post-treatment care and follow-up

Proper cooling of the site after the treatment is helpful to decrease patients' discomfort. Because the two modalities introduced above have inflammation as a sequela, pain and swelling control is necessary. Usually the decrease in sebum production by MFR occurs very fast, and the patient feels dry easily in a dry environment. Proper moisturization is usually necessary. Excessive sebum secretion is something to be controlled, not to be eradicated.

For dark or Asian skin type, cooling after MFR treatment and application of a sunscreen after PDT are essential.

REFERENCES

1. Choi CW, Choi JW, Youn SW. Subjective facial skin type, based on the sebum related symptoms, can reflect the objective casual sebum level in acne patients. Skin Res Technol 2013;19:176-182.
2. Galzote C, Estanislao R, Suero MO, Khaiat A, Mangubat MI, Moideen R, Tagami H, Wang X. Characterization of facial skin of various Asian populations through visual and non-invasive instrumental evaluations: influence of seasons. Skin Res Technol 2014;20:453-462.
3. Janiczek-Dolphin N, Cook J, Thiboutot D, Harness J, Clucas A. Can sebum reduction predict acne outcome? Br J Dermatol 2010;163:683-688.
4. Kim MK, Choi SY, Byun HJ, Huh CH, Park KC, Patel RA, Shinn AH, Youn SW. Comparison of sebum secretion, skin type, pH in humans with and without acne. Arch Dermatol Res 2006;298:113-119.
5. Lee KR, Lee EG, Lee HJ, Yoon MS. Assessment of treatment efficacy and sebosuppressive effect of fractional radiofrequency microneedle on acne vulgaris. Lasers Surg Med 2013;45:639-647.
6. Lee MR, Nam GW, Jung YC, Park SY, Han JY, Cho JC, Suh KD, Hwang JK. Comparison of the skin biophysical parameters of Southeast Asia females: forehead-cheek and ethnic groups. J Eur Acd Dermatol Venereol 2013;27:1521-1526.
7. Pappas A, Johnsen S, Liu JC, Eisinger M. Sebum analysis of individuals with and without acne. Dermatoendocrinol 2009;1:157-161.
8. Roh M, Han M, Kim D, Chung K. Sebum output as a factor contributing to the size of facial pores. Br J Dermatol 2006;155:890-894.
9. Wesley NO, Maibach HI. Racial (ethnic) differences in skin properties: the objective data. Am J Clin Dermatol 2003;4:843-860.
10. Yosipovitch G, Tang M, Dawn AG, Chen M, Goh CL, Huak Y, Seng LF. Study of psychological stress, sebum production and acne vulgaris in adolescents. Acta Derm Venereol 2007;87:135-139.
11. Yosipovitch G, Tang M, Dawn AG, Chen M, Goh CL, Huak Y, Seng LF. Study of psychological stress, sebum production and acne vulgaris in adolescents. Acta Derm Venereol 2007;87:135-139.
12. Youn SW, Na JI, Choi SY, Huh CH, Park KC. Regional and seasonal variations in facial sebum secretions: a proposal for the definition of combination skin type. Skin Res Technol 2005;11:189-195.
13. Youn SW, Park ES, Lee DH, Huh CH, Park KC. Does facial sebum excretion really affect the development of acne? Br J Dermatol 2005;153:919-924.
14. Youn SW. The role of facial sebum secretionin acne pathogenesis: facts and controversies. Clin Dermatol 2010:28;8-11.

Scars

SECTION

04

C / O / N / T / E / N / T / S

General concept for scar remodeling approach

▶ Seung Ha Park, MD, PhD, MBA

Overview of scars

There are many causes of scars, and people with scars that are visible to others want them removed or at least to appear like the surrounding normal skin. Scars commonly occur on the face, and a facial scar may give an unfavorable impression to others and cause negative prejudice. People with a severe facial scar may become reclusive and socially inactive. Scars are noticeable because the surface is elevated or depressed to a greater or lesser degree, and is completely unlike normal skin. Due to the uneven external morphology of scars, they cannot be satisfactorily camouflaged, even with heavy makeup. A scar may appear red in the acute phase, and then remains white in the long term. In some cases, the scar may appear darker than normal skin, and may undergo partial or complete hypopigmentation. In short, a scar is not normal skin. Consisting mostly of fibrotic collagen, a scar is abnormal skin tissue that has been formed by some defect in the wound healing process after some form of skin trauma, accidental or iatrogenic.

After the normal wound healing process has completed, in the best case there is no visible scar: a histological specimen will, however, reveal some extent of abnormal collagen formation in the dermis. To the naked eye, however, the skin appears normal. On the other hand, in the case of hypertrophic scars or keloids, abnormal collagen production and deposition is extended, with an imbalance between the production and lysis and more immature type III collagen being initially laid down resulting in the scar formation. A hypertrophic scar follows the pattern and stays within the boundaries of the original trauma or incision. A keloid scar features scar tissue which extends in a claw-like pattern beyond the borders of the original wound. Keloid formation is seen significantly more often in Fitzpatrick skin type IV-V and type VI than in skin types I and II, and is often shows a genetic disposition.

In the past, scars were treated mostly via scar revision that involved removal of the scar and suture of the resected site; and for residual scars that were not well-treated by scar revision, dermabrasion was also performed. Scar revision and dermabrasion had limitations in the treatment of scars, however, and left a lot of scars incompletely removed, indeed, often caused more extensive scarring and pigmentary changes. With the advancement of medical laser technology, lasers have has been used to treat scars since the early 1980s, and in the past 2 decades, laser resurfacing that encourages the skin regeneration effect has yielded good outcomes for various types of scars. In addition, the application of lasers with wavelengths highly absorbed in hemoglobin (so-called vascular lasers) for removing redness (*e.g.*, the pulsed dye laser and long-pulsed dye laser) and lasers with wavelengths selectively absorbed in melanin (pigmented lasers, *e.g.*, Q-switched ruby, alexandrite and neodymium:yttrium aluminium garnet (Nd:YAG)) for dark-colored scars due to pigmentation have improved the results even further. More recently, fractional laser technology, both nonablative and ablative, has proven successful in improving those scars that are refractory to laser resurfacing, and are thus widely used.

Scars may be caused by trauma, surgery, burns, or even just cutaneous inflammation, so there are many types of scars, including traumatic scars, surgical scars, hypertrophic scars, acne scars, smallpox and chickenpox scars, atrophic scars, hyperpigmented scars, discolored or hypopigmented scars, burn scars, contracture scars, adhesive scars, band-forming scars, and keloids. No single laser can treat all types of scars. Thus, selection of the appropriate laser for the type of scar is required to ensure a good treatment outcome for scars. Tables 01-1 and 01-2 summarize the types and etiology of scars, and Table 01-3 gives an overview of treatment methods.

Table 01-1   **Types of scars**

Item	Description
Scar surface	Flat; elevated; depressed; irregular
Scar morphology	Atrophic; normotrophic; hypertrophic; keloid
Scar color	Depigmented; hypopigmented; hyperpigmented; discolored
Scar chronology	Acute; chronic; immature; mature

Table 01-2   **Etiology of scars**

Origin	Examples
Injury	Accidental trauma; contusion; laceration; burn; surgery
Infection	Bacterial (*e.g.*; *Propionibacterium acnes*); fungal; viral (*e.g.*, chickenpox; smallpox; herpetic)
Inflammation	Acne lesions; poor post-wound management; striae (after obesity or pregnancy)

Table 01-3 **Treatment methods for scars**

Method	Examples
Topical application	Steroids (more for prophylaxis against hypertrophy)
Gel sheet	Silicone gel (more for prophylaxis against hypertrophy)
Compression	Pressure garments
Intralesional injection	Corticosteroid; *e.g.*, triamcinolone acetonide (kenalog®)
Surgical revision	Excision with linear, tension-free closure; split- or full-thickness skin grafting; Z-plasty; W-plasty
Cryotherapy	Liquid N_2 freeze-thaw protocol
Chemotherapy (intralesional)	5-FU; interferon
Laser surgery	Ablative resurfacing laser (CO_2, Er:YAG) Vascular laser (pulsed dye laser) Pigmentation laser (Q-switched laser - ruby, alexandrite, Nd:YAG) Non-ablative fractional laser (Er:glass) Ablative fractional laser (CO_2, Er:YAG)
RF	Microneedle fractional RF (insulated microneedle matrix)
Radiation therapy	Irradiation

5-FU, fluorouracil; CO_2, carbon dioxide; Er:YAG, erbium:yttrium aluminium garnet; Nd:YAG, neodymium:yttrium aluminium garnet RF, radiofrequency.

Scar formation mechanism

Normal wound healing

A wound stabilizes through the normal healing mechanism that comprises three phases: the inflammation phase from day zero till day 3 or 4, the proliferation phase from around day 3 until day 19-21, and the maturation or remodeling phase from around day 19 till 6 months postwound, or even longer. There is no finite border between these three phases, but they overlap slightly. In the inflammation phase, vessels first contract and then dilatate, and the capillary blood flow increases to provide a plentiful supply of platelets. In addition, the levels of white blood cells, mast cells, macrophages, fibrin, lymphocytes, and secretion of various cytokines also increase, with the expression of trophic factors including platelet-derived growth factors and fibroblast growth factor (FGF) from activated macrophages. In the proliferation phase, the inflammatory stage cells drop back to their prewound levels and epithelial cell proliferation increases. The epithelization is triggered and in relation to this, levels of epidermal growth factor (EGF) and plasma protein supporting epithelial movement also increase and consequently re-epithelialization occurs over a layer of granulation tissue, fed by neovascularization driven by higher levels of endothelial cells. An increase in the number of fibroblasts in a wound is stimulated by increases in the level of various growth factors and chemotactic agents laid down by degranulated mast cells. This leads to extensive neocollagenesis, and neoelastinogenesis in the dermis which increases both the shear and tensile strength of the extracellular matrix (ECM), and thus the wound itself. Both neocollagenesis and neoelastinogenesis are driven by the multifunctional fibroblast.

In the long remodeling (maturation) phase, the cells and process that were boosted in the proliferation phase decrease and stabilize. In particular, collagen production decreases and degeneration of excess collagen by the matrix metalloproteinases 1 and 2 (MMP-1 and MMP-2) is promoted by the fibroblasts, the collagenesis process returns to the normal prewound rate and an equilibrium is reached between the production and degeneration of collagen. At the beginning of the remodeling phase there are too many fibroblasts. Some of them transform into myofibroblasts: myo is Greek for muscle, so these are fibroblasts with muscles that form in tufts at the ends of the fibroblasts. These tufts have little barbs that hook onto collagen fibers: the muscles contract and this helps with the linear reorientation of randomly laid-down collagen bundles, thereby tightening up the ECM structure and adding to the tensile strength of the wound. Remodeling is thus an extremely important phase to ensure a normal ECM. Myofibroblasts go into apoptosis once they have completed their task and are phagocytosed by macrophages. Other fibroblasts dedifferentiate into quiescent fibrocytes. These two processes contribute to reaching and maintaining the balance between neocollagenesis and collagenolysis in the normal wound healing process.

Abnormal wound healing: Hypertrophic scars and keloids

The abnormal wound healing mechanism is responsible for hypertrophic scars and keloids. During the normal healing process, collagen deposition discontinues at around 3 weeks and starts to undergo regression during remodeling. In a hypertrophic scar, on the other hand, collagen deposition may continue to up to six months, and in keloids, even longer up to some years, without being controlled. Histologic findings of hypertrophic scars and keloids include dense collagen fiber layers that are thick and arranged irregularly. In the case of hypertrophic scars, the bulk of the scar is due to masses of immature collagen type III, whereas in keloids a mixture of type III and overproduced type I can be seen.

In most cases, hypertrophic scars and keloids can be differentiated based on the clinical findings rather having to resort to histological findings. As noted above, hypertrophic scars follow the wound and remain within the boundaries, gradually flattening with time, whereas keloids extend beyond the wound boundaries and never decrease in size.

Abnormal wound healing is worse when the wound suffers from chronic irritation such as an infection, inflammation, hypoxia, or is subjected to tension, and is more remarkable during the growth period of an individual. It is sometimes related to the individual's propensity to scar formation or a genetic predisposition. In hypertrophic scars, only the levels of collagen fiber bundles and myofibroblasts increase. In keloids, in addition to the increase in the level of the collagen fiber bundles and myofibroblasts, significantly higher levels of mucinous ground substance, eosinophilic-retractile-hyaline-like collagen fibers, α1-antitrypsin (A1A), and α2-macroglobulin (A2M) are also seen. A1A and A2M are powerful protease inhibitors, which also originate from the fibroblasts among other sources, that inhibit collagenolysis by the MMPs, and encourage production of tissue inhibitors of MMPs (TIMPs). High levels of TIMPs have been found in both hypertrophic and keloid scars. The cause of abnormal wound healing has not yet been fully elucidated, but in addition to the MMP-TIMP findings, it has been suggested that a relationship between the SMAD-family protein interaction downstream and the expression of transforming growth factor (TGF)-β1 and TGF-β2 results in overexpression of these growth factors in hypertrophic scars. The TGF family, especially β1 and β2, is associated with the stimulation of fibroblast neocollagenesis.

Scar treatment modalities

Traumatic scars and surgical scars

For post-traumatic scars, the treatment can be adjusted depending on the depth of the scar, the presence of any sutures, the elapsed time since the trauma, and the shape of the scar. If the depth of the trauma is shallow, such as an abrasion, no suture is required. When the wound results in exposure of the dermis, a hydrocolloid dressing or an occlusive dressing is applied to the wound to promote reepithelization over good granulation tissue formation. This type of injury usually heals leaving normal-looking skin without any other intervention except good wound care. Any foreign bodies remaining on an abrasion-type wound can be gently irrigated or brushed off, or removed with forceps. A traumatic tattoo formed by a foreign material stuck in the wound, or post-traumatic hyperpigmentation forming during the wound healing process, can be effectively removed using treatment with a Q-switched laser (ruby, alexandrite or Nd:YAG), which can be performed every 4-8 weeks until the pigment particles have been removed. Mild and low scars following abrasion can be flattened using an ablative laser such as the CO_2 laser or the erbium:yttrium aluminium garnet (Er:YAG) laser after the scar redness disappears, instead of waiting for 6 months. For the re-treatment, a 6-month interval should be allowed. Fractional lasers have more recently proved very useful compared with the conventional total ablative approach with fewer potential side effects and a shorter downtime for the patient.

After the suturing closed of a traumatic wound or post-surgical incision, in the ideal situation a scar is formed that is thin, flat, and whose color is similar to that of its surroundings, and it does not require any particular treatment. Generally, however, the scar associated with such wounds may be accompanied by contracture during the healing process, and the size of the scar may differ between patients or between areas even in the same patient. It is recommended that a scar with contracture be excised or separated from normal tissue. Depending on the case, a Z-plasty can be performed to prevent the recurrence of contracture, the direction of the scar can be changed, the scar can be aligned with the lines of tension of the face, or a fat graft can be performed after the separation from the normal tissue to effectively treat the depression or contracture of the scar. A red traumatic or surgical scar can be treated more effectively using a pulsed dye laser than a coating gel or sheet. For scars that are in the stabilization phase, are narrow, and are expected to heal after ablation, laser ablation can be performed, with fractional ablative lasers providing excellent results in the more recent literature.

Hypertrophic scars and keloids

Red hypertrophic scars indicate that the scar tissue is still in the proliferative phase involving neovascularization and excessive neocollagenesis without the balancing protease-mediated collagenolysis. For red hypertrophic scars, a gel or scar ointment is applied and compression therapy is performed, though the treatment outcome is often not particularly good. For scars with erythema, irradiation with a vascular laser can destroy or shrink the causative vessels, and thereby reduce the blood flow to the scar: this can in turn inhibit collagen synthesis, and thus prevent the enlargement of the scar. Hypertrophic scars which have newly formed can be shrunk using this approach. Vascular lasers are ideal for this treatment, such as the pulsed dye laser (585 and 595 nm) or the frequency-doubled Nd:YAG (532 nm) applied every 2-4 weeks until the erythema disappears.

For more mature elevated, firm and white hypertrophic scars, steroid (triamcinolone) injection into the scar can be more effective. For this type of scar, the ablative laser approach can be indicated after the disappearance of the erythema. For wide hypertrophic scars, recurrence is inevitable after the treatment, and a fractional laser may achieve some degree of improvement. Consistently effective laser treatment methods for keloids have not been reported yet. Unlike hypertrophic scars, keloids exhibit patient-specific features. Usually, the wound stabilizes through the inflammation, proliferation, and maturation phases. For keloids, collagen metabolism is abnormal during the wound healing process, and collagen proliferation continues excessively, which results in the characteristic claw-like keloid formation extending beyond the borders of the original wound. The recurrence rate of keloids after Z-plasty is high, and surgical removal and radiation therapy are reported to be more effective and have less recurrence than post-operative compression therapy and steroid injection. For keloids, laser ablation is contraindicated, and a suture after laser removal of a keloid is ineffective because the recurrence rate is similar to that for the surgical removal. Making pores using laser to induce regeneration is also used but has not proved so effective.

Dyschromic scars: Hypopigmented, depigmented, and hyperpigmented scars

Generally, the suture site first undergoes depigmentation to become white, and then may become darker than the surrounding normal skin. In the case of abrasions, shallow burns, skin graft sites, and trauma, the scar frequently becomes dark brown. Irritation at the dermoepidermal junction of the scar stimulates the melanocytes in the basal layer and increases the amount of melanin in the keratinocytes, which leads to post-inflammatory hyperpigmentation (PIH). The darker Asian skin types are particularly prone to PIH formation. PIH usually becomes lighter over the long term, and rarely remains pigmented. As always, there are exceptions which prove the rule, so earlier treatment is recommended rather than a wait and see attitude.

Pigmented scars can be effectively treated with skin care using bleaching agent preparations and/or laser treatment, as is the case with discrete epidermal pigmented lesions such as freckles. Skin care can be effective if it is performed using a combination of a bleaching agent (4% hydroquinone), exfoliant (0.025-0.05% retinoic acid), and a soothing agent (1% hydrocortisone). Pigmented scars cannot usually be well-resolved with skin care alone but can be effectively treated with one of the Q-switched lasers, with wavelengths that are selectively absorbed by melanin. The use of the Q-switched Nd:YAG at 1064 nm is preferably indicated for the Asian skin types III, IV and darker, because the 694.3 nm and 755 nm wavelengths of the Q-switched ruby and alexandrite lasers are contraindicated in darker skin types owing to their normal higher density of epidermal melanin. A diode laser at an appropriate wavelength or intense pulsed light (IPL) treatment is also effective.

Destruction of the melanocytes due to an injury or burn disables production of melanin, which consequently leads to a partially or completely white scar due to depigmentation or hypopigmentation. Depigmented or hypopigmented scars are more difficult to treat than hyperpigmented ones, and rarely improve. In such cases, various methods have been used to encourage repigmentation. Light therapy to encourage the proliferation and migration of melanocytes and the regular application of exfoliants sometimes improve the condition. In the case of severe depigmentation, the scar can be peeled off using abrasion and a split thickness skin graft (STSG) applied, or a thin STSG can be performed, though the outcome is inconsistent and the scar may be partially mottled. Laser ablation of a depigmented scar is likely to worsen the depigmentation. Laser ablation of a wide and deep scar tends to elevate the scar and make it white and glossy, and is thus contraindicated. Recently, fractional laser treatment, a micro-focal partial ablation procedure, has been used to improve scars with depigmentation or hypopigmentation. The ablative fractional laser forms microablative columns (MACs) into the scar, preserving a good percentage of the scar surface instead of ablating the entire surface of the scar, and consequently induces regeneration of epithelial cells, including, hopefully, melanocytes. Thus, the fractional laser enables rapid healing of wounds and improves their color by encouraging functional melanocytes to migrate into the epidermis of the scar.

Depressed scars: Acne scars, pox scars, and atrophic scars

Acne scars have a depressed appearance. The types of acne scars based on their shape include ice-pick scars, crater-like scars, and the boxcar type. Acne scars may aggregate to form a rolling depressed scar that has a winding depressed shape, and depressed acne scars may form a large conglomerated scar with an irregular shape. In the acute phase of acne, sebum is overproduced and the lesion appears yellow due to the build-up of follicular pus, and red due to inflammation. After the inflammation subsides, the affected site shrinks and forms a depressed scar due to contracture, with a fibrotic tether holding the base of the scar to the deepest reticular layer of the dermis at the dermis-subdermal tissue junction. On gross examination, the acne scar appears depressed, and histopathological examination reveals a band of fibrotic collagen bundles which form an irregular and thick band down to the dermal-subcutaneous tissue junction of the depressed site.

Although there are many procedures for improving acne scars, patient satisfaction with them is low, as it is difficult to improve acne scars because they are deep due to which some form of ablation is required. Mechanical ablation, however, tends to ablate the neighboring normal skin more than the scar; and with mechanical ablation, a depressed scar would not elevate well. Though chemical ablation can ablate a scar area more deeply than can mechanical ablation, there is difficulty in adjusting the ablation depth, which results in inconsistent outcomes. Laser ablation can produce the best outcome, and ablating the scar area more deeply than the neighboring skin tissue will yield a better outcome than ablating the scar area as deeply as the neighboring tissue. If the depressed area is removed using a 2-4 mm biopsy punch, the depressed area will elevate 1-2 weeks later; and after the wound heals, the punched area will become flat and will have the same color as that of the neighboring skin so that it will not be easily noticed. As such, in a published study, based on the 'laser punch-out' concept, the depressed area of a scar was ablated more deeply than the neighboring skin. The best outcomes were achieved using laser ablation for acne scars in 71 patients; 51 patients had excellent (more than 75% improved) outcomes; 19 patients, good outcomes (51-75% improved); one patient, a fair outcome (25-50% improved); and no patient had a poor outcome (less than 25% improved). Of the 71 patients, six underwent a secondary procedure 6-12 months later as they desired.

For acne scars, more recently fractional ablative CO_2 laser and Er:YAG laser have been used. The CO_2 laser can ablate deeply and induce skin contraction well, but it has the disadvantage of inducing erythema that can last for 3-6 months, which would cause inconvenience in social life and could also lead to PIH in the darker Asian skin. The Er:YAG laser has the advantage of causing less thermal damage than the CO_2 laser owing to its significantly higher absorption in tissue water, which can significantly cut down the period of erythema. Multiple pulse-stacking with the Er:YAG laser using a larger spot size and lower fluence can ablate a scar as deeply as can the CO_2 laser, and can thus yield a good outcome that is comparable to that of the CO_2 laser but with less downtime for the patient. Ablative fractional lasers can offer a good outcome even for smallpox and chickenpox scars, which are similar to acne scars. Smallpox disappeared in South Korea after the Korean War. Thus, people with smallpox scars are all 60 years old or older. Fractional laser ablation of smallpox scars increases skin elasticity and straightens wrinkles, yielding a rejuvenation effect. Acne scars or smallpox scars do not completely disappear after laser ablation. After a laser session, 50-70% of the depressed sites improve. Smallpox scars on the forehead and cheek can be improved best, and those at the center of the face such as the nose and mouth areas can be improved least.

If additional laser ablation of a scar is needed, it should be done after the skin stabilizes following the initial ablation, allowing a 2- to 3-month rest period after the erythema has disappeared. As additional laser ablation can ablate scars deeply, further ablation is possible 6-12 months later. After deep laser ablation of acne and smallpox scars, the wound would completely heal within 7-10 days, during which an occlusive hydrocolloidal dressing should be applied to the wound to protect it, promote healing, and reduce the patient's discomfort. As an acne scar is deep, it is difficult to improve with a nonablative laser (1320 nm Nd:YAG, 1064 nm Nd;YAG, or 1450 nm diode) or with a nonablative fractional laser (1540 nm, 1550 nm Er:glass lasers) that is intended to increase skin elasticity. Though less effective than the fully ablative CO_2 or Er:YAG lasers, these fractional ablative lasers may achieve considerable improvement with 3-4 treatment sessions.

Even more recently an energy-based approach using radiofrequency (RF) energy has been developed. Microneedle fractional RF (MFR) systems have appeared in the literature which have attracted a lot of attention in the successful treatment of acne scars in 2-3 sessions, 4-6 weeks apart. These MFR systems deliver RF energy deep into the dermis with a matrix of insulated needles: only the tips of the needles are active, thereby preserving the epidermis from electrothermal damage without the need for skin cooling, and the depth of the precisely-delivered damage in the dermis is controllable by the user. A multicenter study with one such system (INFINI; Lutronic Corp., Goyang, South Korea) in just under 500 patients showed excellent results in even serious acne scars in dark Asian skin (type IV) with no PIH formation.

Many deeper acne scars, including the winding and depressed scars, are tethered to the dermal-subcutaneous tissue junction and the subcutaneous fat volume is decreased due to inflammation. To solve these problems, especially with the larger area aggregated acne scars, the depressed site can be subcised and the adhesive tether split up and disconnected from the base of the scar. The depressed site can then be filled with a fat graft, elevating and flattening the scar in relation to the surrounding normal tissue. Many patients with acne have been prescribed a form of isotretinoin (vitamin A-related retinoid), a sebum secretion inhibitor, because of severe sebum secretion and inflammation. In these cases ablation can be safely performed 3-6 months after the patient has stopped taking the isotretinoin. Otherwise, skin regeneration could be retarded due to vitamin-A-related shrinkage of the skin appendages.

Striae distensae

Striae distensae or stretch marks, form linear but widened scars, which occur most commonly on the abdomen and thighs after pregnancy, or a sudden weight gain. As striae distensae affect the epidermis as well as the dermis, they do not respond well to the usual variety of procedures such as fully ablative laser treatment. Because there are fewer skin appendages in the abdomen and thigh than in the face, the abdomen and thigh do not show satisfactory outcomes with laser ablation, and are highly likely to develop complications after the laser ablation. The fractional laser, both nonablative and ablative, is now being widely used to avoid the disadvantages associated with full ablation and to make the skin more elastic. The fractional laser procedure is safer than other methods and can yield a good outcome. After a fractional laser procedure, however, the sequelae of laser irradiation on the abdomen and thigh tend to last longer than on the face. MFR is now also being explored as a treatment modality for striae distensae.

Burn scars, contracture scars, and band formation

First-degree burns limited to the epidermis or superficial second-degree burns that involve the upper papillary dermis tend to heal well, without leaving a scar. A deep second-degree burn that involves the deeper reticular dermis or a third-degree (full-thickness) burn tends to take a long time to heal and to leave a scar. A deep burn leaves a scar because of the lack of pilosebaceous units, which have been destroyed together with the epidermis and upper layers of the dermis. If total laser ablation is performed on a burn scar, skin regeneration will not occur because of the lack of any basis, and more serious problems such as a hypertrophic scar or a keloid will occur. Thus, full laser ablation is contraindicated for burn scars because the ablative laser ablates the full thickness of the epithelium. However, the fractional ablative laser that only ablates10-30% of the skin surface can be used with care. Fractional laser ablation flattens the surface of a burn scar and can give it a color similar to that of the neighboring area. After the burn heals and the epithelization is complete, low-level light therapy (LLLT) can be performed with laser or light-emitting diode (LED)-based systems to help resolve the inflammatory reaction faster with enhanced healing thereafter. LLLT has proved effective for stabilizing burn scars, inhibiting the formation of hypertrophic scars, and reducing pruritus.

Summary

There are many causes and types of scars and also many methods of scar treatment. In the past, resectioning and suturing were most commonly used to treat scars but this approach had limitations. With the advent of the laser, scars that could not be treated via conventional surgical revision could then be treated, and laser treatment as a stand-alone approach can offer a superior treatment effect. Thus, a laser procedure, or combination of different laser procedures, is the preferred method of scar treatment. There are many types of laser treatment, including ablative laser, vascular laser, pigmentation laser, fractional ablative and nonablative laser, and LLLT with laser and LED systems. MFR has now been added to the non-laser methods of treating a variety of scars, with good results. The use of the appropriate type of laser or energy-based device in the treatment of scars, coupled with consideration of the timing of the treatment together with the stage and type of the scar can offer a superior effect compared with the conventional approaches. Although laser and non-laser energy-based treatments can offer benefits that conventional surgery cannot, the outcome can be better if a combination approach is explored, applying laser surgery, fractional laser, MFR, and LLLT in appropriate combinations. All the methods that are effective for scar treatment, such as non-surgical methods or injection therapy as delineated in Table 01-3 above, should be considered, and the appropriate ones should be chosen and performed.

REFERENCES

1. Abergel RP, Lyons RF, Castel JC, Dwyer RM, Uitto J. Biostimulation of wound healing by lasers: Experimental approaches in animal models and in fibroblast cultures. J Surg Oncol 1987;13:127.
2. Alexiades-Armenakas MR, Dover JS, Arndt KA. The spectrum of laser skin resurfacing: Non-ablative, fractional, and ablative laser resurfacing. J Am Acad Dermatol 2008;58:719.
3. Alster TS, Tanzi EL. Hypertrophic scars and keloids: Etiology and management. Am J Clin Dermatol 2003;4:235.
4. Alster TS, West TB. Treatment of scars: A review. Ann Plast Surg 1997;39:418.
5. Apfelberg DB. A critical appraisal of high-energy scars. Ann Plast Surg 1997;38:95.
6. Calderhead RG, Goo BL, Lauro F, Gursoy D, Savant SS, Wronski. A 2013: The Clinical Efficacy And Safety Of Microneedling Fractional Radiofrequency In The Treatment Of Facial Wrinkles: A Multicenter Study With The Infini System In 499 Patients. Lutronic white paper. Goyang: Lutronic Corporation.
7. Cohen SR, Henssler C, Johnston J. Fractional photothermolysis for skin rejuvenation. Plast Reconstr Surg 2009;124:281.
8. Fisher GH, Kim KH, Bangesh S, Berstein LJ, Skover G, Geronemus RG. Treatment of surgical scars with fractional photothermolysis. Laser Surg Med 2005;36:81.
9. Gaida K, Koller R, Isler C, Aytekin O, Al-Awami M, Meissl G, Frey M. Low-level Laser Therapy: A conservative approach to burn scars? Burns 2004;30:362.
10. Gauglitz GG, Korting HC, Pavicic T, Ruzicka T, Jeschke MG. Hypertrophic Scarring and Keloids: Pathomechanisms and Current and Emerging Treatment Strategies. Mol Med 2011;17:113-125.
11. Goldman MP, Fitzpatrick RE. Laser treatment of scars. Dermatol Surg 1995;21:685.
12. Herascu N, Velciu B, Calin M, Savastru D, Talianu C. Low-level laser theraphy (LLLT) efficacy in post-operative wounds. Photomed Laser Surg 2005;23:70.
13. Johnson WC. Treatment of pitted scars: The punch transplant technique. J Dermatol Surg Oncol 1996;12:395.
14. Kang DH, Park SH, Koo SH. Laser resurfacing of smallpox scars. Plast Reconstr Surg 2005;116:259.
15. Kligman AM, Willis I. A new formula for depigmenting human skin. Arch Dermatol 1975;111:40.
16. Koo SH, Yoon ES, Ahn DS, Park SH. Laser punch-out for acne scars. Aesthetic Plast Surg 2001;25:46.
17. Laubach HJ, Tannous Z, Anderson RR, Manstrein D. A histological evaluation of the dermal effects after fractional photothermolysis treatment. Laser Surg Med 2005;36:86.
18. Lupton JR, Alster TS. Laser scar revision. Dermatol Clin 2002;20:55.
19. Manstein D, Herron GS, Sink RK, Tanner H, Anderson RR. Fractional photothermolysis: A new concept for cutaneous remodeling using microscopic patterns of thermal injury. Laser Surg Med 2004;34:426.
20. Park SH. Laser dermatologic plastic surgery, Ch 13, fractional laser, 2nd Ed. Seoul: Koonja Pub Co.;2014. p.472-502.

02

Hypertrophic scars and keloids

▶ Seung Ha Park, MD, PhD, MBA

Vascular lasers for scar treatment

In its acute stage, a scar appears red, which reflects inflammation, a part of the wound healing process. In the proliferation stage after the acute stage, capillaries proliferate in the scar, which redden the scar. When the scar enters the maturation stage, it stabilizes, and the phenomena that occurred in the inflammation and growth stages disappear. When capillaries proliferate in the scar, fibroblast activity is stimulated, collagen fibers will be deposited in the scar tissue and the scar will become hypertrophic. Then the scar will harden and protrude. Vascular laser treatment of a red scar will reduce capillary proliferation and telangiectasia and decrease blood circulation, which inhibits collagen fiber proliferation by the fibroblasts and advances the onset of the maturation stage. As such, vascular laser treatment is effective for young and red hypertrophic scars. The target chromophore of the vascular laser is oxyhemoglobin, and it has peak absorption points at 400 nm, 533 nm and 577 nm. Light at 400 nm cannot penetrate deeply into living tissue because of very high melanin absorption, making melanin a conflicting chromophore. The green band is highly absorbed in hemoglobin, but is also highly absorbed in melanin so penetration is again limited and epidermal damage is easily caused by lasers in the green waveband. A wavelength in the yellow waveband is ideal for more effective vascular laser treatment, and typically a 585 nm laser was used as it is not possible to find a laser emitting at 577 nm; and for even deeper penetration, a 595 nm laser is ideal. These wavelengths are slightly less well-absorbed by melanin compared with 532 nm, which makes hemoglobin the preferred chromophore. When a laser with a high power density is used for deeper penetration, aggressive skin cooling must be performed to protect the epidermis with its melanin content, particularly so for the darker Fitzpatrick type III–V Asian skin.

For a red hypertrophic scar, a number of wavelengths currently offer potential treatment efficacy: the 532 nm wavelength, obtained by doubling the frequency of the 1064 nm

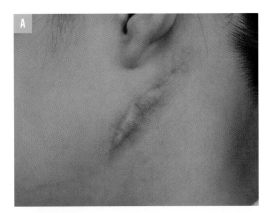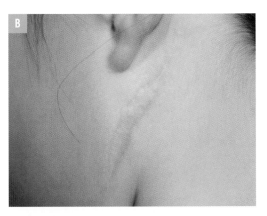

Figure 02-1 **Hypertrophic scar formed after excision of a neck mass.** After application of a vascular laser (Vbeam® pulsed dye laser; Syneron-Candela, Wayland, MA, USA) treatment, the scar elevation and redness improved. For an acute hypertrophic scar, non-ablative fractional laser treatment (Erbium (Er):glass laser, e.g., MOSAIC® at 1550 nm; Lutronic Corp., Goyang, South Korea) has a better outcome than treatment with a vascular laser, because non-ablative fractional laser treatment leaves more of the surrounding tissue to help with swift wound healing, and reaches deeper into the skin than vascular laser treatment, and thus reduces capillary proliferation and inhibits collagen production.

neodymium:yttrium aluminium garnet (Nd:YAG) laser with a crystal, potassium titanyl phosphate (KTP); the flashlamp-pumped pulsed dye laser (FP-PDL; 585 nm); the long-pulsed dye laser (LPDL; 590-595 nm); and intense pulsed light (IPL; polychromatic light 470 nm-1,200 nm).

Pigmentation laser treatment for scars

Scars are commonly redder than normal skin, and occasionally post-inflammatory hyper-pigmentation (PIH) develops, wherein melanin synthesis temporarily increases after trauma or surgery due to excitation of the epidermal melanocytes by inflammation or trauma at the dermo-epidermal junction. If a foreign body is lodged in the skin due to trauma (traumatic tattoo), a black or blue lesion may occur, but this is dermal. In the case of PIH because of abnormal epidermal melanocyte activity, it can take about 6-12 months or more for the scar to return to normal, but this period may be shortened with the use of a whitening (bleaching) agent or peeling cream. Ultraviolet (UV) A/B sunblock application can be recommended for the prevention of hyperpigmentation post-treatment. In some cases, despite these skin procedures, the scar remains dark and thus, easily noticed. To prevent hyperpigmentation or traumatic tattooing of scars, treatment with a pigmentation laser is applied. Furthermore, to prevent damage of the tissue adjacent to any target pigment, the criteria of the theory of

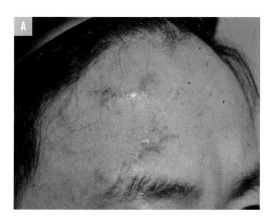 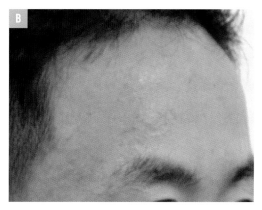

Figure 02-2 **Traumatic tattooing complicated with hypertrophic scarring treated with a Q-switched pigmentation laser.** The Q-switched alexandrite laser treatment (755 nm) was first performed to remove the traumatic tattoo particles, and the irregular skin surface was addressed with a resurfacing laser (Er:YAG laser, 2940 nm).

selective photothermolysis (SPTL) have to be met, namely high peak power, ultrashort pulse width and appropriate wavelength. The Q-switched laser with a pulse width in the nanosecond domain, meets the necessary criteria. Q-switched lasers comprise the ruby laser (694 nm), alexandrite laser (755 nm), and the Nd:YAG laser (532 nm and 1064 nm). All these wavelengths are well absorbed by melanin or tattoo particles, and are therefore effective for pigmented scars.

Resurfacing laser treatment for scars

Scars that are wide and deep, that have contracture, or that are tethered subcutaneously require scar revision with plastic surgery. Scars that cannot be corrected surgically with scar revision may be improved by laser resurfacing, which, in many cases, can improve the scar condition even after the surgical correction. For acne scars that involve small but multiple scars or smallpox scars that cannot be improved with surgical scar revision, the only option is laser resurfacing treatment. Laser resurfacing improves scars via selective vaporization of tissue layers which not only peels off the scar but also tightens the skin, thereby improving the final result. Dermabrasion, which was commonly performed before the development of laser resurfaing, removed normal tissues in addition to the target scar tissues, which caused severe hemorrhage, exudates, and very commonly, pain. Besides, dermabrasion was highly likely to cause inflammation due to its slow healing process. Chemical peeling was introduced later, in which acidic chemical agents were used to destroy the scar. Chemical peeling had the disadvantage of the inability to adjust the ablation depth and consequently causing a bigger scar and serious sequelae. With reports of studies on laser and tissue response appearing in the literature, and when the ability to ablate a scar to the appropriate depth became possible, dermabrasion and chemical peels were replaced by laser resurfacing. In laser resurfacing, the ablation depth can be easily adjusted, and thus the scar can be ablated as deeply as required. Properly applied laser resurfacing can ablate the scar tissue as well as tightening the skin. In addition, use of the laser at appropriate parameters results in only micro focal hemorrhage or the appearance of exudates after the procedure. Wound healing is also fast after laser resurfacing, and compared with other ablation procedures, laser resurfacing causes less swelling, erythema and pain. Because of these advantages, surgeons can perform laser resurfacing safely on patients.

Carbon dioxide laser resurfacing

The carbon dioxide (CO_2) laser emits in the mid-infrared waveband at 10600 nm. As the CO_2 laser wavelength is well-absorbed in tissue water, but not in the hemoglobin in blood and melanin in the skin, it causes non-selective destruction or vaporization and ablation. In addition, the conducted secondary thermal reaction causes secondary thermal damage and contraction of the neighboring tissue that was not vaporized, which has both immediate and delayed effects. In its early days, the CO_2 laser emitted continuous-wave light that caused more coagulation than vaporization, due to which it was mostly used to incise, excise tissue and remove small volumes through ablation and vaporization, but not for the ablation of large areas of tissue. With the development of "superpulsed" CO_2 laser that emitted a train of very short laser pulses, its use in ablative skin resurfacing was developed. The ultrapulsed CO_2 laser, currently the most commonly used CO_2 laser for ablation, was developed to maximize tissue vaporization while reducing thermal damage of nearby tissue. Depending on the system, a CO_2 laser can deliver 100W or more of power, with up to 500 mJ per pulse. As its irradiation time is 1 msec or less, shorter than the thermal relaxation time (TRT) of the skin, it can effectively ablate a scar by irradiating the tissue at a power density and dose (energy density) that are higher than the threshold of vaporization.

Er:YAG laser resurfacing

The erbium:yttrium aluminium garnet (Er:YAG) laser has a 2940 nm wavelength and is very highly absorbed in water, and as skin has a very high percentage of water, the Er:YAG vaporizes cutaneous tissues very efficiently and precisely. Having 10 times greater affinity for

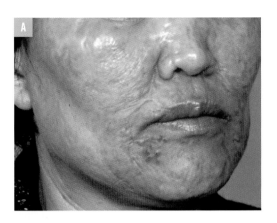 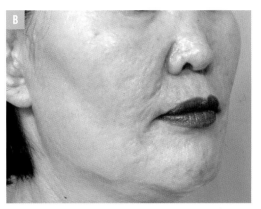

Figure 02-3   **Severe pox scarring.** The skin regeneration effect was achieved after two sessions with a resurfacing laser (Ultrapulse carbon dioxide (CO_2) laser) treatment.

water than the CO_2 laser (coefficient of water absorption: CO_2 laser, 790 μm^{-1}; Er:YAG laser, 13000 μm^{-1}), the Er:YAG laser can induce vaporization of tissue with lower energy densities such as 1.5 J/cm^2, compared with the 5 J/cm^2 vaporization threshold of the CO_2 laser. Though highly effective for ablating and inducing skin shrinkage, the CO_2 laser has the disadvantage of causing long-lasting erythema due to excessive residual thermal damage (RTD) in tissue. The Er:YAG laser, which was introduced in the early 2000s, is now widely used for ablation as is the CO_2 laser, but the degree of RTD deposited by the Er:YAG is significantly less than the CO_2 laser. On the other hand, an adequate degree of RTD was recognized as being essential to kick-start the wound healing process, and too little RTD resulted in less efficacious treatment effects, although downtime was considerably less. Owing to the small zone of RTD normally associated with the Er:YAG laser, it is less hemostatic than the CO_2 and is associated with pinpoint hemorrhage and exudation from the exposed dermis. As both blood and serum have a very high water content, they form a barrier in which the Er:YAG energy is completely absorbed: deep ablation is therefore not usually possible with the Er:YAG laser. To overcome this disadvantage, the long-pulsed mode, much longer than the normal pulse width, has been developed for the Er:YAG laser, which is applied with multiple pulse stacking. This enables depositing adequate RTD to achieve good wound healing with neocollagenesis and remodeling, but still achieving ablation depths similar to the CO_2 without the somewhat disturbing and very uncomfortable sequelae and long downtime associated with the latter. This could be said to make the Er:YAG laser a much safer resurfacing laser than the CO_2.

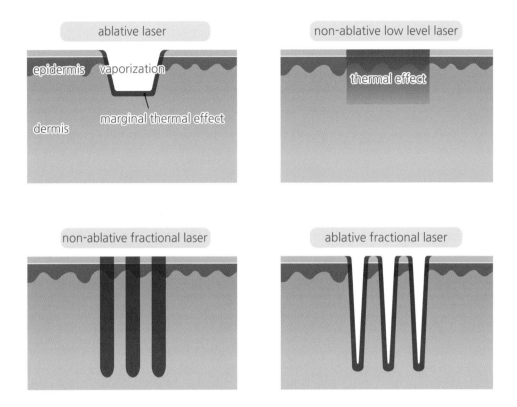

Comparison of the features of the ablative laser (resurfacing laser), nonablative laser (NAR; nonablative rejuvenation), nonablative fractional laser (NAFL), and ablative fractional laser (AFL) (supplement from Lutronic Corp.).

Nonablative laser for scar treatment

The ablative laser is highly effective for skin regeneration and for increasing the contraction and elasticity of the dermis, though it has a long wound healing time and it affects social activity due to the resulting erythema and pigment deposition. To avoid these disadvantages and achieve contraction of the dermis without unwanted side effects, the non-ablative laser was developed. The theory was to deliver controlled heating to the dermis, around 65°C or over, under a chilled epidermis to avoid epidermal damage. Mild coagulation of the collagen fibers in the dermis would occur with contraction and the wound healing process was thus induced. For this purpose, lasers in the near infrared spectrum, the wavelengths of which can penetrate into the dermis, were used as the so-called nonablative rejuvenation (NAR), including the 1320 nm Nd:YAG, 1450 nm diode, and 1540 nm Er:glass. These lasers use a cooling system to protect the epidermis, and needed to be used repeatedly at intervals of 2-6 weeks. Though having the advantage of not affecting the patient's social activity, these lasers were less effective for skin tightening and regeneration even after repeated treatments. When the NAR lasers were first developed, some articles appeared on their use for scar treatment, but results were at best modest and mostly limited to mild to moderate acne scars with multiple treatment sessions required to see any effect. The longer wavelength systems, (e.g., 1450 nm diode laser) had the better effect. The 2004 paper by Tanzi and Alster is typical; comparison of a 1450-nm diode laser and a 1320-nm Nd:YAG laser in the treatment of atrophic facial scars: a prospective clinical and histologic study (Dermatol Surg, 2004; 30:152-157).

A laser delivers coherent light, which comprises the following unique characteristics: all energy is delivered at a single specific wavelength, mono-chromaticity; energy can be delivered in a parallel beam, collimation; and all photons are moving exactly the same in time and in space (phase). Intense pulsed light (IPL) systems on the other hand use a powerful flashlamp to deliver high-powered pulses of non-coherent polychromatic light, with a large waveband stretching from the visible blue at 470 nm all the way to the near infrared at 1200 nm, and every wavelength in between. Because of this, the intrinsic incident power of a laser beam is very high with all incident power concentrated in one wavelength over a small spot size, whereas that of the IPL is comparatively low as it is being delivered over a large waveband and via a coupling crystal with a large treatment area.

A semi-selective effect can be achieved with an IPL using cut-off filters at specific wavelengths to remove the unwanted portion of the visible beam. A yellow filter allows treatment of the hyperactive capillaries in a red hypertrophic scar, and an orange-red or red filter allows treatment of pigmented components in scars. Some IPL systems offer a near-infrared cut-off filter at around 710 nm which will allow penetration of the light energy into the dermis and achieve mild skin tightening in photoaged skin and mild scarring, but it is not effective for severe scars.

Fractional laser treatment for scars

The ablative laser can ablate off layers of scar tissue and lower elevated tissue. The scar, however, can stabilize only when the epithelization is completed swiftly; if the wound healing is delayed and the epidermis fails to cover the wound within 10-14 days, the collagen fibers in the dermis will proliferate and may form a bigger hypertrophic scar.

Not all scars can be ablated using a laser. Laser ablation can be performed only when the scar can be ablated and made smaller, and then epithelization can occur. If there are no residual pilosebaceous units in sparse dermal tissue to assist with island epithelization, a wound cannot be covered by new epithelium except for a small amount from the wound margins, and thus, laser ablation will enlarge such scars. After laser ablation, the scar may become hypopigmented or dyschromic. To avoid these disadvantages and to induce skin contraction, particularly to overcome the inconvenience of post-ablation sequelae and to offer a better outcome than that of the nonablative laser, the fractional approach was next developed whereby the laser beam was fractionated into multiple microbeams with a diameter in the μm range. The microbeams involved a small percentage of the target skin, leaving a large amount of normal, unharmed skin behind to ensure swift wound healing. The first fractional laser was the Er:glass laser at 1,550 nm, at which wavelength there is still reasonable absorption in water but much less so than the CO_2 or Er:YAG, and as a result this wavelength could penetrate more deeply into the dermis than the other two lasers. Up to 400 microbeams could be delivered per square centimeter of skin. The first system was non-ablative, and created microcolumns of coagulation in the dermis under a more or less intact epidermis, which were called micronecrotic columns (MNCs; diameter, 70-100 μm and depth, 350-750 μm). The nonablative fractional approach involved only 10-30% of the skin volume, and any damage to the epidermis over the MNCs was fully repaired within 24 hour after treatment, while the zone of coagulation started the wound repair process to rejuvenate the dermis. With nonablative fractional laser (NFL), the fully ablation related sequelae were prevented, downtime was short and make-up could be used 2-3 days after the procedure. The greatest advantage of the NFL was that it minimally affected social activity.

Although the results of the NFL systems were good and patient downtime was short, patient satisfaction was, however, lower than expected. It was suggested that the lack of damage to the epidermis was a critical factor, and so the first ablative fractional laser (AFL) was developed using the CO_2 laser. Unlike the MNCs delivered by the NFLs, the ablative fractional CO_2 laser delivered microablative columns (MACs) which precisely ablated tissue from the epidermis down into the dermis. In addition, the MACs could have a depth of up to 2 mm or more in the dermis, enabling a potential beneficial effect in the deeper fibrotic collagen bundles of large hypertrophic scars. Each MAC was surrounded by a zone of secondary thermal damage, similar to the delivered thermal damage associated with the fully ablative CO_2 systems, which stimulated a strong wound healing response. Reepithelization was complete 24-48 hour after treatment. Although there was slightly more in the way of side effects and patient downtime compared with the NFL systems, on the other hand the results were much better and patient satisfaction much higher with the AFL approach. Fractional Er:YAG laser next joined the AFL ranks, with very good results. Because they involve a very small area of the skin, including the epidermis, leaving a large volume of the dermis and epidermis intact along with pilosebaceous units, reepithelization is swift. This means that the ablative fractional laser offers a good treatment modality for hypertrophic or acne scars, even those which are hypopigmented, depigmented or hyperpigmented, because neither the CO_2 nor the

Er:YAG laser has blood or melanin as a chromophore, only tissue water.

Figure 02-5 illustrates schematically the principle of ablative fractional resurfacing. Figure 02-6 shows the efficacy of an AFL system on the revision of severe pox scars, and Figure 02-7 shows the ability to follow NFL for a post-thyroidectomy scar with an AFL system at a later stage to give an excellent result with no hypertrophic scar formation.

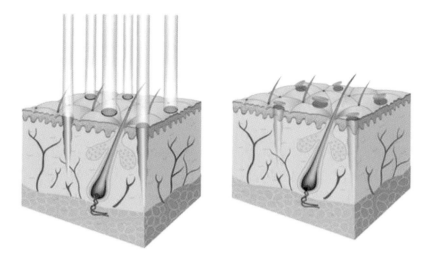

Figure 02-5 The ablative fractional laser creates micro-ablative columns (MACs) into the skin that enables rapid epithelization of the epidermis and remodeling of the collagen in the dermis (supplement from Lutronic Corp.).

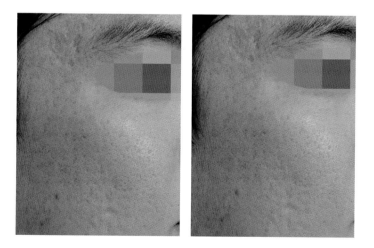

Figure 02-6 **Acne scar.** Two sessions of ablative fractional CO_2 laser (eCO$_2$®; Lutronic Corp, Goyang, South Korea) treatment considerably improved the depressed scarring.

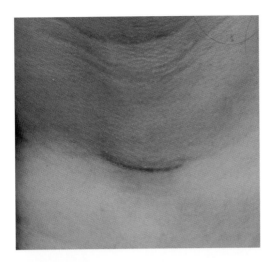 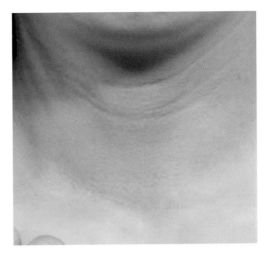

Figure 02-7 Hypertrophic scar on the neck post-thyroidectomy. It was noticeably improved after NAFL (MOSAIC®; Lutronic Corp.) treatment when it was in its immature acute stage, during which it was red. And when in its more mature chronic stage when the redness had disappeared, the scar was treated with AFL (eCO$_2$®; Lutronic Corp.) treatment.

REFERENCES

1. Alster TS, Tanzi EL. Hypertrophic scars and keloids: etiology and management. Am J Clin Dermatol 2003;4:235.
2. Alster TS, West TB. Treatment of scars: a review. Ann Plast Surg 1997;39:418.
3. Cohen SR, Henssler C, Johnston J. Fractional photothermolysis for skin rejuvenation. Plast Reconstr Surg 2009;124:281.
4. Fisher GH, Kim KH, Bangesh S. Berstein LJ, Skover G, Geronemus RG. Treatment of surgical scars with fractional photothermolysis. Lasers Surg Med 2005;36:81.
5. Herascu N, Velciu B, Calin M, Savastru D, Talianu C. Low-level laser theraphy(LLLT) efficacy in post-operative wounds. Photomed Laser Surg 2005;23:70.
6. Hunzeker CM, Weiss ET, Geronemus RG. Fractionated CO2 laser resurfacing; our experience with more than 2000 treatments. Asthetic Surg J 2009;29:317.
7. Koo SH, Yoon ES, Ahn DS, Park SH. Laser punch-out for acne scars. Aesthetic Plast Surg 2001;25:46.
8. Laubach HJ, Tannous Z, Anderson RR, Manstein D. Skin responses to fractional photothermolysis. Laser Surg Med 2006;38:142.
9. Laubach HJ, Tannous Z, Anderson RR, Manstrein D. A histological evaluation of the dermal effects after fractional photothermolysis treatment. Lasers Surg Med 2005;36:86.
10. Lawrence WT. Physiology of the acute wound. Clin Plast Surg 1998;25:321.
11. Lupton JR, Alster TS. Laser scar revision. Dermatol Clin 2002;20:55.
12. Manstein D, Herron GS, Sink RK, Tanner H, Anderson RR. Fractional photothermolysis: a new concept for cutaneous remodeling using microscopic patterns of thermal injury. Laser Surg Med 2004;34:426.
13. Rokhsar CK, Tse Y, Fitzpatric R. Fractional photothermolysis on the treatment of scars. Lasers Surg Med 2005;36:30.
14. SH Park. Laser Dermatologic Plastic Surgery. Ch 14, Laser treatment of Scars. Seoul: Koonja Pub Co;2014. p504-532.

Keloids

▶ Won Serk Kim, MD, PhD

Definition

A keloid is diagnosed when the wound tissue continues to grow beyond the wound area, unlike in a normal or hypertrophic scar. The cause of a keloid remains uncertain. It develops immediately or delayed after the damage. As it is common in Blacks and Asians but rare in Caucasians, the genetic factor is believed to be closely related to the etiology of keloids. Other factors such as hormones and skin elasticity are also involved in the etiology.

Tips for diagnosis

Keloids are known to occur mostly in humans, though they have been reported to have occurred in higher-level animals such as horses, cows, and dogs. They are most common in Blacks, followed by Asians and Caucasians. Their incidence rate does not differ between men and women. They are common in young people; and in women, in whom the lesion tends to decrease after menopause.

The histopathological findings in cases of keloids are included in Table 03-1.

The two most common types of keloids in Asians are ball-shaped lesions that occur in a site pierced in the ear, and acne keloids where the acne site becomes itchy and hard.

Table 03-1   The histopathological findings

Normal skin	Hypertrophic scar	Keloid
Moderate level of extracellular matrix between collagens that are parallel to the epidermis	Nodal structure and amorphous arrangement of collagen	Haphazard collagen and whirlpool or nodal collagen fibers

Tips for treatment

For hypertrophic or atrophic scars, various forms of laser treatment have been performed, with some degree of efficacy, varying by report. For keloids, however, laser treatment is still not considered as a primary treatment.

- Carbon dioxide (CO_2) laser ablation make less bleeding and pain than simple conventional excision, but does not differ greatly in its recurrence rate compare to excision. As this procedure has a higher risk of keloid recurrence or exacerbation, adjunctive radiation or steroid injection therapy must be performed after the procedure (Figure 03-1).

- Pulsed dye laser (PDL): This is used mostly for vascular disease. It induces tissue necrosis by causing tissue hypoxia, and is considered effective for the treatment of keloids (Figure 03-2). On the other hand, given its high cost and the great difference in its treatment effect by the size and location of the keloid, it cannot be considered a main treatment method. Complications such as a burning sensation, itchiness, or hyperpigmentation may occur after the procedure.

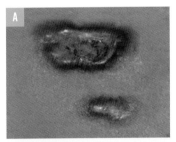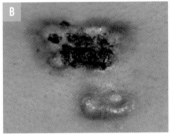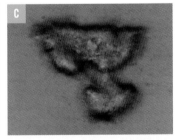

Figure 03-1 Aggravation of keloids after carbon dioxide laser ablation.

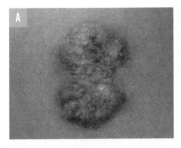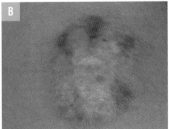

Figure 03-2 Example of the application of pulsed dye laser on a keloid.

- Fractional laser: This laser has been reported to be somewhat helpful for keloid treatment, but has not been extensively studied.
- Laser toning: In recent studies, laser toning was reported to be effective for the treatment of keloids, but its applicability is considered limited.
- Appropriate treatment methods should be selected based on the location, size, and number of lesions, the patient's age, and the convenience of visiting the hospital. Generally, for a large lesion, it is recommended that the size of the lesion be reduced by surgery, and then an adjunctive non-surgical procedure be performed. For young patients or elderly patients in which the wound healing process is likely to be slow, treatments such as cryotherapy that involves severe pain and high risk of complications should be avoided. For patients who cannot visit a hospital frequently, prescription of topical applications or compressive treatment using a dressing is recommended. Before the treatment, it is good to explain to the patient the possible treatment outcome. Clinicians should avoid telling patients that the lesion is incurable without giving a good reason for it, and care must be taken not to give patients the illusion that their skin could become normal. Even if the treatment outcome is good, regular checkup for at least 1 year is recommended. It is more important to make patients aware of the importance of prevention of keloids. As psychological issues among patients with keloids may be more serious than thought, sufficient communication is necessary before and after the treatment; and if a psychological problem arises, the clinical treatment should be accompanied by psychological treatment.

REFERENCES

1. Akasaka Y, Fujita K, Ishikawa Y, Asuwa N, Inuzuka K, Ishihara M, Ito M, Masuda T, Akishima Y, Zhang L, Ito K, Ishii T. Detection of apoptosis in keloids and a comparative study on apoptosis between keloids, hypertrophic scars, normal healed flat scars, and dermatofibroma. Wound Repair Regen 2001;9:501-506.
2. Alster TS, Tanzi EL. Hypertrophic scars and keloids: etiology and management. Am J Clin Dermatol 2003;4:235-243.
3. Alster TS. Laser treatment of hypertrophic scars, keloid and striae. Dermatol Clin 1997;15:419-429.
4. Shaffer JJ, Taylor CC, Cook-Boddin F. keloidal scars: a review with a critical look at therapeutic options. J Am Acad Dermatol 2002;46:S63-97.

04

Stretch marks (striae distensae)

◗ Sung Bin Cho, MD, PhD & Sang Ju Lee, MD, PhD

Introduction

Striae distensae (stretch marks) are linearly depressed atrophic patches of the skin that usually appear along the anatomical cleavage lines. They can develop under various physiologic or pathologic conditions, including pubertal growth spurts, rapid weight changes, pregnancy, obesity, and excessive endo- or exogenous steroid hormone levels. Striae gravidarum refer to the striae distensae occurring in pregnant women that usually develop after the 24th week of gestation. Striae distensae occur in all age groups, but more commonly in women than in men.

Although the precise pathogenesis of striae distensae has not been fully elucidated, it has been suggested that the stretching of the skin results in ruptures in the connective tissue leading to dermal atrophy. Additionally, mast cell degranulation, including elastases, and macrophage activation in the early stage of striae distensae have been suggested to result in elastolysis of the mid-dermis. A comparative study on the biophysical properties of striae distensae demonstrated that there were no significant differences in skin barrier function and hydration when compared to the adjacent normal skin. However, striae distensae presented a significantly lower melanin concentration and light scattering value than normal skin. Additionally, mechanical properties, including skin firmness and elasticity, were remarkably decreased in striae distensae.

Tips for diagnosis

Generally, striae distensae can be divided into 'striae rubrae' and 'striae albae' according to their clinical features. Also, two additional types of striae distensae have been suggested including striae nigrae and striae caerulea that occur in patients with darker skin resulting from increased melanization of the lesions. The early stage of striae distensae, which is called striae rubrae, presents as asymptomatic or mildly pruritic flat to slightly raised red-to-violaceous lesions. Histopathologically, striae rubra show significant inflammatory reactions in the dermis with elastolysis and mast cell degranulation, but with a normal or flattened epidermis.

Over time, the lesions of striae rubrae gradually become atrophic and white, which are then called striae albae. The histologic features of striae albae include a flattened or atrophic epidermis with blunted rete ridges, decreased dermal thickness, especially caused by the thinning of collagen bundles in the upper dermis, and the absence of skin appendages. The differential diagnosis of striae albae includes those cutaneous disorders presenting with skin atrophy of connective tissues, especially linear focal elastosis, mid-dermal elastolysis, and anetoderma.

Tips for treatment

It is difficult to predict or prevent striae distensae. Although striae distensae have a tendency to spontaneously regress over time, they commonly result in significant cosmetic problems, especially when they are large in size and located in exposed areas. There have been several therapeutic modalities for treating striae distensae, including topical agents, various laser or light sources, and radiofrequency devices, however, standard treatment recommendations remain to be established.

Topical agents

Topical agents for treating striae distensae include topical tretinoin, hydrating creams, topical silicone, and topical oil. Treatment of striae rubrae with 0.1% tretinoin cream, which has an affinity for fibroblasts and induces collagen synthesis, effectively improves the overall appearance by decreasing length and width of the lesions. However, the clinical efficacy of topical tretinoin for treating striae albae is unsatisfactory.

Previous studies evaluated various products, including Trofolastin®, cocoa butter, Alphastria®, Verum®, and olive oil, for their efficacies in the prevention of striae distensae; however, no statistically significant evidence was reported. The efficacy of topical silicone has been shown in treating striae distensae by increasing collagen and decreasing melanin compared with a placebo.

Chemical peels

Chemical peels using acid substances, including glycolic acid and trichloroacetic acid, have been reported to increase collagen synthesis. Topical therapy using 70% glycolic acid for treating striae rubrae significantly decreased the width of the lesions as well as hemoglobin, whereas in striae alba lesions it decreased the width of lesions and increased levels of melanin. However, care must be taken when using acids with high concentration to prevent irreversible dyspigmentation and/or scarring.

Laser or light source devices

Recently, laser or light devices have become widely used for treating striae distensae. Several laser or light source devices have been introduced, including the carbon dioxide (CO_2) laser, intense pulsed light (IPL) systems, pulsed-dye laser (PDL), long-pulsed neodymium-doped yttrium aluminum garnet (Nd:YAG) laser, non-ablative erbium:glass fractional laser, and ablative fractional CO_2 laser.

Pulsed-dye laser

The 585- or 595-nm PDL, which mainly targets dilated blood vessels, has been used most frequently for treating striae distensae, especially striae rubrae. In addition to its therapeutic effects on the pathologic vascular structures in striae rubrae, PDL treatment is known to increase collagen and elastin structures that theoretically improve either striae rubrae or striae albae lesions. The reported laser settings for PDL treatment showed a range of therapeutic outcomes with a 10 mm spot size and a laser fluence of 3.0-4.25 J/cm^2 using a 585-nm PDL, or a 10 mm spot size, pulse duration of 500 μs, and a laser fluence of 2.5 J/cm^2. Because PDLs have a superior treatment response in striae rubrae compared with striae albae, combination therapy with topical agents and/or other lasers, light-based, and radiofrequency devices as described below has also been recommended.

Fractional laser; ablative and non-ablative

Fractional lasers have been effectively used for the treatment of various dermatologic diseases. Additionally, the U.S. Food and Drug Administration has approved non-ablative 1,540 nm erbium:glass (Er:glass) fractional lasers for use in striae distensae. Several studies demonstrated that non-ablative Er:glass fractional lasers were effective for treating both striae rubrae and striae albae without any remarkable major side effects. After 5-10 sessions of non-ablative fractional laser treatment at 1-month intervals, epidermal and dermal thicknesses can be increased with the up-regulation of type 1 procollagen. Increased levels of melanin pigment can also be expected in striae albae lesions of after non-ablative Er:glass fractional laser treatment.

In Asian patients, the risk of post-treatment pigmentary disorders after ablative laser therapy is relatively high, especially when treating lesions in locations other than the face. Because of this consideration, patients with Fitzpatrick's skin phototypes of IV to VI had been recommended to avoid CO_2 laser treatment of striae distensae. However, several investigations have reported that the treatment of striae albae using an ablative CO_2 fractional laser was objectively effective and satisfactory without any major side effects. Additionally, the ablative CO_2 fractional laser has been found to provide better immediate tissue tightening and collagen stimulation than the non-ablative Er:glass fractional laser. Moreover, the CO_2 laser treatment results in adequate inflammation in the treated areas that starts the wound healing process, eliminating fragmented collagenous matrix through macrophage activity, promoting neocollagenesis and leading to the remodelling process.

An example of fractional CO_2 laser settings for treating striae includes a spot size of 1-10 mm depending on the width of the lesions, with a microbeam diameter of 120 μm, a pulse energy of 10 mJ, a density of 10% coverage, and a single pass. Noticeable overall clinical improvements have been reportedly achieved with 1-3 sessions of ablative CO_2 fractional laser treatment at 1-2-month intervals, and hypopigmented lesions of late-stage striae distensae have been reported to return to the skin color of the adjacent non-lesional skin within 3 months after the final treatment (Figure 04-1). Post-therapy erythema can be noticed at the treatment site for approximately 4 weeks and spontaneously disappears within 4-8 weeks. Minor short-term side effects, including pruritus, crusting or scaling, and oozing, also can be observed. Additionally, post-treatment hyperpigmentation is frequently encountered in Asian patients treated with the ablative CO_2 fractional laser that has almost completely resolved within 1-2 months.

Others

IPL systems can be effectively used to reduce the width of striae distensae and increase collagen expression that is comparative to PDL treatment. However, it has been found that post-treatment collagen I expression is superior in PDL treatment compared with IPL treatment. In the treatment of striae rubrae, the cut-off filter blocking the shorter wavelengths for the better treatment of vascular lesions is preferentially chosen.

The 308 nm XeCl excimer laser provides good therapeutic outcomes for treating the hypopigmented lesions of striae albae. The 308 nm excimer laser emits in the ultraviolet waveband, the efficacy of which has been proved in the treatment of vitiligo and psoriasis by reducing dermal inflammatory reactions and restoring epidermal melanin production. When

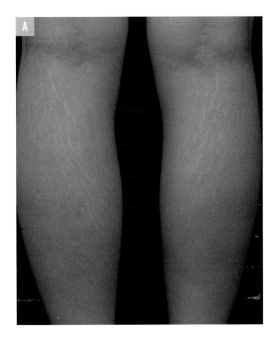
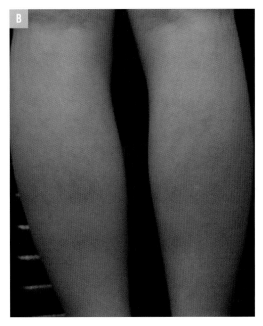

Figure 04-1   Striae distensae on the calves of a 24-year-old Korean woman before **A** and 3 months after **B** one session with an ablative 10600 nm carbon dioxide fractional laser system.

the XeCl laser is used for treating striae albae, the hypopigmented lesions can be reportedly improved by over 70% by delivering a maximum of 10 sessions of 308 nm excimer laser treatment with treatment sessions ranging from twice weekly to once every two weeks.

The 1064-nm long-pulsed Nd:YAG laser can be effectively used for treating striae rubrae by targeting the striae vasculature. Additionally, as has been shown in other long-pulsed laser devices, the long-pulsed Nd:YAG laser induces new collagen formation which clinically results in the improvement of skin atrophy. One reported example of laser settings for striae treatment with the 1064-nm long-pulsed Nd:YAG laser suggested as a spot size of 2.5 mm, fluences of 80-100 J/cm^2, and 3-5 sessions with an interval of 3-6 weeks. However, adjustment of the treatment parameters should be made according to the individual device. Owing to the absorption characteristics of the 1064 nm wavelength, the risk of major side effects in the treatment of striae distensae using the 1064 nm long-pulsed Nd:YAG lasers is low.

Radiofrequency devices

Radiofrequency current can be delivered to skin with either the unipolar or bipolar mode using surface electrodes, or more recently, insulated microneedle electrodes to deliver the

RF energy directly into the dermis. A unipolar superficial radiofrequency device has been used for rejuvenating dermal structures while preserving the epidermis with cooling. This radiofrequency device has shown to be effective for treating striae distensae in combination with the pulsed-dye laser by inducing new collagen production. The reported parameters for striae treatment with a unipolar non-invasive radiofrequency device were fluences ranging from 53-97 J/cm^2 and 2-3 passes. However, adjustment of the treatment parameters should be made according to the individual device.

More recently, a bipolar fractionated radiofrequency device using insulated microneedle electrodes was introduced for treating atrophic scars, wrinkles and lax skin. Fractional microneedle radiofrequency can efficiently deliver a higher level of RF current into the deeper layers of the dermis compared with the superficially-delivered devices. Only the tip of the microneedles is live, and the penetration depth of the microneedles can be precisely controlled to effectively deliver RF energy at preset depths in the dermis, while the epidermis is spared from any electrothermal damage by the insulation on the needle shafts, and therefore does not require cooling. The RF-induced fractionated electrothermal tissue reaction usually results in generating water-drop or cocoon-shaped coagulation zones around the tip of the needle electrodes in the dermis surrounded by normal undamaged tissue, whereas the ablative fractional CO_2 laser delivers a conical zone of ablation, the microablative column (MAC) surrounded by photothermal coagulation. The MACs are widest at the epidermis and get narrower as they go deeper the dermis. The suggested treatment settings for the fractional microneedling radiofrequency were depths of from 1.5 to 3 mm, a power level of 7.5 to 12.5 W,an exposure time of 100 to 300 msec , and single or double passes. However, the RF parameters should be selected according to the individual device and the condition being treated. The fractional bipolar microneedling radiofrequency treatment can be used alone with 2 or more sessions at 1- to 2-month intervals, but synergistic effects could be achieved by combination treatment with topical agents, and laser or light devices. Fractional radiofrequency treatment for striae distensae is generally well tolerated without remarkable side effects, except for transient and minimal post-treatment pin-pointbleeding, followed by oozing, crusting, and scaling. These sequelae improve spontaneously within 5 days.

REFERENCES

1. Al-Himdani S, Ud-Din S, Gilmore S, Bayat A. Striae distensae: a comprehensive review and evidence-based evaluation of prophylaxis and treatment. Br J Dermatol 2014;170:527-547.
2. Alexiades-Armenakas MR, Bernstein LJ, Friedman PM, Geronemus RG. The safety and efficacy of the 308-nm excimer laser for pigment correction of hypopigmented scars and striae alba. Arch Dermatol 2004;140:955-960.
3. Bak H, Kim BJ, Lee WJ, Bang JS, Lee SY, Choi JH, Chang SE. Treatment of striae distensae with fractional photothermolysis. Dermatol Surg 2009;35:1215-1220.
4. Cho S, Park ES, Lee DH, Li K, Chung JH. Clinical features and risk factors for striae distensae in Korean adolescents. J Eur Acad Dermatol Venereol 2006;20:1108-1113.
5. Cho SB, Lee SJ, Lee JE, Kang JM, Kim YK, Oh SH. Treatment of striae alba using the 10,600-nm carbon dioxide fractional laser. J Cosmet Laser Ther 2010;12:118-119.
6. Elsaie ML, Baumann LS, Elsaaiee LT. Striae distensae (stretch marks) and different modalities of therapy: an update. Dermatol Surg 2009;35:563-573.
7. Goldman A, Rossato F, Prati C. Stretch marks: treatment using the 1,064-nm Nd:YAG laser. Dermatol Surg 2008;34:686-691.
8. Hernandez-Perez E, Colombo-Charrier E, Valencia-Ibiett E. Intense pulsed light in the treatment of striae distensae. Dermatol Surg 2002;28:1124-1130.
9. Jimenez GP, Flores F, Berman B, Gunja-Smith Z. Treatment of striae rubra and striae alba with the 585-nm pulsed dye laser. Dermatol Surg 2003;29:362-365.
10. Kang S, Kim KJ, Griffith CE, Wong TY, Talwar HS, Fisher GJ, Gordon D, Hamilton TA, Ellis CN, Voorhees JJ. Topical tretinoin (retinoic acid) improves early stretch marks. Arch Dermatol 1996;132:519-526.
11. Katz TM, Goldberg LH, Friedman PM. Nonablative fractional photothermolysis for the treatment of striae rubra. Dermatol Surg 2009;35:1430-1433.
12. Kim BJ, Lee DH, Kim MN, Song KY, Cho WI, Lee CK, Kim JY, Kwon OS. Fractional photothermolysis for the treatment of striae distensae in Asian skin. Am J Clin Dermatol 2008;9:33-37.
13. Lee SE, Kim JH, Lee SJ, Lee JE, Kang JM, Kim YK, Bang D, Cho SB. Treatment of striae distensae using an ablative 10,600-nm carbon dioxide fractional laser: a retrospective review of 27 participants. Dermatol Surg 2010;36:1683-1690.
14. Nouri K, Romagosa R, Chartier T, Bowes L, Spencer JM. Comparison of the 585-nm pulsed dye laser and the short pulsed CO2 laser in the treatment of striae distensae in skin types IV and VI. Dermatol Surg 1999;25:368-370.
15. Orringer JS, Voorhees JJ, Hamilton T, Hammerberg C, Kang S, Johnson TM, Karimipour DJ, Fisher G. Dermal matrix remodeling after nonablative laser therapy. J Am Acad Dermatol 2005;53:775-782.
16. Ryu HW, Kim SA, Jung HR, Ryoo YW, Lee KS, Cho JW. Clinical improvement of striae distensae in Korean patients using a combination of fractionated microneedle radiofrequency and fractional carbon dioxide laser. Dermatol Surg 2013;39:1452-1458.
17. Stamatas GN, Lopes-DaCunha A, Nkengne A, Bertin C. Biophysical properties of striae distensae evaluated in vivo using non-invasive assays. Skin Res Technol 2014; in press.

05

Scar prevention

Won Serk Kim, MD, PhD

Introduction

Scars are a very common cosmetic concern in the Asian aesthetic market. Scars are closely related to skin features, and their presentation varies from individual to individual due to genetic and racial factors. Predicting a hypertrophic scar or keloid tissue at a surgery site is known to be difficult, and their treatment is recognized as being even more difficult. With the recent increase in the incidence of surgical intervention, surgery-related scars have become common, and their treatment is very complex and difficult.

Tips for diagnosis

Surgical scars are mostly diagnosed with gross examination. In a surgical scar, the skin in the surgical site normally swells or grows over time. A surgical scar is diagnosed as hypertrophic when the skin in the surgical site has grown excessively and deviated from the normal skin color or configuration. In some cases, it is observed that the skin in the surgical site grows beyond the borders of the surgical wound, and this overgrowth is diagnosed as a keloid. Basically, a keloid occurs in the wound or ulceration during the healing process. Histological examinations show that keloids consist mostly of fibrous tissue generally with a thin epidermis but without skin wrinkles and appendages. Pathological findings include abnormal activity of fibroblasts, increased production of hyaluronate, an increased level of cytokines, the absence of apoptosis in fibroblasts, and excessive neovascularization.

Tips for treatment

Recently, there have been various attempts to treat hypertrophic, atrophic, or flat scar tissue. Available treatments for hypertrophic scars and keloids include surgical removal of the lesion, intralesional injections of steroids or bleomycin, local application of a highly potent steroid ointment, cryosurgery, application of silicon gel or a silicon sheet, and intermittent radiation therapy. Treatments for flat or atrophic lesions include laser ablation, chemical ablation, filling, and autologous fat tissue grafting. Each treatment method has its own advantages and disadvantages. Of these methods, surgical removal, cyrosurgery, and ablation are invasive, with many side effects reported.

For laser treatment of scars, various types of lasers have been used with ablation of acne scars, of which the carbon dioxide (CO_2) laser is the most commonly used. Recent reports have suggested that the pulsed dye laser at a wavelength of 585 nm or 595 nm, which has usually been used for vascular diseases, was effective for scars or keloids. As a result, various types of laser can be used for the minimally invasive treatment of scars, which produce good outcomes. The pulsed dye laser has the disadvantages, however, of high cost, slow treatment effect, and ineffectiveness for large and old scars. As such, numerous ways to predict the occurrence of a scar immediately after surgery have been proposed, and new methods of laser treatment of scars have been suggested.

It has been reported that lasers based on fractional technology and the 532 nm KTP laser were effective for the prevention of scars, and since then, various methods that use these lasers have been utilized to treat scars. The authors have used the nonablative fractional 1,550-nm erbium-doped fiber (Er:glass) in the effective prevention of scarring after a thyroidectomy, and we have reported our experience. We performed two sessions of treatment with an energy level of 4-120 mJ and a density of 50-500 spots/cm^2 at an interval of 2 weeks (Figure 05-1). We also found that the 532 nm potassium titanyl phosphate (KTP) laser produced a similar treatment outcome. We performed two sessions of treatment with a 10 mm spot size, a 25-millisecond pulse duration, an 8 J/cm^2 fluence, and a 1.5-Hz frequency at an interval of 2 weeks. It is known that starting treatment 2 weeks after surgery is most effective because at this time, the wound can regenerate and a scar can form simultaneously.

Low level light therapy with light-emitting diode systems (LED-LLLT) at the near-infrared wavelength of 830 nm has begun to attract a great deal of attention in accelerating and improving wound healing, with an increasing number of reports in the literature, including some from the author's team, illustrating its efficacy both in the healing of normal and compromised wounds, and as an adjunctive modality in aesthetic and cosmetic surgery. The indication of LED-LLLT for scar prevention would appear to be a logical step forward. A recent

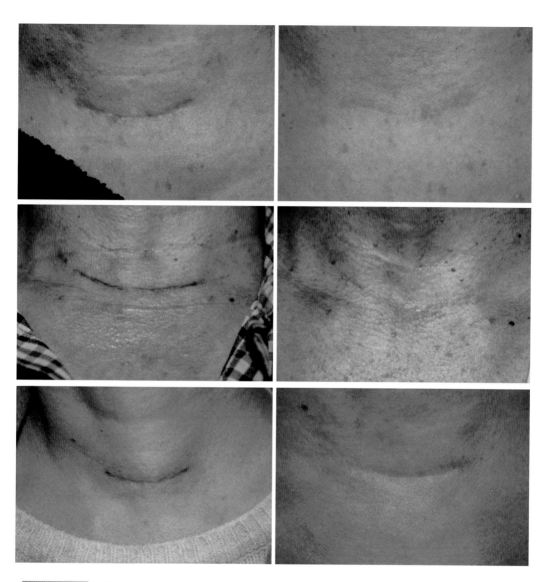

Figure 05-1   **Clinical results of the nonablative laser treated group post thyroidectomy. Left:** pictures of each patient taken 2 to 3 weeks after surgery (pre-treatment). **Right:** pictures taken 6 months after surgery (post-treatment). Note the preventive effect in pigmentation, redness, and hypertrophic scar change. See text for treatment parameters.

report has shown good efficacy of an 830 nm LED-LLLT system (HEALITE, Lutronic Corp., Goyang, South Korea) in the prevention of hypertrophic scars in a controlled study on post thyroidectomy wounds. This easy-to-apply modality must therefore be seriously considered when thinking of strategies to prevent hypertrophic scar formation in anatomical areas prone to hypertrophy post-trauma.

Tips for post-treatment care and follow-up

Even if laser treatment or LED-LLLT for scar prevention has been performed, apart from the usual wound management strategies, close monitoring of the wound area is required up to 6 months after the surgery, as a scar may occur up to 6 months after the surgery.

REFERENCES

1. Alam M, Pon K, Van Laborde S, Kaminer MS, Arndt KA, Dover JS. Clinical effect of a single pulsed dye laser treatment of fresh surgical scars: randomized controlled trial. Dermatol Surg 2006;32:21-25.

2. Alster TS. Laser treatment of hypertrophic scars, keloid, and striae. Dermatol Clin 1997;15:419-429.

3. Baryza MJ, Baryza GA. The Vancouver Scar Scale: an administration tool and its interrater reliability. J Burn Care Rehabil 1995;16:535-538.

4. Baugh WP, Kucaba WD. Nonablative phototherapy for acne vulgaris using the KTP 532-nm laser. Dermatol Surg 2005;31:1290-1296.

5. Berman B, Perez OA, Konda S, Kohut BE, Viera MH, Delgado S, Zell D, Li Q. A review of the biologic effects, clinical efficacy, and safety of silicone elastomer sheeting for hypertrophic and keloid scar treatment and management. Dermatol Surg 2007;33:1291-1302.

6. Bouzari N, Davis SC, Nouri K. Laser treatment of keloids and hypertrophic scars. Int J Dermatol 2007;46:80-88.

7. Butler EG 2nd, McClellan SD, Ross EV. Split treatment of photodamaged skin with KTP 532-nm laser with 10 mm handpiece versus IPL: a cheek-to-cheek comparison. Lasers Surg Med 2006;38:124-128.

8. Chan HH, Wong DS, Ho WS, Lam LK, Wei W. The use of pulsed dye laser for the prevention and treatment of hypertrophic scars in Chinese persons. Dermatol Surg 2004;30:987-994.

9. Choe JH, Park YL, Kim BJ, Kim MN, Rho NK, Park BS, Choi YJ, Kim KJ, Kim WS. Prevention of thyroidectomy scar using a new 1,550-nm fractional erbium-glass laser. Dermatol Surg 2009;35:1199-1205.

10. Chowdhury MM, Harris S. Lanigan SW. Potassium titanyl phosphate laser treatment of resistant port-wine stains. Br J Dermatol 2001;144:814-817.

11. Kang JM, Cho HK, Lee KH, Lee JB. The effect of TCA chemical peel on acne scars. Korean J Dermatol 1996;34:919-923.

12. Keller GS. Use of the KTP laser in cosmetic surgery. Am J Cosmet Dermatol 1992;9:177-180.

13. Kim WS, Calderhead RG. Is light-emitting diode low level light therapy (LED-LLLT) really effective? Laser Ther 2011;20:205-215.

14. Lee MW. Combination 532-nm and 1064-nm lasers for noninvasive skin rejuvenation and toning. Arch Dermatol 2003;139:1265-1276.

15. Min PK, Goo BCL. 830 nm light-emitting diode low level light therapy (LED-LLLT) enhances wound healing: a preliminary study. Laser Ther 2013;22:43-49.

16. Mustoe TA. Evolution of silicone therapy and mechanism of action in scar management. Aesth Plast Surg 2008;32:82-92.

17. Nouri K, Elsaie ML, Vejjabhinanta V, Stevens M, Patel SS, Caperton C, Elgart G. Comparison of the effects of short- and long-pulse durations when using a 585-nm pulsed dye laser in the treatment of new surgical scars. Lasers Med Sci 2010;25:121-126.

18. Nouri K, Jimenez GP, Harrison-Balestra C, Elgart GW. 585-nm pulsed dye laser in the treatment of surgical scars starting on the suture removal day. Dermatol Surg 2003;29:65-73.

19. Nouri K, Vidulich K, Rivas MP. Lasers for scars: a review. J Cosmet Dermatol 2006;5:14-22.

20. Park YJ, Kim SJ, Song HS, Kim SK, Lee JH, et al. Prevention of thyroidectomy scars in Asian adults with low-level light therapy. Dermatol Surg 2016. (Accepted, In press)

21. Vaccaro M, Borgia F, Guarneri B. Treatment of hypertrophic thyroidectomy scar using 532-nm potassium-titanyl-phosphate (KTP) laser. Int J Dermatol 2009;48:1139-1141.

Hair

C / O / N / T / E / N / T / S

Hair removal

▶ Woo Seok Koh, MD, PhD

Introduction

People have been removing their unwanted body hair since prehistoric times, as seen in paintings that are thousands of years old. Nowadays, in civilized cultures, people tend to dislike more showing their body hair to others, and even men now dislike having body hair. Not all women who have undergone laser removal of their unwanted body hair had more hair than normal. People who have experienced sudden increased growth of their hair or who have excessive hair, however, need to find the cause (Table 01-1).

Tips for the treatment

Laser hair removal started in 1996, when the long-pulsed ruby laser was introduced. The wavelength range of hair removal lasers is between 600 to 1,100 nm. Laser energy within this waveband can be absorbed mostly by the melanin pigment in the hair shaft and in hair bulb, thereby limiting damage to the hair and its follicle, to prevent hair production or to make hair invisible. For laser hair removal, the long-pulsed ruby laser (694 nm), the long-pulsed alexandrite laser (755 nm), the long-pulsed Nd-YAG laser (1,064 nm), and IPL (intense-pulse light) are currently being used. It is assumed that hair is removed or becomes thin and thus, invisible, after the stem cells in the hair bulge (Figure 01-1) and the dermal papilla cells (Figure 01-2) are disabled or destroyed by the photothermal reaction as light energy is absorbed in melanin and converted to heat, but the exact mechanism of action involved remains uncertain. The shape and thickness of the hair shaft varies by race and location in the body, and the thickness of the hair follicle with its bulge where the stem cells are highly concentrated is also diverse, thus making the selection of the most effective pulse duration for hair removal difficult. Most clinical and

Table 01-1 **Etiologies of hirsutism**

Local	Peripheral (hair follicle) androgen sensitivity
Ovarian	Polycystic ovary syndrome Insulin-resistance syndromes Hyperandrogenism, insulin resistance, acanthosis nigricans (HAIR-AN) Hyperthecosis Familial ovarian hyperplasia Hilus cell hyperplasia Ovarian tumors
Adrenal	Classical congenital adrenal hyperplasia Nonclassical (late-onset) congenital adrenal hyperplasia Cushing's syndrome Adrenal virilizing tumors (adenomas and carcinomas)
Pituitary	Cushing's disease Acromegaly Hyperprolactinemia
Idiopathic	Occult functional hyperandrogenism (detectable with combined stimulation tests) Increased peripheral 5a-reductase activity Altered androgen receptor function
Pregnancy	Aromatase deficiency in the fetus Luteoma of pregnancy Hyperreactio luteinalis

Drug-induced hirsutism	Androgenic medications
	   Testosterone
	   Danazole
	   ACTH
	   Metyrapone
	   Phenothiazine
	Anabolic steroids
	Androgenic progestins
	   Levonorgestrel
	   Norgestrel
	   Norethindrone
	Acetazolamide
	Valproic acid
	Nonandrogenic medicationsa
	   Cyclosporine
	   Phenytoin
	   Diazoxide
	   Minoxidil
	   Minocycline
	   High-dose glucocorticoids
	   Hexachlorobenzene
	   Penicillamine
	   Psoralens

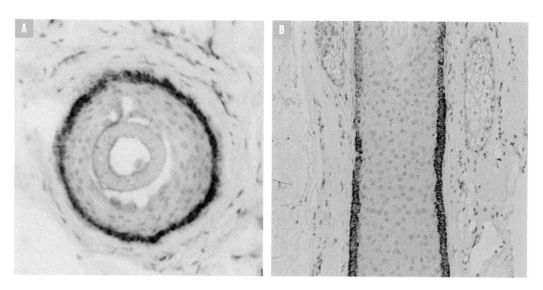

Figure 01-1   (A) Stem cell staining of the transverse section of a hair follicle (CD8/144B). Hair stem cells are located away from the hair shaft, at the margin of the outer root sheath. (B). Stem cell staining of the vertical section of a hair follicle (CD8/144B).

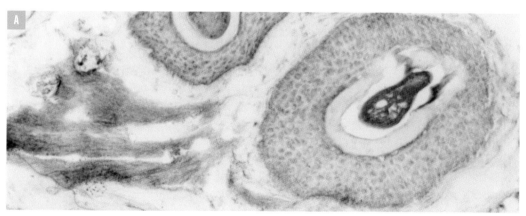

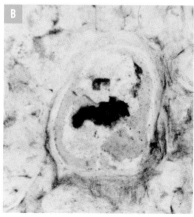

Figure 01-2   (A) Vialbility stain (NBTC) after Ruby laser 30 J/cm², 3 ms, 10 mm spot size. The arrector pili are shown and parts of the outer root sheath are damaged. (B) In the same hair strand, the hair bulb and the papilla cell show overall viability loss.

ex vivo studies have reported that 3-200 ms is effective so far. The hair follicle extends from the epidermis up to 5 mm below the skin surface. As it is deeper than other cutaneous targets, the spot size should be 7 mm or more. If all other mechanical properties are equal, the larger the spot size is, the more effective the hair removal will be, as large spot sizes are associated with better scattering contained within the beam, and thus deeper penetration.

Pre-procedure precautions

1. Sufficiently moisturize the skin to prevent dryness.
2. Take care to avoid treating patients who are suntanned or who have been attending tanning salons.
3. Do not pluck or wax the hair.
4. If eczema or a wound exists, it should be treated first.

Procedure protocol

1. The condition of the hair (i.e., its thickness, density, and color) should be recorded before the procedure.
2. Shave the hair as cleanly and closely to the skin as possible, while taking care not to damage the skin. If hairs are not shaved and lie or are pressed on the skin surface, they will absorb the laser energy and the potential for a skin burn is quite high.
3. The fluence (J/cm^2) should be selected based on the color, thickness, and density of the hair (as applying topical anesthesia may make the skin color temporarily lighter, the skin color must be checked before the anesthesia is administered). When unsure about the appropriate fluence setting, test treatments at 3-4 different fluence levels should be performed, and 2 days later, the fluence that caused the least complications should be selected for the actual treatment.
4. For patients who are sensitive to pain, topical anesthesia should be administered (general anesthesia is not recommended as serious complications may occur because the patient's response cannot be detected).
5. Ensure that the skin-cooling device works well.
6. The treatment should be started at the site where the pain is felt less (e.g., for the calf, first at the back and then in front).
7. Ensure that all areas that need to be treated are irradiated.
8. Apply a cold pack on the treated skin after the treatment to soothe redness and swelling.
9. Depending on the treated site, apply an antibiotic.

Tips for improving the permanent hair removal rate.

No skipped area
Method for delivering laser light to 100% hair follicles (no skipped area)
Practice on white leather.

ex. If the effective spot size is 1 cm x 1 cm, to cover 10 cm without any skipped area we need 10 shots.

10 cm

	10 cm								
1	2	3	4	5	6	7	8	9	10

Use as high a fluence as possible
Higher fluences have been correlated with greater permanent hair removal.

Use as large a spot size as possible
The larger, the better if other specs are the same.

Select an appropriate wavelength
For the Asian skintype, the alexandrite or diode laser (800-810 nm) is preferred.

Use an apprpriate pulse duration
30-40 ms gives better results in Asian patients.

Skin Cooling
Proper skin cooling is essential to minimize epidermal damage, while permitting treatment with higher fluences. (e.g., Contact parallel cooling, DCD, Cold air cooling, Lower Room temperature)

Regular treatment (4-8 weeks interval)

Asians have more melanin pigments in their epidermis than Caucasians, and thus, are more prone to having such complications as hyperpigmentation or crust formation. Asian hair, however, absorbs light better, as it has more melanin pigments than Caucasian hair. As such, laser hair removal can be more effective for Asians than for Caucasians. As the energy from the ruby laser is highly absorbed by the epidermal melanin, however, the risk of skin complications due to the ruby laser is higher in Asians than in Caucasians. Thus, the ruby laser is not suitable for hair removal in Asians. As laser hair removal must be repeated and it is difficult to check skipped areas in each session, care must be taken. Calculating the irradiation area and the number of irradiations per second before the irradiation to prevent skipped areas is more helpful for reducing skipped areas than finding out skipped areas after the irradiation. Asian hair tends

(continued)

to stick to the tip of a contact cooling device because it is thicker than Caucasian hair. Thus, the tip should be regularly wiped. A study has reported that alternating the use of lasers with different wavelengths did not have a further hair removal effect. The current consideration is that constant treatment with a laser that is believed to be most effective can have a better hair removal outcome on average.

Tip for post-treatment care and follow-up

The most important thing in pre- and post-laser hair removal management is to manage the skin to prevent its tanning by ultraviolet light through regular application of a UVA/B sunscreen. If hyperpigmentation unavoidably occurs following laser hair removal, a whitening agent should be used or the next session should be postponed to several months later. In most cases, no particular management is required after the treatment, but a moisturizer, antibiotic ointment, or steroid ointment can be used depending on the treated site. If the redness and rash-like response persists for 2 days or more, taking oral steroids for 5-7 days can be helpful. If the treated site has a history of herpes, an oral antiviral agent should be administered. Regular application of a UVA/B sunscreen should also be recommended.

As hair-removal-related complications mostly occur in the epidermis, a scar very rarely occurs if the fluence and wavelength are appropriate. Even crust or blister formation would not matter if secondary infection is avoided, as the wound would not be dirty. Though rare, redness may become worse 2-5 days later. Studies have reported that this may be an allergic reaction to the patient's own hair. If the redness is severe, an oral steroid can be helpful. If hyperpigmentation occurs in an Asian patient after laser hair removal, postpone the treatment. Even if hyperpigmentation does not occur, the fluence should be lowered in summer when there is a higher risk of sun exposure, or in tropical regions. There is a controversy about the permanent outcome of laser hair removal. This controversy has arisen because hair follicles that are temporarily resting look as if they were removed. The U.S. FDA has defined permanent hair reduction as a state wherein the condition of the hair is maintained for 4-12 months without further hair removal treatment. For Asians, laser hair removal can have a permanent effect if the wavelength, pulse duration, spot size, fluence, and treatment interval are appropriate and if no areas are skipped. In clinics that do not meet any of these conditions, the permanent hair reduction rate appears to be low.

Dilemmas of laser hair removal

Low Fluence = Less Side Effects = Less Pain = Less Effect
High Fluence = More Side Effects = More Pain=More Effect

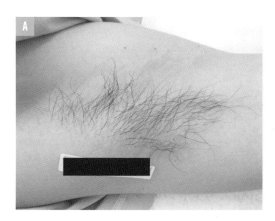 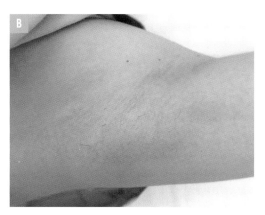

Figure 01-3 **A.** Before Laser hair removal. **B.** 6 months later post 3rd tx (805 nm, 40 ms, 5℃ Contact cooling, 26 J/cm^2 × 3, Spot size; 1 cm × 3 cm)

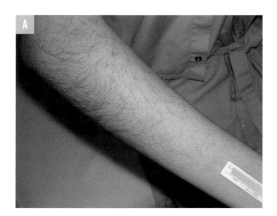 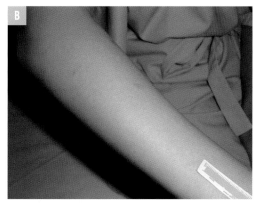

Figure 01-4 **A.** Before Laser hair removal. **B.** 3 years 2months later post 5th tx (no shaving post 5th tx, 805 nm, 30 ms, 5℃ Contact cooling, 25 J/cm^2 × 2, 26 J/cm^2 × 1, 25 J/cm^2 × 1, 24 J/cm^2 × 1).

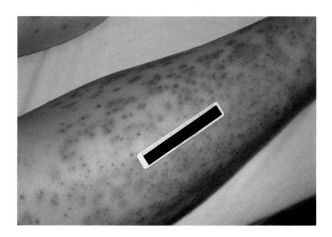

Figure 01-5 **Persistent erythema after laser hair removal.** In this case an oral corticosteroid was erythema subsided in two weeks prescribed, and the without any permanent change.

REFERENCES

1. A Gerardo et al .Side-Effects After IPL Photodepilation. Dermatol Surg 2002;28:1131–1134.

2. A Omar, et al. Laser hair removal. Dermatologic Therapy 2011;24; 94–107.

3. B Finkel, et al. Pulsed alexandrite laser technology for noninvasive hair removal. J Clin Laser Med Surg 1997;15:225–229.

4. C Dierickx CC, et al. Permanent hair removal by normal-mode ruby laser. Arch Dermatol 1998;134:837-842.

5. C Dierickx, et al. Comparison between a long pulsed ruby laser and a pulsed infrared laser system for hair removal. Lasers Surg Med 1998(suppl);10:199.

6. C Dierickx, et al. Hair removal by a pulsed, infrared laser system. Lasers Surg Med 1998;10:198(suppl).

7. C Raulin C, et al. IPL technology: a review. Lasers Surg Med 2003;32:78–87.

8. CL Goh, et al. Comparative study on a single treatment response to long pulse Nd : YAG lasers and intense pulse light therapy for hair removal on skin type IV to VI – is longer wavelengths lasers preferred over shorter wavelengths lights for assisted hair removal. J Dermatolog Treat 2003;14:243–247.

9. DJ McGill, et al. A randomised, split-face comparison of facial hair removal with the alexandrite laser and intense pulsed light system. Lasers Surg Med 2007;39:767–772.

10. EL Tanzi EL, et al. Long-pulsed 1064-nm Nd: YAG laser assistedhair removal in all skin types. Dermatol Surg 2004;30: 13–17.

11. G Lask G, et al. Laser-assisted hair removal by selective photothermolysis. Dermatol Surg 1997;23:737-739.

12. J Khoury, et al. Comparative evaluation of long-pulse alexandrite and long-pulse Nd : YAG laser systems used individually and in combination for axillary hair removal. Dermatol Surg 2008;34:665–670. Discussion 670–661.

13. J Rao, et al. Prospective, comparative evaluation of three laser systems used individually and in combination for axillary hair removal.Dermatol Surg 2005;31:1671–1676. Discussion 1677.

14. Jo, et al. Efficacy and Safety of Hair Removal with a Long-Pulsed Diode Laser Depending on the Spot Size: A Randomized, Evaluators-Blinded, Left-Right Study. Ann Dermatol 2015;7: 517-552.

15. JR Lloyd, et al. Long-term evaluation of the long pulsed alexandrite laser for the removal of bikini hair at shortened treatment intervals. Dermatol Surg 2000;26:633–637.

16. K Nouri, et al. Comparing 18- vs 12-mm spot size in hair removal using a gentlease 755-nm alexandrite laser. Dermatol Surg 2004;30:494–497.

17. M Hussain, et al. Laser-assisted hair removal in Asian skin: efficacy, complications, and the effect of single versus multiple treatments. Dermatol Surg 2003;29:249–254.

18. MJC Van Gemert, et al. Time constants in thermal laser medicine. Lasers Surg Med 1989:9:405–421.

19. N Bouzari, et al. Hair removal using an 800-nm diode laser: comparison at different treatment intervals of 45, 60, and 90 days. Int J Dermatol 2005;44:50–53.

20. N Somani, et al. The clinical evaluation of hirsutism. Dermatologic Therapy 2008;21:376–391.

21. Noh, et al. BioMedical Engineering OnLine Tool to visualize and evaluate operator proficiency in laser hair-removal treatments 2014, 13:40.

22. NS Sadick, et al. High-intensity flashlamp photoepilation: a clinical, histological, and mechanistic study in human skin. Arch Dermatol 1999:135:668–676.

23. R Weiss, et al. Hair removal with a noncoherent filtered flashlamp intense pulsed light source. Lasers Surg Med 1999;24: 128–132.

24. RR Anderson, et al. Selective photothermolysis: Precise microsurgery by selective absorption of pulsed radiation. Science 1983;220:524–527.

25. S Eremia, et al. Laser hair removal with alexandrite versus diode laser using four treatment sessions: 1-year results. Dermatol Surg 2001:27:925–929.

26. SM Davoudi, et al. Comparison of long-pulsed alexandrite and Nd:YAG lasers, individually and in combination, for leg hair reduction: an assessorblinded, randomized trial with 18 months of follow-up. Arch Dermatol 2008:144:1323–1327.

27. T Alster, et al. Long-pulsed Nd : YAG laser-assisted hair removal in pigmented skin: a clinical and histological evaluation. Arch Dermatol 2001;137:885–889.

28. V Campos VB, et al. Hair removal with an 800-nm pulsed diode laser. J Am Acad Dermatol 2000;43:442–447.

29. V Campos, et al. Ruby laser hair removal: Evaluation of long term efficacy and side effects. Lasers Surg Med 2000;26:177-185.

30. W Koh, et al. Effects of very long pulses on human hair follicles. Lasers Surg Med 2000(supp)12:86.

31. W Lou, et al. Prospective study of hair reduction by diode laser (800 nm) with long-termfollow-up. Dermatol Surg 2000;26:428–432.

32. WP, et al. Hair reduction using a scanning 800 nm diode laser. Dermatol Surg 2001;27:358–364.

02

Laser-assisted approach in hair transplantation

Hyung Uk Choi, MD, Jin Soo Kang, MD & Gu-Il Seo, MD, PhD

Introduction

Hair transplantation is a technique employing surgical approaches whereby hair follicles are moved from one area (the donor site) to another part of the body (the recipient site). Although male pattern baldness (MPB) is one of the main reasons why people elect to undergo transplantation, it is not the only reason. In MPB, a special consideration must be given to the genetic resistance of the donor site to balding so that the transplanted follicles are predisposed against balding.

Modern transplantation methods more often than not are based on 'follicular units' (FUs) containing groupings of hairs, from 1–4, the follicle being extracted complete with a small full-thickness epidermal and dermal graft, so that transplantation of the entire FU results in more natural-looking hair in the recipient site. FUs may be harvested in a strip of skin, so-called strip harvesting, which is a more invasive surgical approach requiring sutures to be placed and then removed. Alternatively, the individual follicular unit extraction (FUE) harvesting approach obtains individual FUs using small punches. These are reinserted in the balding area with micro-incisions. This approach does not require suturing so recovery is much faster than strip harvesting.

As an integral part of hair transplantation, the final shape of the hairline is of paramount importance. The adjunctive role of the laser in hair transplantation as performed by the author is focused on depilation procedures on the brow to obtain a more natural-looking hairline in conjunction with transplantation, so it is important to think about the hairline and its appearance before discussing the use of the laser.

Considerations regarding a natural-looking hairline

Everyone wants to have a hairline that suits their individual appearance. Those who want to have a nice hairline that will make them look young, but is natural-looking, may consider hair transplantation. Anyone who is to undergo a hair transplantation procedure to have a nice hairline, or an epilation procedure for a wide brow, must consider the following.

First, the age of the person who is to undergo the procedure must be considered. As people age, their hairline gradually retreats, and their hair gets thinner. Thus, consideration should be given to the hairline that is suitable for the age of the person who is to undergo the procedure.

Second, the features of the person should also be considered, such as density expressed as follicular units (FUs) /cm^2, coarseness (dependent on a combination of the hair diameter and the number of hair strands per FU), color, and degree of curl of the hair. People who have high-density hair usually think that they have thick hair, but they may actually need more hair to be transplanted. If a person has thin hair, it is more difficult to create a natural-looking hairline for him/her, and black hair tends to make the hair look denser. A combination of fair skin and dark black hair, however, may make the hair look less dense than it really is. Curly hair may look denser than straight hair, even when the same amount of hair is transplanted.

Third, the facial form should be considered. The hairline that suits the facial form can satisfy both the clinician and the patient who is to undergo the hair transplantation procedure. For example, for a wide and round face, a higher and flatter hairline may bring about better results.

Fourth, the patient's expectations should be considered. The clinician should make an effort to meet the patient's expectations by explaining to them the best- and worst-case scenarios.

Fifth, gender difference should be taken into account. In male patients with a hairline which has receded, a triangular recession that becomes larger in the frontotemporal junction is usually observed, and in female patients without alopecia, the hairline is normally bent towards the temple, without any triangular recession.

Sixth, racial differences also need to be considered. For example, blacks, Asians, and Hispanics often have wide, flat hairlines. As the hairline created via hair transplantation is likely to last for the patient's lifetime, it is recommended that sufficient consultation with the patient be made to decide the type of hairline that the patient can aesthetically accept.

For hair transplantation, a suitable transplantation method should be decided for each zone of the scalp (e.g., frontal, midscalp, vertex, occipital, parietal, and temporal zones). For the hairline, however, a natural-looking design must be considered for only two zones: the frontal and temporal zones. A natural-looking hairline is created at the 1- to 2-cm-wide transitional zone that lies between the area where no hair exists and that where the hair is dense. The transitional zone can be more natural-looking when the change is gradual than when the change is abrupt. For this zone, it is important to make what are known as "irregularly irregular border patterns," for the creation of which macro-irregularities (macropatterns) and micro-irregularities (micropatterns) are commonly used (Figures 02-1 & 02-2) .

Macro-irregularities include frontal protruding mounds (known as peaks) and temporal peaks, and micro-irregularities include clusters and random single hair grafts (sentinel hairs). The frontal hairline has one to three naturally distributed peaks, and about 50% of men and

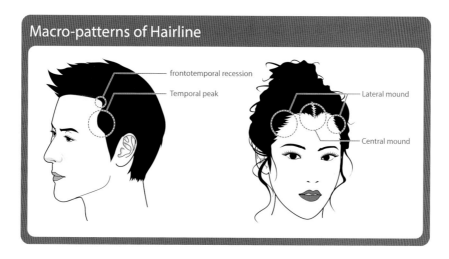

Figure 02-1 Macro-patterns of the Hairline. (supplement from Lutronic Corp.)

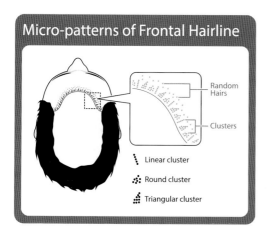

Figure 02-2 Micro-patterns of the Frontal Hairline. (supplement from Lutronic Corp.)

women have at least one peak. The peak in the central area (the so-called widow's peak), makes the face look less round. For the central peak in male-pattern alopecia, transplantation of a small amount of hair is sufficient to slightly lower the hairline. Lateral peaks make up an important design that allows the face of a female patient to look more feminine, particularly when hair is transplanted. The temporal peak, which is a post-temporal boundary, is important for estimating the severity of alopecia in a male patient. It is less conspicuous in females than in males, but it is important in determining the facial form and the area of the brow.

Brandy classified temporal peak baldness in males into four categories: (1) no loss; (2) slight recession of the peak, with early diffuse thinning; (3) significant posterior recession of the peak, with the remaining area being overtly thin; and (4) loss of the peaks and remaining area, except for the remaining vellus hair. Mayer and Perez-Meza, on the other hand, classified temporal peak baldness into the following four categories: (1) no thinning or recession, with the upper margin usually convex; (2) thinning and mild recession; (3) upper margin parallel to the anterior sideburn line; and (4) recession with a reversed angle (concave).

As for the temporal peak in females, Bernard et al reported that the concave triangular type accounts for 61% of the cases, the concave oval type 26%, the concave type 9%, and the straight type 3%, with the concave oval or concave triangular type accounting for 87% of all temporal peaks (Figure 02-3). Although temporal peak morphological statistics have never been reported in South Korea, the temporal peak is considered an important structure in the design for hair transplantation or epilation, and if it is omitted from the design, an awkward impression and a doll-like appearance may occur.

In the micro-irregularities, a 3- to 6-mm-long cluster, protruding anteriorly at an angle of about 45°, consists of several to around ten hair strands and mostly shows a triangular, round, or linear arrangement. Each cluster lies at certain intervals, in which hair is rare.

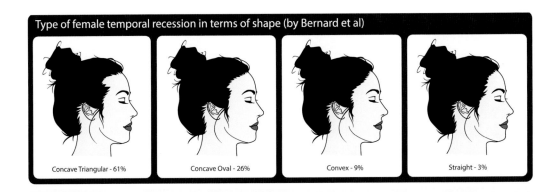

Type of female temporal recession in terms of shape (by Bernard et al)

Concave Triangular - 61%　　Concave Oval - 26%　　Convex - 9%　　Straight - 3%

Figure 02-3　Type of female temporal recession in terms of shape. (After Bernard et al) (supplement from Lutronic Corp.)

Random single hair grafts exist around the cluster, and they contribute to the formation of a more natural-looking hairline. Although in the hair transplantation or narrow-brow epilation procedure, the hairline is designed taking into consideration the aforementioned various factors, fine (thin) hair is necessary in the transitional zone to create a natural-looking hairline. When the hairline is to be created using fine hair in hair transplantation, single hair grafts in the donor site are separated or transplanted, and bisected hair follicles are also used. Even when the hairline looks natural after the hair transplantation procedure, if fine hair is lacking in the hairline, the patient (particularly female patients) may feel that their hairline looks awkward, and may hesitate to expose their brow. In this case, even retransplantation may not correct the problem. If fine hair is formed using laser epilation, however, a natural-looking hairline can be conveniently created, without surgery. This will be explained in the section on narrow-brow epilation (hairline correction method). For male patients who have undergone hair transplantation, if the irregularity of the transitional zone is low, even if the hairline is appropriate, creating undulation in the hairline using laser epilation can solve the problem. If the hairline is too low due to the progression of male-pattern alopecia over time, although a frontal forelock was created, the height and shape of the hairline can be remodeled via laser epilation.

Laser epilation for a narrow forehead

For epilation of unwanted hair, the areas to be depilated are very diverse. In particular, narrow-brow epilation (hairline correction) to make the brow wider is a unique procedure performed in South Korea. In South Korea, some people shave or pluck their hair or resort to conventional folk remedies without scientific basis because the brow is considered associated with a person's personality, nature, and fortune. Unlike epilation of other areas, in narrow-brow epilation (hairline correction), the design aspect plays an important role because a hairline that suits each individual has to be created. In particular, for women, a natural-looking hairline can be created only when fine hair exists. Thus, a technique that creates fine hair using laser epilation is an important issue.

Treatment tips for narrow-brow epilation (hairline correction)

1. An irregularly patterned hairline should be the ultimate goal. Specifically, the macro- and

micro-irregularities are appropriately distributed by area.

2. The difference in density is considered.

3. The temporal peak is not removed.

4. Fine hair is achieved.

Female patients

The height of the brow should be decided using the rule of thirds (dividing the distance from the end of the brow to the end of the chin into three equal segments), and the entire contour should be decided so that the shape of the brow can resemble part of a circle, taking into consideration the facial form. Considering the widow's peak or bilateral mounds, caution should be taken so that the temporal peak will not disappear, and the shape of the temporal peak should be designed according to the facial form. As a rule, macropatterns should be made with an "irregularly irregular" pattern in mind, and then micropatterns should be made along the hairline. Considering the difference in density of the hair near the hairline, the areas to be depilated and the areas where fine hair has to be created during laser treatment should be determined in advance.

Male patients

The overall procedure is similar to that for female patients, but the overall contour line should be close to the shape of the letter 'M', and the temporal peak should be designed such that it will be more distinct and conspicuous than in women.

Considerations in and procedure of laser depilation

The area to be depilated should be designed such that it will not be too wide. Following the rule of thirds, a conservative approach should be used (this is because the patient's mind may change over time, depending on the views of her family or friends). It is more difficult to make the brow narrower than to make it wider. The procedure should be performed with separation achieved between the area to be depilated and the transitional zone, where fine hair will be created. During the design step, the patient should be seated, and red ink that can be easily removed should be used.

The designed area should first be rid of hair using a hair remover. After this, it is recommended that the clinician explain the design to the patient and solicit the patient's opinion with the patient looking into a mirror (if the clinician and patient will first talk about the shape of the area to be treated, the patient's trust in and compliance with the clinician can be enhanced because even the smallest change in the hairline may actually radically change the patient's appearance).

The area to be treated should be anesthetized for about one hour using topical anesthesia, such as EMLA. During the laser depilation, the patient should be in a supine position and should be wearing some form of eye protection. For laser depilation, the use of a system that can provide various spot sizes (i.e., 3, 5, 7, and 10 mm) is advantageous because it is more effective for creating an irregular hairline, such as for macro- and micro-irregularities. The laser used by the author is a long-pulsed 1064 nm Nd:YAG system, used at spot sizes from 3-10 mm, pulse durations from 5-10 msec and fluences of 3-40 J/cm², varied depending on each patient's circumstances. The author performs depilation first using a large spot size, and then designs the overall hairline, taking into account the central peak or the lateral mounds for the transitional zone. Then, micro-irregularities between the peaks are created each time treatment is performed. For female patients, it is important to transplant fine hair in the transitional zone. During depilation, thick hair strands naturally change into fine hair, or fine hair is intentionally made.

When fine hair is the treatment goal, the thicker hair is removed using parameters that can remove finer hair. For example, if treatment is repeated three to five times using 3-10 mm spot sizes, a pulse duration of 5-10 msec, and 3-40 J/cm² fluence, sufficiently fine hair can be obtained. As the statistical data on the use of the clinical laser for transplanting fine hair are currently not sufficient, further studies on laser parameters and on the relation between the thickness of the hair and the number of laser treatments are needed. For women who have undergone hair transplantation, the hairline may look unnatural even though it was transplanted with single hair grafts. In this case, fine-hair creation treatments can make the hairline look natural, as seen in Figure 02-4. In this case, the treatment interval can be about three months. After laser treatment, the treatment site can be cooled down using an icepack, and can be locally treated with steroids followed by administration of oral antibiotics or steroids for two to three days. The patients should be advised that the treatments should be done five times or more, and at six- to eight-week intervals.

There is one more thing that should be explained to the patient when depilation for a narrow brow is to be performed: the volume of the temple, and the malar area under the eye. If the volume of the brow, temple, or area below the eye is decreased, or if the wrinkle lines are conspicuous, the brow cannot be beautiful or look good even if the hairline has become natural-looking and beautiful after the depilation. Thus, for hairline correction, it is necessary to explain to the patient the volume of the brow or the area below the eye, or the necessity of

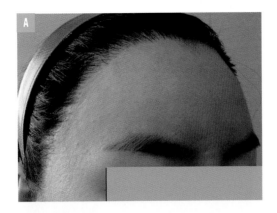 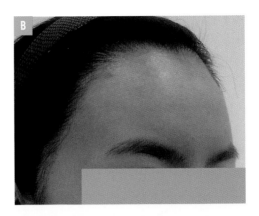

Figure 02-4 **Using laser depilation to create fine hair. A.** Before treatment. **B.** After treatment, with a much more natural appearance.

the correction of wrinkles. If it is considered appropriate, fat graft, filler or Botox treatment can be recommended to the patient.

Side effects of narrow-brow epilation (hairline correction) (Figure 02-5)

The most serious side effect of narrow-brow epilation (hairline correction) is an unnatural look. An asymmetrical or overly wide brow is common after epilation. For women, the common side effects include (1) a masculine hairline; (2) a hairline consisting only of thick hair, without any difference in density; (3) absence of a temporal peak; and (4) loss of areas where vellus, intermediate, and terminal hair is naturally distributed (i.e., areas with fine hair). These side effects result in an unnatural-looking hairline. For men, the side effects include a feminine hairline and loss of the temporal peak. Caution is thus required.

Other side effects that may occur after narrow-brow epilation include transient erythema and a stinging sensation. Although most of the side effects are transient, folliculitis, pigment deposition, blister, burn, or depression of the skin may occur. Caution is thus required during treatment.

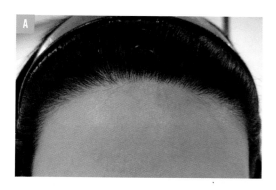
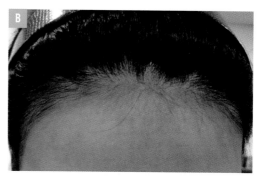

Figure 02-5   **Hairline re-correction of narrow-brow epilation to achieve a natural forehead line. A.** Before treatment. **B.** After treatment, 4 sessions every 6 weeks. A more natural effect has been achieved.

REFERENCES

1. Brandy DA. A Method for Evaluating and Treating the Temporal Peak Region in Patients with Male Pattern Baldness. Dermatol Surg 2002;28:394-401.
2. Marritt E. Single-Hair Transplantation for Hairline Refinement: A Practical Solution. J Dermatol Surg Oncol 1984;12:962-966.
3. Moreno-Arias GA, Navarra E, Vilalta A, Ferrando J. Corrective Photoepilation for Improper Hairline Placement After Hair Transplantation. Dermatol Surg 2000;26:790-792.
4. Norwood OT, Taylor BJ. Hairline Design and Placement. J Dermatol Surg Oncol 1991;17:510-518.
5. Nusbaum BP, Fuentefria S. Naturally Occurring Female Hairline Patterns. Dermatol Surg 2009;35:907-913.
6. Parsley WM. Hair transplantation goals based on natural hair patterns. In: UngerWP, Shapiro RS, editors. Hair transplantation. New York: Marcel Dekker, Inc.;2004. p151-63
7. Parsley WM. Natural hair pattern. Facial plast Surg Clin N Am 2004;12:167-180.
8. Rose PT, Parsley WM. The science of hairline design. In: Haber RS, Stough DB, editors. Procedures in cosmetic dermatology. Hair transplantation. Philadelphia: Elsevier Saunders;2006. p55-72.
9. Swinehart JM. "Cloned" Hairlines: The Use of Bisected Hair Follicles to Create Finer Hairlines. Dermatol Surg 2001;27:868-872.
10. Unger WP, Marritt E. General Principles of Recipient Site Organization and Planning. In Unger WP, Nordstrom R(eds): Hair Transplantation. 2nd edition. New York:Marcel Dekker;1988. p107.
11. Villlnow MM, Feriduni B. Update on Laser-assisted Hair Transplantation. Dermatol Surg 1998;24:749-754.

Body & Facial sculpting

SECTION

06

C/O/N/T/E/N/T/S

General concept of interstitial laser

Chan Yeong Heo, MD, PhD & Ji Hoon Kim, MD

Introduction

Body contouring is a major area in the field of dermatologic and plastic surgery. Operative methods, including surgical lipectomy, and less invasive methods, including various liposuction techniques, are mainly used for the purpose of reducing fat. Liposuction can be accomplished using various methods. Widely used methods are suction-assisted liposuction (SAL), ultrasound-assisted liposuction (UAL), power-assisted liposuction (PAL), and laser-assisted liposuction (LAL). Efforts in the search for alternatives and new tools primarily seek to reduce downtime, decrease operative fatigue, reduce bleeding, and promote skin contraction.

Laser-assisted liposuction

Laser-assisted liposuction was developed to improve the removal of fat cells and to affect the underlying collagen with the goal of skin tightening. Previous clinical studies in human fat tissue after treatment with pulsed Nd:YAG lasers at 1064 nm have shown areas of reversible cellular damage (tumefaction), irreversible tissue damage (lysis), and a reduction in bleeding when compared to conventional liposuction . In addition, another experimental study in the pig model has shown that the subdermal laser irradiation can stimulate collagen deposition in the reticular dermis .

The Nd:YAG and diode lasers are the lipolytic lasers currently being clinically used for LAL. Nd:YAG laser lipolysis was first described in 1994 and today, it has become one of the most popular laser lipoplasty methods in the world.

Laser lipolysis

The mechanism of action of laser lipolysis is through the generation of photohyperthermia. The heat generated through absorption of the laser energy by the target chromophore results in lysis of the adipocyte membranes as well as of dermal collagen. In lipolysis with the interstitial laser, the energy delivered via an optical fiber through a thin cannula (Figure 01-1) is converted to heat energy within the subcutaneous layer. Adipocytes absorb the energy, resulting in apoptosis and necrosis (Figure 01-2).

Up to the present, several interstitial Nd:YAG laser systems have been developed with the wavelengths of 1064 nm, 1320 nm and 1444 nm, and their clinical application has been reported. Each wavelength targets different chromophores with different levels of affinity. The lipolytic effect of the micropulsed laser is manifested by its photothermal effect on water and the combined photothermal and photoacoustic effects on fat. Among these wavelengths, 1444 nm delivered by the micropulsed AccuSculpt™ system (Lutronic Co., Goyang, South Korea) is highly effective in many aspects of laser-assisted lipolysis for both body and facial contouring. 1444 nm is a wavelength with inherent safety when used in laser-assisted lipolysis because of its high duality of absorption in fat and water with resulting low thermal diffusion to the tissue surrounding the target area. It has been argued that more effective laser lipolysis can be achieved with the 1444 nm wavelength (Figure 01-3) because its affinity to fat is more than 10 times greater than that associated with the 1064 nm wavelength (Figure 01-4).

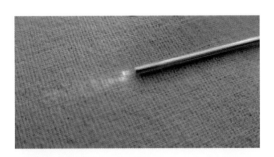

Figure 01-1 One-millimeter cannula containing a 600 µm optical fiber extending approximately 2 mm from the distal end and emitting a visible red aiming beam for the invisible near infrared laser energy.

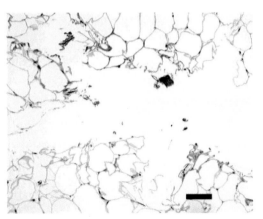

Figure 01-2 Photomicrograph of human fat in a laser-treated specimen showing hollows with denatured cell membranes. Scale bar: 100 µm. (Hematoxylin eosin, original magnification: x200).

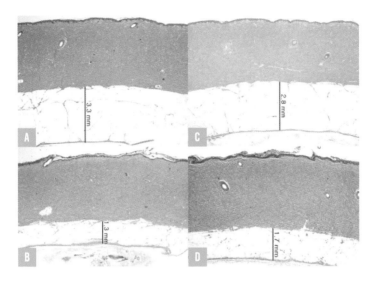

Figure 01-3   **Comparison of fat reduction between 1444 nm and 1064 nm wavelengths.** There was 60.6% decrease of the thickness in the mantle fat layer between the immediate biopsy (**A**) and 3 month biopsy (**B**) after the irradiation with 1444 nm. On the other hand, 1064 nm EL3 laser lipolysis showed a 39.2% decrease of the thickness in the mantle fat layer between the immediate postop biopsy (**C**) and 3 month biopsy (**D**).

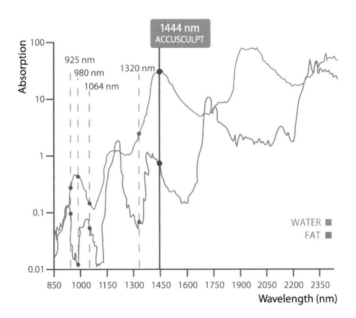

Figure 01-4   **The fat absorption coefficient at 1444 nm is much higher than 1064 nm or 1320 nm providing 8 times more absorption than other wavelengths.** This translates into much quicker fat emulsification with very low peripheral thermal damage, coupled with the added safety due to the very high water absorption coefficient thus delivering thermal containment at the fiber tip. Wavelengths other than 1444 nm rely on higher power levels to increase fat emulsification but the downside is that this also increases peripheral thermal damage which increases the chance for complications and produces a much less predictable procedure.

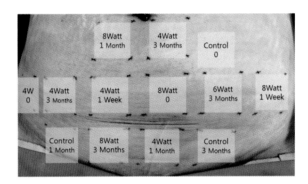

Figure 01-5   Parameters for a clinical in vivo/ex vivo study in human abdominal skin.

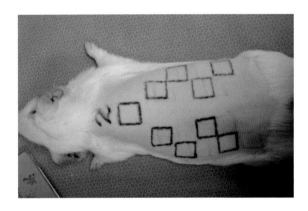

Figure 01-6   Guinea pigs experimental study model for Long-term collagen remodeling after 1444nm interstitial laser lipolysis.

The greater selectivity of the 1444 nm lipolysis laser provides improved efficiency and greater thermal confinement (energy relatively more localized near the fiber tip) which are extremely important features that enable safe use of this technology for subregional facial contouring, where the skin is much thinner and more liable to secondary thermal damage through conducted heat.

In addition to removal of fat using laser lipolysis, heating of the subdermal and dermal tissues can theoretically be used to treat skin laxity. The action time of the laser varies according to the area to be treated and tissue resistance. All subjects suitable for a traditional liposuction method can also be treated with laser-assisted lipolysis. In a previous experimental study by the authors in human abdominal skin (Figure 01-5) and guinea pig model (Figure 01-6) with the 1444 nm interstitial laser, the thickness of the dermis was found to increase, regardless of the power settings used, three months after laser treatmenet (Figure 01-7). Histopathological examinations revealed alteration to the dermal structure. One month after the laser treatment the collagen bundles were found to be thicker and well-organized, oriented parallel to the skin (Figure 01-8). Using different kind of stains. The levels of muco-,els-,and fibro-proliferation were evaluated.

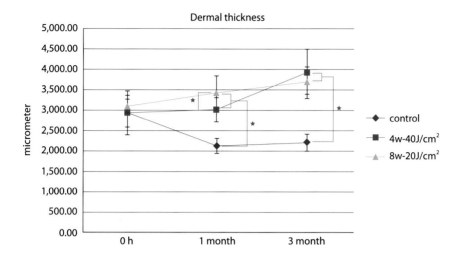

Figure 01-7 Dermal thickness of human abdominal skin

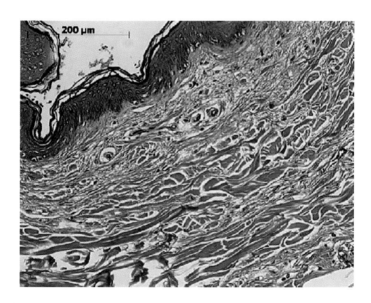

Figure 01-8 **One month after laser treatment using a setting of 4 W and 40 J/cm². ** dense collagen bundles were found to be rearranged parallel to the direction of skin.

LAL vs other approaches

A variety of surgical and medical interventions have been reported to assist fat reduction including ultrasound, vibration, carbon dioxide injection and mesotherapy for prevention of complications associated with traditional liposuction and lipectomy. With the advent of laser lipolysis many authors advocate that this method has many advantages compared to the traditional liposuction procedure. The skin laxity might worsen after conventional liposuction, but with laser lipoplasty skin laxity may be successfully treated. The main advantages of laser lipolysis are less bleeding, less pain, minimal tissue damage, early recovery, and dermal tightening.

Since the introduction of interstitial laser lipolysis, many clinicians have used the procedure for the removal of local fat and for skin tightening. Many new indications have been developed. It is ideal for areas such as the as the cheeks, jowls, under the chin, hips, thighs, knees, bra line, arms, and chest. Interstitial laser lipolysis is a useful tool for the treatment of local lipodystrophy, and the laser has proved to be effective for cellular lysis and neocollagenesis.

REFERENCES

1. Apfelberg DB, Rosenthal S, Hunstad JP, Achauer B, Fodor PB. Progress report on multicenter study of laser-assisted liposuction.Aesthetic Plast Surg 1994;18:259-264.
2. Celik A, Ersoy OF, Ozkan N, Kayaoglu HA, Ozugurlu F, Cakir EA, Lordlar N, Omeroglu S. Comparison of the effects of troxerutin and heparinoid on flap necrosis. J Plast Reconstr Aesthet Surg 2010;63:875-883. Epub 2009 Apr 5.
3. Collawn S. Skin tightening with fractional lasers, radiofrequency, smartlipo. Ann Plast Surg 2010;64:526-529.
4. Goldman A, Gotkin RH. Laser-assisted liposuction. ClinPlast Surg 2009;36:241-260.
5. Goldman A. Submental Nd:Yag laser-assisted liposuction. Lasers Surg Med 2006;38:181-184.
6. Ichikawa K, Tanino R, Wakaki M. Histologic and photonic evaluation of a pulsed Nd:YAG laser for ablation of subcutaneous adipose tissue. Tokai J Exp Clin Med 2006;31:136-140.
7. Katz B, McBean J, Cheung JS. The new laser liposuction for men. Dermatol Ther 2007;20:448-451.
8. Kim JH, Min KH, Heo CY, Back RM, Park HJ, Youn SW, Kim EH. Histological evaluation of dermal tissue remodeling with the 1444-nm neodymium:yttrium-aluminum-garnet laser in an in vivo model. J Dermatol 2013;40:706-710.
9. Levi JR, Veerappan A, Chen B, Mirkov M, Sierra R, Spiegel JH. Histologic evaluation of laser lipolysis comparing continuous wave vspulsed lasers in an in vivo pig model. Arch Facial Plast Surg 2011;13:41-50.
10. Mann MW, Palm MD, Sengelmann RD. New advances in liposuction technology. SeminCutan Med Surg 2008;27:72-82.
11. Min KH, Kim JH, Park HJ, Chung HS & Heo CY. The Skin-Tightening Effects of 1,444-nm Nd:YAG Laser on Human Skin: An In Vivo Study. Aesthetic Plastic Surgery 2014;38:585-591.
12. Prado A, Andreades P, Danilla S, Leniz P, Castillo P, Gaete F. A prospective, randomized, double-blind, controlled clinical trial comparing laser-assisted lipoplasty with suction-assisted lipoplasty. Plast Reconstr Surgery 2006;118:1032-1045.
13. Reszko AE, Magro CM, Diktaban T, Sadick NS. Histological comparison of 1064 nm Nd:YAG and 1320 nm Nd:YAG laser lipolysis using an ex vivo model. J Drugs Dermatol 2009;8:377-382.
14. Reynaud JP, Skibinski M, Wassmer B, Rochon P, Mordon S. Lipolysis using a 980-nm diode laser: a retrospective analysis of 534 procedures. Aesthetic Plast Surg 2009;33:28-36.
15. Tark KC, Jung JE, Song SY. Superior lipolytic effect of the 1,444 nm Nd:YAG laser: comparison with the 1,064 nm Nd:YAG laser. Lasers Surg Med 2009;41:721-727.

Body sculpting: abdomen, flanks, buttocks & thighs, gynecomastia, arms, calves & ankles, 2nd lipoplasty

▶ Jae-Woo Park, MD, PhD

Introduction

As part of our modern life style, concern regarding the form of the body is becoming more and more apparent, and not only among women. As an approach to reforming body shape, liposuction has developed rapidly as far as associated skills, technique and equipment are concerned, and results have improved remarkably over the last few decades. In Asia, lipoplastic surgery has become one of the most common procedures in aesthetic plastic surgery. The instrumentation used for liposuction has evolved extremely rapidly from simple curettage to the classic negative pressure cannula-based instruments, ultrasound assisted systems, water-jet assisted systems and power assisted instruments. These developments have resulted in shortening the procedure time, decreasing the physical effort required for the procedure, minimizing side effects and increasing procedure safety. These developments have also brought benefits in faster wound healing and the better recovery of skin tone and texture. The laser as an adjunctive tool in lipoplasty or liposuction has a comparatively short history and is used as an auxiliary instrument for a very limited purpose, namely to assist the lipolysis process: the procedure name has correctly evolved as 'laser-assisted lipolysis', or LAL. The lasers and wavelengths commonly used for LAL are the continuous wave diode laser at 980 nm, and the micropulsed Nd:YAG laser at 1064 nm and 1320 nm.

Laser assisted liposuction, as it was originally termed, was introduced with the pulsed 1064 nm Nd:YAG laser and this technique was developed in Europe and Middle- and South America. Laser-assisted lipoplasty as a procedure was approved by the FDA in 2006, and this technique showed the most marked development in the USA and Korea. The basis of the technique was to lyse or melt fat with laser energy at a wavelength offering absorption in fat, and then remove the liquefied lipid: this could be done sequentially, or with specially developed cannulae, simultaneously. Refinement of the LAL technique made it possible to remove small localized areas of fat accumulation, especially in the face and neck for which classic liposuction was not well indicated, with decreased bleeding, fewer skin irregularities and faster and better recovery of the skin tone and texture.

As already mentioned, 1064 nm was the first Nd:YAG wavelength used for LAL to selectively remove fat and minimize the physical effort associated with classic liposuction. However, the initial results were not as good as had been expected due to inefficient lipolysis with low power and low energies. Increasing the power and delivered energy certainly enhanced the lipolysis effect, as with the continuous wave (CW) 980 nm diode laser, but at that wavelength the selectivity in fat was reasonable but water absorption was minimal, so there were potentially more serious issues associated with overtreatment and safety. The 1320 nm line of the Nd:YAG had increased selectivity in both fat and water compared with the 1064 nm line and 980 nm and offered more efficient, faster and safer LAL. Most recently, however, a new line of the micropulsed Nd:YAG at 1444 nm (AccuSculpt™, Lutronic Corporation, Goyang, South Korea) has been developed which has absorption coefficients in fat and especially in water which are orders of magnitude higher than the existing wavelengths. This system has ushered in a much faster and safer approach to LAL, especially for areas of finer and thinner tissue such as the face.

Mechanisms of laser lipolysis

Laser-assisted lipoplasty or lipolysis (LAL) consists of the following technique. A very small entry point is made in the skin under local anesthesia. In the case of the 1444 nm AccuSculpt system used in the face, the entry point can be made with an 18 G hypodermic needle. The area to be treated is then infiltrated with a small amount of tumescent solution containing a local anesthetic with epinephrine to assist hemostasis via a blunt cannula inserted through the entry point. An optical fiber, usually 600 μm in diameter, is then introduced through the entry point, either with or without a cannula, and placed in the subcutaneous fatty tissue. While the fiber is continuously moved to and fro in the subcutaneous tissue in a fan-like pattern, laser energy is delivered to the tissue via the fiber, and melts fatty tissue at the fiber tip through a photothermal reaction induced by the duality of absorption of 1444 nm in both fat and water. Simultaneously with the photothermal reaction, the extremely high peak power over the 300 μs pulse causes an explosive reaction in the tissue which results in the creation of a photoacoustic/photoosmotic shock wave that helps to disrupt the membranes of nearby lipocytes, further releasing lipid into the target area. Then, with the fiber tip raised towards the junction between the dermis and sub-Q layer, the laser energy can be directed up into the lower layers of the dermis to stimulate collagen fiber regeneration in the interstitial tissue and reticular dermis which, followed by remodeling, can effect tightening of the skin and improved texture. If appropriate, the melted fat is then sucked out with a small blunt cannula. This LAL technique has received FDA approval for safety and efficacy. In addition to its use purely for LAL, it is clear that this technique will be used more widely and more frequently in many surgical fields, such as aesthetic plastic surgery, as an adjunctive process to other surgical procedures, such as rhytidectomy.

As mentioned above, the mechanisms on which LAL is based in fatty tissue are selectively photothermal and nonselectively photoacoustic/photoosmotic, i.e., photomechanical. Both these effects act on the target simultaneously, but not separately. The wavelength of the light coupled with the beam mode (pulsed or CW) will determine which one of these two effects will be dominant, and the other one less dominant in the overall tissue reaction, or if they occur fairly equally as is the case with LAL using the micropulsed 1444 nm Nd:YAG laser. Tissue at, and immediately adjacent to, the fiber tip will undergo irreversible destructive photothermal and photomechanical changes, whereas the more distant area will be stimulated indirectly through conducted heat, and the changes will be reversible. These changes are correlated with the wavelength and the total energy in a linear manner.

When laser energy is delivered in a pulsed mode, i.e., at pulse widths of less than one millisecond (1 ms), the interplay between two other parameters has to be considered, namely the wavelength and the peak power per pulse. The wavelength of a laser is usually associated with one or more particular tissue targets, or chromophores. Tissue may contain more than one target, for example blood, melanin, fat and water, and in general each target can act as a chromophore for a different wavelength. The wavelengths currently popular for LAL are 980 nm (CW diode laser), 1064 nm, 1320 nm and 1444 nm (all Nd:YAG laser lines, pulsed mode). The different wavelengths are associated with different effects in tissue, based both on their absorption characteristics and also on the beam mode, i.e., pulsed or CW. Of these wavelengths, in general the longer the wavelengths, the better the absorption rate in fat, but the lasing medium, usually giving its name to the laser type, and the beam mode also govern the ultimate tissue effect. The continuous wave 980 nm diode laser, for example, delivers more power than the pulsed 1064 nm Nd: Yag laser, more than 25 W with a very high energy efficiency of around 30% due to the nature of its laser diode. Compared to the diode laser, the pulsed 1064 nm Nd:YAG laser generates around 6 W, with an energy efficiency of only a few percent because it is flashlamp-pumped. Due to these characteristic, the pulsed 1064 nm Nd:YAG laser has become less widely accepted in the LAL field due to its low power and lower energy efficiency. The CW 980 nm diode laser therefore became more popular and was more frequently selected as the laser of choice for laser assisted lipolysis due to its power and higher efficiency. On the other hand, the very low selectivity of the 980 nm diode laser in the water in tissue was a pitfall, although it is slightly better absorbed in fat. Water can act as a 'safety net' in tissue, so coupled with the high power and CW beam of the diode laser, this meant that great care had to be taken when using this wavelength in LAL, to avoid overheating tissue and causing burns, including underlying vital structures and the overlying epidermis. In this respect, the 1064 nm Nd:YAG wavelength was better than 980 nm. On the other hand, the pulsed 1444 nm Nd:YAG laser has been shown experimentally to be 10 times more efficient at lysing fat tissue compared to the pulsed 1064 nm Nd:YAG laser, and over 2 orders of magnitude better absorbed in water: fat is known to contain around 45% water, and the interstitial matrix has a much higher concentration. This combination of fat and water selectivity means that, with the 1444 nm pulsed Nd:YAG, the same amount of fat as the 1064 nm laser can be lysed with lower pulse energy, thus reducing the potential for side effects such as epidermal and other tissue burns and neurovascular damage.

The other factor for a pulsed laser is the peak power of the laser. In the case of the CW laser, used at low powers, there is only a thermal effect over a long irradiation time with a minimal or no photomechanical effect. Only a limited volume of fatty tissue near the tip of the fiber is lysed, with very little damage being caused to surrounding tissues and no photo-thermal activation. To lyse larger volumes of fat, the power has to be turned up. This does increase the thermal effect in the adjacent tissues, but if the power is too high, or the irradia-tion time is too long, this can cause excessive damage with the concomitant increased risk of side effects, such as burns. Basically, this means a CW laser is not an optimum system for laser-assisted lipolysis. On the other hand, if the energy per pulse of a pulsed laser is too low, however, then the end result is the same as the CW laser because the photoacoustic/photo-osmotic effect is minimal, and the photothermal effect is the main LAL reaction. However, when a short pulse width is combined with a higher pulse energy and peak power, then the optimum synergy between photothermal and photomechanical effects is achieved and direct lysis of a 1-4 ml volume of tissue can be achieved around the tip. A wave of conducted heat can also beneficially affect the collagen fibers in the deeper dermis, stimulating collagenesis so that skin tightening can be combined with efficient volume reduction through LAL. This is why the 300 μs 1444 nm AccuSculpt system is more effective for LAL compared to the other pulsed systems (1064 nm and 1320 nm), because of its high duality of absorption in fat and water combined with short pulse width and high peak power. The average power of the AccuSculpt can be as high as 12 W, but at the 600 μm fiber tip with an energy per 300 μs pulse of 200 mJ, the actual peak power per pulse is over 6.50 W giving a power density at the tip of around 230 kW/cm². That is certainly high enough to achieve excellent laser-assisted lipolysis with a concomitantly powerful photomechanical effect.

Indications of laser-assisted body sculpting

Laser assisted lipolysis for the body is ideal for skin with moderately decreased skin tension and localized fibrotic areas such as cellulite, the back, buttocks, thighs and flank, so-called buffalo hump, lipomas, arms, calves, gynecomastia, and secondary liposuction. The laser can melt the fat tissue and simultaneously bring about tissue shrinkage and ultimately tightening. LAL can also improve the skin texture and tension without skin excision after classic liposuction. It is very difficult to perform classic liposuction in fibrotic areas because the fat is trapped between tough fibrotic septae. With the interstitial LAL approach via a fine optical fiber, the laser energy can melt the fat between the fibrous septae, facilitating liposuction with minimum effort and without bleeding. It also improves the texture through incising closed fibrous septae in areas of cellulite formation while simultaneously achieving regeneration of interstitial and overlying collagen fibers. When used as secondary liposuction, LAL can cut through scar tissue and melt the fat between scars. After LAL, it is very easy to perform liposuction in scarred areas.

Tips for the diagnosis & design

Abdomen & Flanks

Laser assisted lipolysis is most effective for subjects who have minimal or moderate skin tension, especially in young or middle aged patients. During the consultation, the maximum points of sagging or bulging on the belly or flanks should be marked with circles. Depressed areas should be marked with a series of oblique diagonal lines. If a patient wants to add definition to the rectus muscles, markings should be made along the muscles and indentations. For the flanks, the narrowest point should be marked (Figure 02-1, 02-2).

Buttocks & Thighs

The buttocks are associated with the underwear line, bulging gluteal folds and the so-called saddle bags: all of these should be marked. If there is any depressed area on the upper buttock, it is also marked with a series of oblique parallel lines for a fat graft. The marking on the medial thigh is designed for the liposuction and preserved areas. Usually, the middle of the medial thigh is depressed and liposuction in this area must be avoided. The 5 cm-wide area should be marked in the central portion of the posterior thigh as an area for preservation.

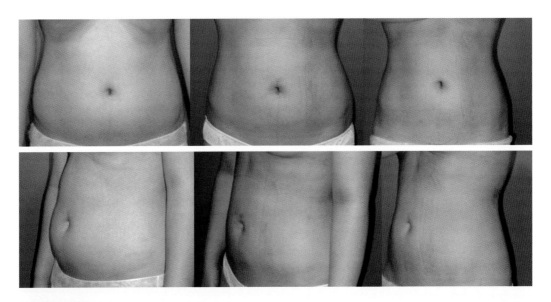

Figure 02-1 Left: A 25-year-old woman with abdominal obesity. Middle: Two months after laser assisted lipoplasty. Right: Ten months after LAL.

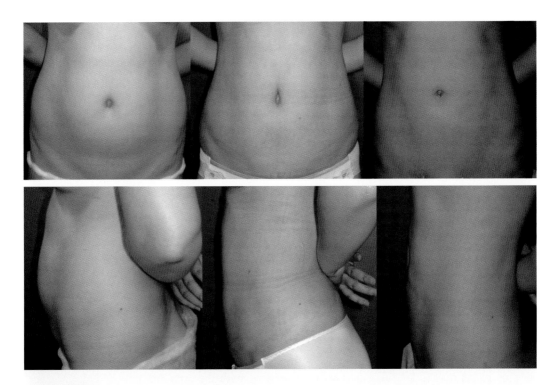

Figure 02-2 Left: A 42-year-oldwoman with abdominal obesity. Middle: Two weeks after laser assisted lipoplasty. A change in the umbilical shape is observed due to skin tightening after LAL. Right: Twenty-three months after LAL.

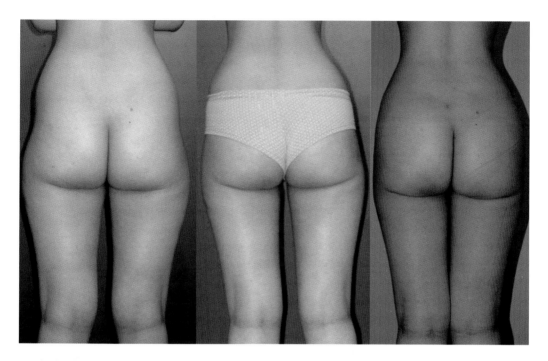

Figure 02-3   Left: A 22-year-old woman requiring correction of fat in the abdomen and thigh. Middle: Six months after conventional lipoplasty. Right: Ten months after undergoing a secondary lipoplasty with LAL.

If this area is damaged, the buttock will droop downwards and it is very difficult to correct this once it occurs. Localized bulging areas around the knees are also marked for LAL (Figure 02-3).

Gynecomastia

If the gynecomastia consists more of fatty and less of glandular tissues, it is a good indication for LAL. The breast area and surrounding area should be marked taking the eventual smooth contouring into consideration. After laser lipolysis, it can be determined if the remaining glandular tissue should be removed through the axillae or a small periareolar Z-plasty (Figure 02-4, 02-5).

Arms

Bulging areas on the lateral arm should be marked with the arms held at the side, and the most sagging portion should be marked with the arm elevated laterally. Bulging areas around the elbows are also marked. The depressed areas around the spiral groove, brachial artery

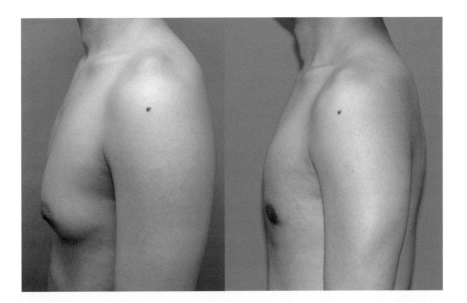

Figure 02-4 Left: A 27-year-old man with gynecomastia. Right: One month following correction with LAL removal of the remaining glandular tissue through a minimal periareolar incision.

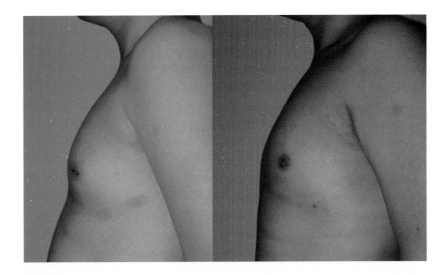

Figure 02-5 Left: A 23-year-old man with gynecomastia. Right: One month following correction with LAL and fat aspiration on its own.

and medial arm are marked for preservation. The whole arm should be treated with LAL to achieve maximum elevation of the drooping skin (Figure 02-6).

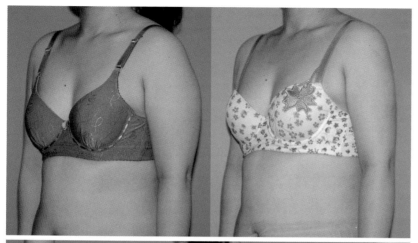

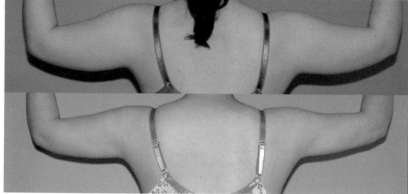

Figure 02-6
Upper panel, left & lower panel, upper: A 29-year-oldwoman with localized obesity of the arm. Upper panel, right & lower panel, lower: Six months following correction with LAL and liposuction.

Calves & Ankles

Localized bulging areas should be marked, especially at both the medial and lateral border areas. The area over the lateral malleolus and the anterior tibial area should be preserved to avoid skin damage that might result in skin necrosis with exposure of the bone. The posterior central area is also preserved for a better aesthetic result. If this area is too flat after liposuction, the results can be bad with the underlying neurovascular structures becoming visible, and a less narrowed diameter due to the atypical flat appearance (Figure 02-7).

2nd lipoplasty

Secondary liposuction can be very difficult to perform because there are so many scars that prevent the introduction of the cannula and the inability to suction the fat trapped between the scar tissue. For the abdomen, any depressed areas and bulging of the remaining fat should be marked. The entry point is decided depending on the scars and presence of any adhesion

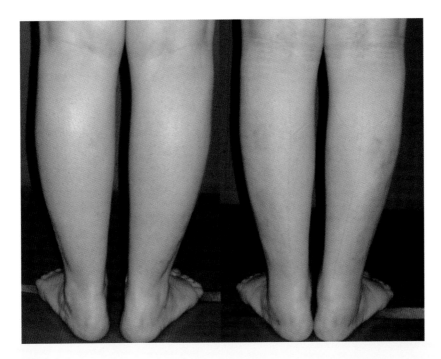

Figure 02-7 Left: A 40-year-old woman with localized obesity of the calves. Right: One week after correction with LAL and liposuction.

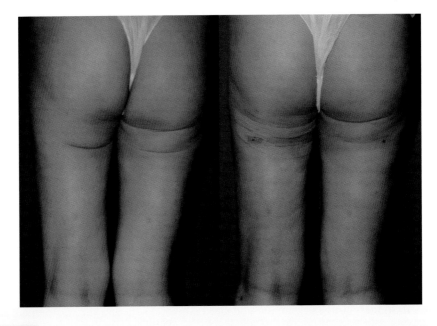

Figure 02-8 Left: A 35-year-old woman with a double (banana) roll deformity after conventional liposuction. Right: Two weeks following secondary correction with LAL and a fat graft.

between the skin and the abdominal wall. Other areas on the body indicated for secondary liposuction are also marked in the same way (Figure 02-8).

Tips for treatment

Abdomen & Flanks

After local infiltration for the entry points (at the pubic area or both inguinal areas, the navel area and the submammary area), the surgical field is then infiltrated with the tumescent solution. The infiltration step is very important to maximize the effect of the laser irradiation and subsequent liposuction. It must be done very meticulously to achieve more efficient anesthesia and a better procedure. Ten to 15 minutes after infiltration, the laser cannula is introduced into the surgical field. The parameters are usually a frequency of 40 Hz, pulse energy of 300 mJ and 12 W output power. The superficial layer is melted first with a total of about 500 J per 10×10 cm area. The cannula is then inserted more deeply layer by layer in 1 cm increments with a total energy of 500 J per 10×10 cm area per layer. The total energy for each 10×10 cm area will be 1000-2000 J depending on the number of layers treated, which in turn is determined by the thickness of the target tissue. A two-way cannula has been designed with which liposuction and lasing can be performed simultaneously, or separately, which helps the clinician save both time and effort. After the procedure is complete and all liquefied lipid has been aspirated, the surgical field is washed with diluted triamcinolone and hyaluronidase solution (1:10000). The entry point is left uncovered to allow the tumescent solution to drain out.

Buttocks & Thighs

For the buttocks and thigh, the parameters are usually the same as for other parts of the body, namely frequency of 40 Hz, pulse energy of 300 mJ and output power of 12 W. The total energy per 10×10 cm area remains at 1000-2000 J, depending on the thickness. The area between the underwear line and gluteal fold should be stimulated with the skin tightening technique, with minimal liposuction. If too much fat is lysed and aspirated from this area, the definition of the buttocks will be decreased, accompanied with downward sagging. For the saddle bags, the bulging fat is melted and the skin over them is tightened to avoid sagging that might occur after excessive liposuction. The lateral border of the thigh is then tapered taking the decreased volume of the saddle bags into account. The depressed area over the tensor fascia lata must be preserved to prevent any deformity due to over-depression and lax skin there. The medial thigh should be marked with a straight line from the upper thigh to medial knee. To ensure the natural beauty of this line, LAL should be performed so as to avoid any depressed area in the middle. Sometimes, there are localized bulging areas of fat around the knees. These are very difficult to remove with conventional liposuction and can result in very noticeable scars on a highly visible area. If these areas of fat are removed via an inguinal incision, they can end up looking worse than before. In such cases, correction and sculpting can be achieved with LAL through an almost invisible entry point created with a hypodermic needle on the medial knee. The process following LAL for these areas is the same as for other areas.

Gynecomastia

With laser assisted lipolysis, gynecomastia can be treated without scarring or with minimal scars. The fat between the fibrotic tissues can be melted through small incisions on the axillary area and submammary area on the anterior axillary line. In addition to the breast area, the surrounding chest area should be tapered to achieve a smooth margin. If hard glandular tissue remains after liposuction, it can be removed through a small axillary or periareolar incision.

Arms

With the patient in the prone position, the posterior, lateral, and medial aspects of the arm can be treated through a small incision on the medial end of the elbow crease. Efficacy is greatest in those cases with very loose skin and too much fatty tissue. After laser treatment, the melted fat can be aspirated with the classical method or by manual syringe liposuction. During the procedure, the laser probe must be accurately placed in the subcutaneous layer, and must not be allowed to penetrate the muscular fascia and brachial neurovascular structures in the axillae. After the posterior aspect has been treated, the patient should be placed in the supine position for treatment of the anterior aspect. Fat in this area is melted and the tissue tightened through a small entry point created in the axillary fold. Removal of the melted fat should be extremely minimal in this area. If the arm is treated as a whole, better results can be achieved than if areas of the skin are skipped. The remaining procedures for these areas are the same as for the others already mentioned.

Calves & Ankles

After local infiltration on both sides of the heel, small slits are made at the junctional area of the skin of the calf and the sole. The incision must be placed away from the Achilles' tendon to avoid skin necrosis over this structure. During tumescent infiltration, the supramalleolar area should be over-infiltrated to avoid damage to the skin and tendinous structures. The fat on both sides should be melted and removed while avoiding the central area. If too much fat is removed over the central area, the deep sural neurovascular structures can be seen through the thin skin and it is very difficult to correct this coverage defect. In addition to this deformity, a flattened posterior aspect is not attractive, as already discussed previously, and looks wider than untouched cases. The area anterior to the lateral malleolus can be treated through the supramalleolar area. The remaining post-LAL procedures are the same as for other areas.

2nd lipoplasty

Areas indicated for secondary lipoplasty contain very dense scar tissue, and it is difficult to advance the cannula through such areas. There may be much more bleeding and more irregularities in the area after treatment. LAL makes fat removal easier during secondary lipoplasties, and also has some benefits as far as achieving tightened skin and a smooth surface. The total energy for the area should be reduced in accordance with the thickness of the fat tissue. For skin tightening, the fiber tip should be aimed up towards the reticular dermis. The other procedures following the LAL are the same as mentioned before.

Tips for post-treatment care and follow-up

The entry point can be left open for drainage of the tumescent solution, and a compression dressing can be applied in all areas except the face and neck. The garment could be applied from the day following the operation and kept in place for 2-3 months. If sutures have been used, they should be removed after 7 days. From the second postsurgical day, the treated area can be gently massaged for several weeks to improve lymphatic drainage. As for exercise, jogging can be resumed after 2 weeks, and more strenuous excercises after 4 weeks.

Side effects

As with facial sculpting with LAL, the possible complications following body sculpting with LAL are also very rare. The side effects usually seen after any other kind of surgery can occur, such as bleeding, hematoma formation, burns, infection, scarring, and so on. Injury of major neurovascular structures is rare because the LAL procedure is usually restricted to the subcutaneous layer, always providing that the laser probe has been properly placed in the subcutaneous layer, parallel to the skin surface, and not in the deeper tissue. The subcutaneous layer is free from major neurovascular structure. Care, however, must be exercised regarding superficial cutaneous nerves, particularly in the case of the superficial peroneal nerve, superficial radial nerve, and medial or lateral cutaneous nerves of the arm. Burns are very rare, and can be avoided completely by keeping the probe moving through the tissue in a to-and-fro manner, never allowing the fiber tip to remain in one spot for any length of time, certainly not more than 5-10 seconds. The most common problem after laser lipolysis is either over- or under reduction. In the case of over reduction, correction must be performed as soon as possible with a fat graft or filler.

REFERENCES

1. Apfelberg DB, Rosenthal S, Hunstad JP, Achauer B, Fodor PB. Progress report on multicenter study of laserassisted liposuction. Aesthetic Plast Surg 1994;18:259–264.
2. Badin AZ, Gondek LB, Garcia MJ, Valle LC, Flizikowski FB, de Noronha L. Analysis of laser lipolysis effects on human tissue samples obtained from liposuction. Aesthetic Plast Surg 2005;29:281-286.
3. Badin AZ, Moraes LM, Gondek L, Chiaratti MG, Canta L. Laser lipolysis: Flaccidity under control. Aesth Plast Surg 2002;26:335-339.
4. Collawn SS. Skin tightening with fractional lasers, radiofrequency, smartlipo. Ann Plast Surg 2010;64.
5. Goldman A, Gotkin RH, Sarnoff DS, Prati C, Rossato F. Cellulite: A new treatment approach combining subdermal Nd:YAG laser lipolysis and autologous fat transplantation.Aesthetic Surg J 2008;28:656-662.
6. Goldman A. Submental Nd:YAG laser-assisted liposuction. Laser Surg Med 2006;38:181-184.
7. Ichikawa K, Miyasaka M, Aikawa Y. Subcutaneous laser treatment of axillary osmidrosis: a new technique. Plast Reconst Surg 2006;118:170-174.
8. Ichikawa K, Miyasaka M, Tanaka R, Tanino R, Mizukami K, Wakaki M. Histologic evaluation of the pulsed Nd:YAG laser for laser lipolysis. Lasers Surg Med 2005;36:43-46.
9. Katz B, McBean J, Cheung JS. The new laser liposuction for men. Dermatol Ther 2007;20:448–451.
10. Khoury JG, Saluja R, Keel D, Detwiler S, Goldman MP. Histologic evaluation of interstitial lipolysis comparing a 1064, 1320 and 2100 nm laser in an ex vivo model. Lasers Surg Med 2008;40:402–406.
11. Kim KH, Geronemus RG. Laser lipolysis using a novel 1064 nm Nd:YAG Laser. Dermatol Surg 2006;32:241-248; discussion 247.
12. Koechner W. Nd:lasers. In: Schawlow AL, editor. Solid-state laser engineering. 4th ed. New York: Springer;1996.
13. Mordon S, Eymard AF, Wassmer B, and Ringot J. Histologic evaluation of laser lipolysis: Pulsed 1064 nm Nd:YAG laser versus CW 980 nm Diode laser. Aesthetic Surg J 2007;27:263-268.
14. Mordon S, Plot E. Laser lipolysis versus traditional liposuction for fat removal. Expert Rev Med Devices 2009;6:677-688.
15. Prado A, Andrades P, Danilla S, Leniz P, Castillo P, Gaete F. A prospective, randomized, double-blind, controlled clinical trial comparing laser-assisted lipoplasty with suctionassisted lipoplasty. Plast Reconstr Surg 2006;118:1032–1045.

16. Sasaki GH. The significance of shallow thermal effects from a 1064nm/1320nm laser on collagenous fibrous septae and reticular dermis: Implications for remodeling and tissue tightening through coagulation. Cynosure White Paper 2008;1-7.

17. Tark KC, Jung JE, and Song SY. Superior Lipolytic Effect of the 1,444nm Nd:YAG Laser: Comparison With the 1,064nm Nd:YAG Laser. Lasers in Surgery and Medicine 2009;41:721–727.

18. Wassmer B, Zemmouri J, Rochon P, and Mordon S. Comparative study of wavelengths for laser lipolysis. Photomedicine and Laser Surg 2009;1-4.

19. Youn JI. A comparison of wavelength dependence for Laser-Assisted Lipolysis effect using Monte Carlo Simulation. White paper of Lutronic 2009;1-4.

20. Youn JI. Ablation efficiency measurement for Laser-Assisted Lipolysis effect using optical coherence tomography. White paper of Lutronic 2009;1-4.

03

Facial sculpting (Approach for the individual aesthetic unit)

▶ Jae-Woo Park, MD, PhD & Sung Jong Baek, MD

Introduction

Facial sculpting with laser-assisted lipolysis (LAL) is an upcoming surgical procedure for correction of facial deformity or for facial contouring. In some of those patients who have a large volume of fat or soft tissue, it can be very difficult to improve the facial contour with maxillofacial bony reconstructive surgery on its own. In such patients reduction of the facial soft tissue volume with liposuction is required, sometimes together with botulinum toxin treatment. Traditional liposuction, however, is not effective in the fine tissues of the face, and is moreover hard to perform. Owing to the smaller-sized cannulas associated with LAL, or the use of the bare fiber in some cases, LAL could help to reduce the facial soft tissue volume and achieve facial contouring without having to resort to facial bone surgery. LAL must be performed according to the facial aesthetic units. The laser parameters appropriate for each area are very important for the first-time users. Careful assessment for each patient is mandatory before and during the intraoperative period in order to achieve the best results.

Ideal Indication for laser assisted facial sculpting

The ideal patients for laser assisted facial sculpturing (LAFS) are those who have areas of thick subcutaneous tissue with reasonable skin tightness. LAFS has successfully reduced the volume of affected areas such as protruding fat pads of the lower eyelids, and for excessive subcutaneous fat in the malar, nasolabial and lower cheek area, but not for buccal fat, and for correction of double chin deformity, retrusive chin, thick neck, blunt neck angle, and deformities after the injection of certain fillers.

Tips for the diagnosis & design

Nasolabial fold

After marking the border of the nasolabial prominence, the area is marked up with circles to figure out the differences in the volume of the protrusive fat. The midline is marked along the midportion of the long axis. When LAFS is performed with suction, the lysed fat below this line will be sucked out and the fat over this line will only be melted with laser, without suction. Depressed areas like the nasojugal groove, tear trough and others should be marked as "no go" areas to avoid laser or suction in these areas. If LAFS were to be performed in these areas, the depressed area would be even more obvious.

Malar prominence

After discussion with the patient, the area to be reduced in volume and prominence is marked with circles. The vertical line from the lateral canthus represents the medial border of the surgical area. If a noticeable tear trough line exists, the approach has to be made from the sideburn to avoid crossing or touching the tear trough. The lateral fat protruding over the zygomatic arch is also marked up to the preauricular area.

Drooping cheeks

On the primary standard position of the face, the first line is drawn bilaterally from the lower pole of the ear to the tip of the chin. This line represents the future mandibular border. The second line is marked along the marionette lines. These two lines intersect and divide the area into four sections on both sides of the face. The entry point is placed in the medial lower sector, and about 1 cm distant from the protruding and drooping fat in the cheek. It is virtually visible post-procedure and is an effective entry point from which to perform LAFS. With the patient in the supine position, the most prominent areas of descending fat are marked with circles to identify them during the procedure. A 3rd line is then marked parallel to the 1st line and about 1 cm below it, representing the lower margin of the mandibular border.

Double chin, submandibular area and neck

The anterior and posterior margin of the sternocleidomastoid (SCM) muscle, the bilateral margins of the trachea, neck wrinkle lines, and the uppermost neck line should be marked. In addition, the expected cervical angle must be marked situated between the midportion of the lower mandibular border and the uppermost neck line. The middle & lower neck lines and clavicular bony margin should also be marked if wide LAFS for the lower neck is to be performed. There are some areas in which LAFS must not be performed, namely the area just above the point where the facial artery crosses the mandibular border. If too much suction is performed in this area, a severely depressed deformity will develop after LAFS. Because of that, this area is marked with many hashed lines as a "no go" area for laser or suction. Any other depressed areas should be similarly marked as areas where LAFS must be avoided.

Tips for treatment

The areas to be treated can be divided into "power units". The volume of the nasolabial prominence, 3×5 cm^2 and 2 cm thick, represents the basic unit for the irradiated energy. For this area, the total energy delivered might be 200 J with a repetition rate of 40 Hz, 150 mJ per pulse, and an output power of 6 W as the laser parameters. The total surgical area is divided into basic power units, so that 200 J multiplied by the total number of power units for each patient will give the total energy to be delivered during the procedure. The concept of the basic power unit makes the procedure easier for the novice practitioner and reduces the surgical time because the surgeon does not need to check frequently for the endpoint. According to some practitioners, the endpoint is when lipid can be seen leaking out from the entry point after LAFS. However, this is a variable reaction and can differ case by case depending on the volume of tumescent solution or local anesthetics infiltrated, the volume of fat to be lysed, the presence of bleeding, and so on. Because of that a more standardized guide is required for LAFS. A consistent surgical effect can be achieved if a standard format is followed for the procedure to achieve an even surgical condition with the same emerging condition of the fat, the same laser parameters and the same laser energy for the same amount of fat. If a standard protocol is in place, the endpoint for the laser part of an LAFS procedure need not be constantly considered. It is the authors' belief that the concept of the basic power unit makes this consistent result possible.

If only one localized area needs to be treated, such as fat-related laxity of only the cheeks, a wider treatment area must be considered from the earlobe to the marionette line and from the zygomatic arch to the submental area, divided into power units. This wider laser treatment improves the skin laxity more effectively. If a limited localized treatment is performed, localized depression of the treated area might occur, or highly localized tightening giving a mismatch with the surrounding area.

Local anesthesia and tumescent solution

There are three different methods for the injection of local anesthetics and the tumescent solution. The first is the dry technique in which the surgical field is injected with only 2-3 cc of 2% lidocaine with 1:100,000 epinephrine solutions, less than 5 cc per one area such as the cheek. This approach can maximize the laser effect for the skin tightening, achieving lysis of the target fat without wasting energy to boil the infiltrated tumescent solution. In the authors' opinion, however, the dry technique has some limitation for a procedure involving multiple layers and a wide area for tightening. The wavelength of 1444 nm is quite highly absorbed in water, and blood comprises over 85% water. If there is some bleeding in the treatment area, it is possible that the laser absorption could be confined to the area of the hemorrhage with results which could be different from those expected. It is very difficult to perform suction after LAFS with the dry technique. Because of that, some surgeons follow the second method, known as the double tumescent technique consisting of post-LAFS re-infiltration with tumescent solution about 2-3 times the volume of the first local anesthetic injection. The re-infiltration makes it easier to perform liposuction with the cannula without bleeding. The third technique, the tumescent technique, also known as the wet technique, is the authors' recommended technique in which the surgical field is infiltrated with differing amounts of tumescent solution depending on the area to be treated: about 5-10 cc over the nasolabial or malar prominence, 20-30 cc in each cheek and 50-100 cc in the neck area. The fluid infiltrating the tissue expands the volume of the tissue to several times the volume of the original. With this volume of expansion of the area of interest it is possible to do multi-layered LAFC and remove the fat more easily and evenly. The wet technique reduces the chance of bleeding, increases the safety of the procedure by limiting collateral damage to the surrounding tissue and avoiding other complications such as burn formation.

After proper preparation with adequate draping of the surgical field, the entry point is covered with 3M surgical tape to prevent skin damage from friction between the cannula and tissue with maceration and possible scarring. The entry point is injected with 2% lidocaine and 1:100,000 epinephrine solution. The sites are punctured with an 18 G hypodermic needle and an 18 G blunt cannula is placed for the tumescent injection.

Nasolabial fold and malar prominence

The nasolabial area is infiltrated with tumescent solution about 5-10 cc on the each nasolabial prominence. After 10 min LAFC is performed with the laser set at a repetition rate of 40 Hz, 150 mj per pulse, 6 W output power, and a total energy of about 200 J. The superficial subdermal areas are irradiated with about 50 J. The subcutaneous area is divided into 3 layers

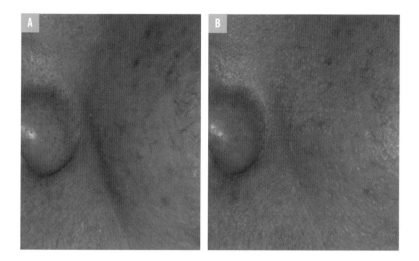

Figure 03-1 **A.** Minimal drooping of the nasolabial fold seen at baseline. **B.** The post-treatment findings at 6 months after a single procedure. The nasolabial fold has become shallow after LAFS without any fat removal. The parameters used were 40 Hz rep rate, 150 mj/pulse, 6 W power, and 200 J.

and each layer is treated with about 50 J. After use of the laser, about 1-2 cc lysed fat per side should be removed from the area with a 19 G single hole cannula. With the patient in the sitting position, both sides of the nasolabial area should be checked for an even shape. Finally, the surgical field is flushed out with diluted hyaluronidase and triamcinolone solution. The entry point is usually opened and dressed with small sponge and skin tapes. Along the long axis, multiple skin tapes are applied for compression of the prominence (Figure 03-1).

The same procedure is performed in the same way and at the same parameters for the malar eminence. The procedure will, however, be limited to the area lateral to the vertical line from the lateral canthus. The anterior malar area should be preserved for the stereotypic facial shape. The cannula and fiber must be inserted into the subcutaneous area parallel to the skin surface to avoid nerve damage especially in the area where the frontal nerve crosses the zygomatic arch (Figure 03-2).

Cheek laxity, double chin & submandibular area

Tumescent placement in the surgical field for laser lipolysis and lifting is as follows: 20-30 cc in each cheek, and 50-100 cc in the submental area and the neck area above the uppermost neck line. After tumescent solution infiltration, 10-15 minutes should be allowed for the epinephrine-mediated hemostasis effect. The multiple layer LAFS method can be used because of the increased volume of the target tissue due to the infiltration of the tumescent into the

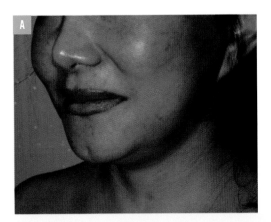 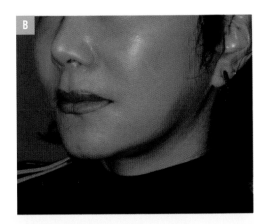

Figure 03-2 **A.** The baseline findings in a patient who had a classic facelift surgery about 4 years previously. **B.** Eight months after LAFC and interstitial fractional radiofrequency treatment. The displaced fat has been reduced through LAFS with removal of the lysed fat on the malar eminences, nasolabial folds, cheek, and submental area.

target tissues. the parameters for the face are about 40 Hz, 150-200 mj/pulse, 6-8 W power. The total energy for the area is calculated by 200 mJ multiplied by the total number of the power units. For example, if the surgical area is divided into 15 basic units, then the total delivered energy will be 3,000 J (200 J × 15 units = 3,000 J).

- Using the entry point as the fulcrum, move the cannula and fiber steadily to and fro in the target tissue in a fan-like pattern. Avoid bringing the tip of the fiber within 5 mm of the entry point.
- Always keep the cannula or fiber moving evenly and steadily during the procedure to avoid overheating any particular area and causing a burn.
- The appearance of the red guide beam through the skin is helpful for the beginner when performing the multiple layered approach. In the superficial layer, the beam is small and bright, and gets progressively larger and less bright as the deeper layers are irradiated..
- The irradiated area should be as wide as possible to achieve optimum results because the final lifting effect depends on the summation of the micro-area lifting around the laser tip.

After laser irradiation, the melted fat is removed with a single hole blunt cannula 1-1.5 mm in diameter. Lysed fat can be suctioned out using the multiple layer technique, and the orientation of the cannula aperture can be controlled to prevent nerve or vascular damage. The fat volume for evacuation is around 2-5 cc per side for the cheeks and 5-10 cc per side for the neck and submental area, or more if the fat deposition in the neck is very thick. If this is the case, with very thick fat deposits in the neck an additional entry point will be needed at the suprasternal area for both LAFS and liposuction. Usually the extra entry point is located

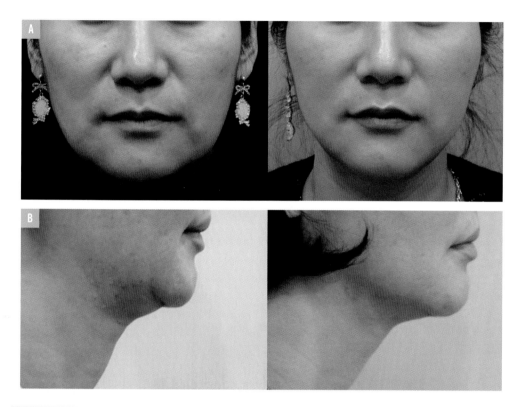

Figure 03-3   **A.** Left: Baseline findings in a patient with lower jowl laxity after Botulinum toxin injection for masseter muscle reduction. Right: The result at 2 months postoperation with LAFS. **B.** Left: Baseline findings in a patient with double chin. Right: The result at 1 month postoperation with LAFS.

to either side of the suprasternal notch.

After LAFS is complete, the surgical field is irrigated with diluted hyaluronidase and triamcinolone solution to assist an early recovery. The hyaluronidase irrigation after LAFS could potentially decrease the swelling by increasing the absorption of fluids and decrease the potential for bruising. Triamcinolone increases the local fluid absorption through altering the water and salt balance and decreases the anti-inflammatory reaction through decreasing immune cell activity (Figure 03-3).

Tips for post-treatment care and follow-up

After irradiation of the treated area, a small sheet of gauze is taped over the entry point. No other dressing is needed. No compression bandage should be applied in the case of LAFS of the face and neck because compression around the ears and submental neck can prevent lymphatic drainage from the treated area, causing severe edema of the face and neck and potentially prolonging the recovery time. The dressing can be removed on the day after treatment and the entry point can be dressed simply with ointment without gauze or skin tape. The patient should avoid washing the face until the 2nd postoperative day. From the day after surgery, treatment with HEALITE ™, an 830 nm LED-based phototherapy system from Lutronic, Goyang City. South Korea, is good to reduce pain, swelling, recovery time and to accelerate the resolution of bruising. If a patient should complain about remaining swelling on the treated area(s) after the 2nd postsurgical day, a gentle RF massage might be helpful for them. The patient should be followed-up for 2 to 4 weeks after treatment. During the healing, some hardness or induration may appear in the submental area that can be managed with diluted hyaluronidase and triamcinolone solution. Pain in the treated area should disappear spontaneously within 2-3 months without any kind of medication. Some patients, however, experience levels of pain that require prescription of a painkiller or tranquilizer. Application of HEALITE LED phototherapy post-LAFC has also been shown to accelerate the resolution of pain and other post-LAFS sequelae.

Side effects

Possible complications of LAFS on the face and neck are very rare. These are those that might happen after other any kind of laser surgery such as bleeding, hematoma, burn, infection, scar, and so on. Injury to the major neurovascular structures is rare because, if the cannula and/or fiber are correctly placed in the subcutaneous layer, and maintained parallel to the skin surface and not in the deeper layers, the laser energy is confined to the subcutaneous layer which is free from major neurovascular structures. Major nerve damage-related complications are usually caused by mechanical injury during the liposuction process. Burns are very rare if the cannula and fiber are kept in smooth motion all the time and not allowed to remain in the one position for too long, for example, over 5-10 sec. When the probe is kept in continuous motion during an LAFS procedure, burns should not happen. The most common problem after laser lipolysis is over- or under-reduction. Under-reduction can be corrected with a secondary LAFS procedure, but over-reduction must be corrected with a fat graft or similar as soon as possible. If an area of under-reduction is left untreated for too long, abnormal adhesion will occur between the damaged dermis and the underlying muscular fascia. It is very difficult to correct any such problem after adhesion has occurred. Because of that, under-reduction should be corrected as soon as possible with an autologous fat graft, or with a hydroxyapatite (HA) filler if a depressed area is noted on movement of the facial muscles.

REFERENCES

1. Apfelberg DB, Rosenthal S, Hunstad JP, Achauer B, Fodor PB. Progress report on multicenter study of laser-assisted liposuction. Aesthetic Plast Surg 1994;18:259–264.
2. Badin AZ, Gondek LB, Garcia MJ, Valle LC, Flizikowski FB, de Noronha L. Analysis of laser lipolysis effects on human tissue samples obtained from liposuction. Aesthetic Plast Surg 2005;29:281-286.
3. Badin AZ, Moraes LM, Gondek L et al. Laser lipolysis: Flaccidity under control. Aesthetic Plast Surg 2002;26:335-339.
4. Badin AZ, Moraes LM, Gondek L, Chiaratti MG, Canta L. Laser lipolysis: Flaccidity under control. Aesth Plast Surg 2002;26:335-339.
5. Dong Y-Y, Ren Q-S, Liu H-X, et al. Comparison of histologic, biochemical, and mechanical properties of murine skin treated wth the 1064-nm and 1320-nm Nd: YAG lasers. Exper Dermatol 2005;14:876-882.
6. Goldman A, Gotkin RH, Sarnoff DS, Prati C, Rossato F. Cellulite: A new treatment approach combining subdermal Nd:YAG laser lipolysis and autologous fat transplantation. Aesthetic Surg J 2008;28:656-662.
7. Goldman A. Submental Nd: YAG laser-assisted liposuction. Laser Surg Med 2006;38:181-184.
8. Ichikawa K, Miyasaka M, Aikawa Y. Subcutaneous laser treatment of axillary osmidrosis: a new technique. Plast Reconst Surg 2006;118:170-174.
9. Ishikawa K, Miyasaka M, Tanaka R, et al. Histologic evaluation of the pulsed Nd: YAG laser for laser lipolysis. Lasers Med Surg 2005;36:43-46.
10. Katz B, McBean J, Cheung JS. The new laser liposuction for men. Dermatol Ther 2007;20:448–451.
11. Kim KH, Geronemus RG. Laser lipolysis using a novel 1,064 nm Nd: YAG laser. Dermatol Surg 2006;32:241-248.
12. Melega J. Liposuction using neodymium:yltrium:aluminium:garnet laser. Plast Reconstr Surg 2003;111:2497.
13. Mordon S, Eymard AF, Wassmer B, and Ringot J Histologic evaluation of laser lipolysis: Pulsed 1064 nm Nd:YAG laser versus CW 980 nm Diode laser. Aesthetic Surg J 2007;27:263-268
14. Mordon S, Plot E. Laser lipolysis versus traditional liposuction for fat removal. Expert Rev Med Devices 2009;6:677-688.
15. Prado A, Andrades P, Danilla S, Leniz P, Castillo P, Gaete F. A prospective, randomized, double-blind, controlled clinical trial comparing laser-assisted lipoplasty with suction-assisted lipoplasty. Plast Reconstr Surg 2006;118:1032–1045.
16. Sasaki GH The significance of shallow thermal effects from a 1064nm/1320nm laser on collagenous fibrous septae and reticular dermis: Implications for remodeling and tissue tightening through coagulation Cynosure White Paper, October 31, 2008:1-7
17. Tark KC, Jung JE, and Song SY. Superior Lipolytic Effect of the 1,444nm Nd:YAG Laser: Comparison With the 1,064nm Nd:YAG Laser. Lasers in Surgery and Medicine 2009;41:721–727.
18. Youn JI. A comparison of wavelength dependence for Laser-Assisted Lipolysis effect using Monte Carlo Simulation. White paper of Lutronic 2009;1-4.
19. Youn JI. Ablation efficiency measurement for Laser-Assisted Lipolysis effect using optical coherence tomography. White paper of Lutronic 2009;1-4.

Vascular lesions

SECTION

07

C/O/N/T/E/N/T/S

Flushing

Sang Ju Lee, MD, PhD

Introduction

Flushing is a transient reddening of the face and frequently other areas, including the neck, ears, and upper chest. Blushing is a subset of flushing reactions associated with emotions, such as embarrassments or anxiety. Flushing is a phenomenon associated with transient vasodilation. Dual control of vascular smooth muscle is affected both by the autonomic nervous system and by circulating vasoactive agents. The autonomic system also controls the eccrine sweat glands, so that whenever vasodilation is mediated by the autonomic system, it is accompanied by eccrine-mediated sweating.

Tips for diagnosis

Two mechanisms of flushing can be distinguished at the bedside or in the office (Table 01-1): autonomic neural-mediated flushing, which includes eccrine sweating ("wet flushing"), and flushing from circulating agents that act directly on vascular smooth muscle ("dry flushing"). Accordingly, the first step in the diagnosis of a flushing reaction is to decide whether the reaction is due to events at some level in the neural control of vascular smooth muscle or to a circulating direct-acting vasodilator.

Tips for treatment

There is no broad-spectrum medication or regimen which can combat or treat flushing. Treatment should be targeted at the specific cause of the flushing reaction. Previous reports have

Table 01-1	Two classes of flushing and the responsible mediators

I. Autonomic neural-mediated (wet flushes)
II. Direct vasodilator-mediated (dry flushes)
   A. Antidromic sensory neural-mediated (dysesthesia)
   B. Circulating vasodilator agent (no dysesthesia)
      i. Exogenous (elicited in history)
      ii. Endogenous (associated features)

shown variable clinical outcomes for treatments such as sunscreen use or sun avoidance, topical medications (such as metronidazole, clindamycin, erythromycin, tretinoin, benzoyl peroxide, azelaic acid, pimecrolimus and tacrolimus), or oral antibiotics (such as tetracyclines, macrolides, and metronidazole), and oral isotretinoin.

Recently, for flushing and rosacea-related erythema, IPL and laser treatment are reportedly preferred to drug treatment. The most widely used forms of laser treatment for flushing are 585 nm or 595 nm flashlamp-pumped pulsed-dye laser (PDL) treatment, 532 nm potassium-titanyl-phosphate (KTP) laser treatment, and long-pulse 1064 nm neodymium-doped yttrium aluminum garnet (Nd:YAG) laser treatment.

The PDL approach treats blood vessels through the principle of selective photothermolysis. If the wavelength is matched to a specific target with an adequately short pulse width, the light energy will be maximally absorbed by the target and minimally by the surrounding structures, thereby reducing the risk of adverse events, especially scarring.

The first PDL emitted laser light at 577 nm, coinciding with the last peak of the oxyhemoglobin absorption spectrum (418 nm, 542 nm, 577 nm). By lengthening the wavelength to 585 nm, the PDL offered deeper penetration into the dermis without compromising vascular selectivity, and with a slightly lower absorption in melanin to help remove that as a competing chromophore.

The first PDL emitted light at a wavelength of 585 nm in a comparatively short pulse (0.45 ms), and had no separate cooling device. Because of its high vascular selectivity, it had a better treatment effect than lasers at other wavelengths, but it required multiple treatments for vessels with a diameter of 0.2 mm or more, and had a poor treatment effect for vessels with a diameter of 0.4 mm or more. In addition, due to its skin penetration depth of less than 1.2 mm, it could not treat vessels located deep in the tissues, and had the disadvantage of causing purpura after the treatment due to extravasation of blood through the damaged vessel wall. To improve these shortcomings, three major changes were made to the PDL. A longer wavelength (595 nm) than 585 nm was introduced thereby increasing the depth of penetration, the pulse duration was extended (long-pulsed dye laser, LPDL), and a cooling device was employed.

PDLs with longer wavelengths such as the V-Beam (Syneron medical, USA) or Cynergy operating at 595 nm appear to achieve greater depth of penetration of the light energy and therefore target deeper vessels more effectively. Although there is deeper penetration of energy at 595 nm compared to 585 nm, the absorption by oxyhemoglobin is lower than at 585 nm. In order to compensate for decreased absorption, the longer wavelength PDL systems require an additional 20-50% fluence compared to 585 nm PDL systems.

The treatment of flushing with 585-nm PDL with a short pulse duration was effective but left prominent, long-lasting purpura. This purpuragenic setting was also related to the formation of hyperpigmentation and atrophic scarring, and patients were frequently unable to tolerate treatment due to unacceptable cosmetic side-effects.

Adding the longer pulse duration has lessened the incidence of purpura after the treatment and is effective for the treatment of larger-caliber vessels. Due to these advantages, the LPDL is commonly used at subpurpuric doses for treatment of flushing. After LPDL treatments, however, swelling may occur for several days. Epidermal cooling devices allow the use of higher fluences (Figure 01-1).

The KTP laser emits light at 532 nm with high absorption in both blood and melanin, and can be therefore be effective for both vascular and pigmented diseases, though it may cause more post-procedure erythema and swelling. Particularly, as KTP treatment has a higher risk of causing postinflammatory pigmentation (PIH) in Asians than PDL treatment, care must be taken with parameter selection. The long-pulsed Nd:YAG laser emits a wavelength of 1064 nm where there is comparatively less absorption in melanin, but a minor absorption peak in oxyhemoglobin, therefore it is effective for the treatment of deep vascular anomalies. It is also effective for larger-diameter vessels because it uses a long pulse. As flushing normally arises due to the superficial thin-walled microvascular plexus, the 1064 nm Laser Genesis technique that uses a shorter pulse duration and is performed repeatedly at low fluences is commonly used

In the Laser Genesis approach, the handpiece of the laser is held approximately 1-2 cm away from the skin and passes are made over the skin in a painting motion till the clinical end-point is reached. The clinical end-point is moderate erythema and a heating sensation over the treatment area. Multiple treatments at an interval of 2 to 6 weeks (average of 4 weeks), are required. Table 01-2 gives examples of the lasers commonly used for the treatment of flushing.

Intense pulsed light (IPL) is a comparatively new technology using a broad-spectrum flashlamp that emits a continuous polychromatic and noncoherent spectrum in the range of 500–1,200 nm to target pigment chromophores, blood vessels and pilosebaceous structures. Low-end cut-off filters are used to eliminate shorter wavelengths, depending on the applica-

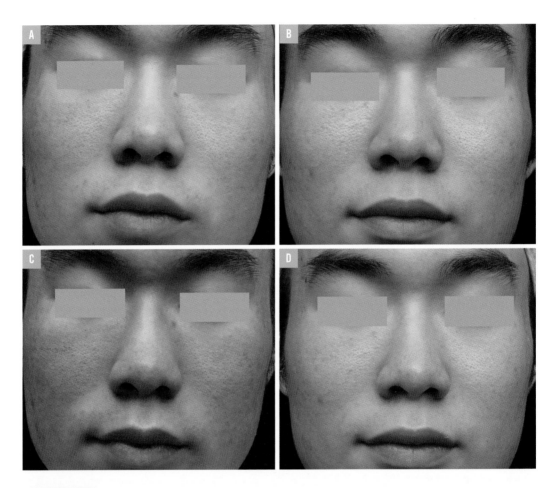

Figure 01-1 Clinical photos taken prior to the application of topical niacin cream showing the face of a Korean male before (A) and after (B) three sessions of 595-nm pulsed-dye laser using topical niacin cream. Facial appearance 20 minutes after the application of topical niacin cream before (C) and after (D) three sessions of 595-nm pulsed-dye laser using topical niacin cream.

tion. IPL is mainly used for non-ablative photorejuvenation and hair removal. IPL has been successfully used in the treatment of facial vascular lesions, including rosacea-associated erythema and telangiectasia of < 0.1 mm, without any reported permanent side-effects. Generally, there is a difference in the treatment of flushing between Asians and Caucasians. First, treatment of flushing in Asians is known to be less effective than in Caucasians. It is postulated that the undesired absorption of laser energy by the melanin in the epidermis reduces the laser energy to be delivered to the oxyhemoglobin in the target vessels, which results in such difference between Asians and Caucasians. Besides, Asians are more likely to develop post-inflammatory hyperpigmentation than Caucasians. Particularly, as the occurrence of secondary pigmentation after purpura is common in both Caucasians and Asians, the treat-

Table 01-2	Different lasers used in the treatment of flushing						
Laser	λ (nm)	Spot size (mm)	Pulse duration (ms)	Rep. rate (Hz)	Fluence (J/cm²)	Crygen spray / delay (ms)	Clinical endpoint
V beam laser	595	7	6, 10	-	8~11	medium, 30/20	transient intravascular purpura, which will disappear and become bluish pink dusky erythema
V beam laser	595	10	10	-	5~7	medium, 30/20	
Vantage (Laser Genesis)	1064	5	0.3	5~7	13~14	off	diffuse erythema, feeling of heat
G-max (Laser Genesis)	1064	6	0.3	5~7	16~18	off	diffuse erythema, feeling of heat
Gemini	532	10	25~30	-	8~10	contact cooling	diffuse erythema, feeling of heat
Clarity (Quatro Technique)	1064	8	0.3~1	10	8~14	off	diffuse erythema, feeling of heat
Clarity (Innerlift Technique)	1064	12	20	2	20~26	off	diffuse erythema, feeling of heat

V-Beam, Gmax, Syneron/Candela, USA; Vantage, Cutera, USA; Gemini; Laserscope, USA; Clarity, Lutronic Corp, South Korea

ment should be performed at a subpurpuric dose, if possible. A recent study has reported that to overcome these shortcomings, erythema was induced using vasodilators such as niacin, and then laser treatment was performed. As this treatment method is performed at a subpurpuric dose, it involves less pigmentation complications and can deliver a higher energy level, which enhances the treatment effect.

- The erythema treatment effect is lower in Asians than in Caucasians, and the risk of secondary pigmentation after the treatment is higher in Asians than in Caucasians.
- Because the cheeks of Asians are prone to flushing and melasma, the existence of underlying melasma should be checked before the treatment.
- A purpuric dose may have a good treatment effect but may cause a bruise that can last for 1-2 weeks or a month. Thus, an effective and safe treatment is to use a long pulse duration at a subpurpuric dose.

Tips for post-treatment care and follow-up

The recently developed PDL and IPL are equipped with some form of cooling device, and thus anesthesia is generally not required during the treatment. Furthermore, as application of a topical anesthesia may induce vasoconstriction, which will weaken the treatment effect by removing the target chromophore, it is desirable not to administer anesthesia if possible. When the treatment will be performed using the long-pulsed Nd:YAG laser and the Laser Genesis technique, the skin should not be anesthetized, as the patient would be unable to feel any burning sensation or pain, which would make him/her susceptible to burns. The use of high-level energy may cause pain or bruising during the treatment. In this case, the application of an ice roller or gauze-wrapped ice on the treatment site may be helpful.

After laser or IPL treatment, cooling the skin may be helpful. Simply using a cooling spray on the skin surface would be good. If the treatment was performed at high fluences, a cooling mask or pack should be used for 15 minutes or more to soothe the skin and possibly reduce the post-treatment pain, erythema, or swelling, as well as such secondary adverse events as purpura, blistering, or burning. As post-treatment swelling or erythema may last for several days, it is recommended that the patient's head be raised during sleep. In some cases, bruising may occur; and though rarely, a blister or crust may also form. In this case, the patient must visit the hospital to receive the appropriate dressing. Although wearing makeup or washing the face is possible immediately after the treatment if there is no blister or crust, irritating or rubbing the face while washing it should be avoided. Generally, follow-up monitoring for about 1 week is required to reduce adverse events. In general, 3-5 treatment sessions are performed with 1-month intervals.

- As Asians are more likely to develop adverse events such as pigmentation, blistering, or scarring after the treatment than Caucasians, adequate cooling is required to reduce these events.

REFERENCES

1. CA Schroeter, et al. Effective treatment of rosacea using intense pulsed light systems. Dermatol Surg 2005;31:1285-1289.
2. EF Bernstein, et al. Rosacea treatment using the new-generation, high-energy, 595 nm, long pulse-duration pulsed-dye laser. Lasers Surg Med 2008;40:233-239.
3. IM Neuhaus, et al. Comparative efficacy of nonpurpuragenic pulsed dye laser and intense pulsed light for erythematotelangiectatic rosacea. Dermatol Surg 2009;35:920-928.
4. R Odom, et al. Standard management options for rosacea, Part 1: overview and broad spectrum of care. Cutis 2009;84:43-47.
5. S Laube, et al. Laser treatment of rosacea. J Cosmet Dermatol 2002;1:188-195.
6. S Lee, et al. Topical niacin cream-assisted 595-nm pulsed-dye laser treatment for facial flushing: retrospective analysis of 25 Korean patients. J Eur Acad Dermatol Venereol 2011;26:54-58.
7. SB Cho, et al. Treatment of facial flushing by topical application of nicotinic acid cream followed by treatment with 595-nm pulsed-dye laser. Clin Exp Dermatol 2009;34:e405-406.
8. TG Kim, et al. Enhancing effect of pretreatment with topical niacin in the treatment of rosacea-associated erythema by 585-nm pulsed dye laser in Koreans: a randomized, prospective, split-face trial. Br J Dermatol 2011;164:573-579.

02

Telangiectasia

▶ Sang Ju Lee, MD, PhD

Introduction

Telangiectasias consist of chronically dilated capillaries or small venules. They appear on the skin and mucous membranes as small, dull red, linear, stellate or punctate markings either as discrete vessels or as conglomerates of vessels occupying an area of tissue. Telangiectasias are caused by the dilatation (expansion, stretching) of pre-existing vessels without any apparently new vessel growth (angiogenesis) occurring.

Tips for diagnosis

Telangiectasias are commonly seen on the face, occurring in at least 10-15% of Caucasians. Simple telangiectasias comprise small, dilated vessels that are 0.1–1.0 mm in diameter. They are commonly located on the midface region and appear as linear red or blue vessels. Spider telangiectasias ('spider nevi') consist of red, radial branches emanating from a central feeding arteriole that blanch with pressure. They are especially common in children.

Tips for treatment

Treatment of telangiectasia differs according to the location, size, and depth of the lesions, though they can mostly be addressed with laser or intense pulsed light (IPL) treatment. Small individual vessels can be treated via electrocautery or with a carbon dioxide (CO_2) laser. To treat small vessels, an epilating needle is inserted into the dilated portion of the vessel, and then electrocauterization is performed. Longer vessels can be treated at 5-mm intervals along the dilatated vessel. For clearly circumscribed spider telangiectasia, electrocauterization of the central arteriole leads to removal of nearby vessels, but it is better to treat from the outside of the 'spider', working towards the feeder vessel, otherwise blood may remain in the radiating vessels resulting in eventual hemosiderin deposition. CO_2 laser treatment can be performed in a manner similar to electrocauterization. The vessels can be coagulated using a laser along the vessel at regular intervals, working from outside towards the central feeder. Care must be taken not to use too high a pulse energy or output power, however, as this may leave a small scar. It must always be remembered that neither electrocautery nor CO_2 laser treatment is pigment selective, and in the case of the CO_2, tissue water is the chromophore. Too aggressive treatment will almost certainlyleave a small scar, and the potential for postinflammatory hyperpigmentation (PIH) is very strong in the Asian skin types III and higher.

For vessels that are small but are numerous and distributed over a wide area, a vascular laser or IPL treatment is commonly used. The most representative lasers for this type of vessel include, by increasing wavelength, the 532-nm potassium-titanyl-phosphate (KTP) laser, the 585 nm or 595-nm flashlamp-pumped pulsed-dye laser (PDL), the 578-nm copper bromide laser, the long-pulsed 755-nm alexandrite laser, and the long-pulsed 1064-nm neodymium-doped yttrium aluminum garnet (Nd:YAG) laser. Particularly for superficial telangiectasia on the face, a laser emitting in the green-yellow spectrum has high vascular selectivity and is safe, and thus, widely used. Care must be taken with the KTP laser treatment when treating telangiectasia in Asian skin types, however, as it is very highly absorbed in both blood and epidermal melanin, with the potential for causing more epidermal damage and PIH formation. Though such lasers as the alexandrite (755 nm), diode (810 nm and 940 nm), and Nd:YAG (1064 nm) in the near-infrared range can also be used for superficial telangiectasia, they are more effective for thicker or deeper vessels. As the PDL has a wide range of pulse durations, from 0.45 to 40 ms, it is highly effective for the treatment of various types of telangiectasia. An IPL system used with a yellow cutoff filter can also treat certain types of telangiectasia.

In the past, severe purpura due to the extravasation of blood from a damaged vessel and pain after PDL treatment were inevitable due to the short pulse duration of the previous laser systems, and the absence of a cooling device. These days, however, long pulse durations and advanced cooling systems have considerably reduced post-procedure pain and purpura formation. In the more recent PDL systems, the fluence, pulse duration, spot size, and degree of skin cooling can be adjusted. Given the same fluence, shorter pulse durations will deliver a better treatment effect, though the risk of purpura formation is higher. For the same incident laser parameters, the larger the spot size is, the deeper the penetration of the laser will be.

Cooling the skin surface protects the epidermis while allowing the laser energy to penetrate to the target dermal vessels. Thus, it is important to select the appropriate parameters according to the depth of the lesion and the thickness of the vessels, and to be aware of the ideal endpoints.

Generally, for telangiectasia, the disappearance of the vessels right after the laser irradiation indicates a good treatment outcome. Recently, due to the pulse stacking technique at a lower fluence, adverse events such as purpura have been reduced and the treatment effect has been enhanced. With some laser protocols, treatment with the PDL is followed with a session using the long-pulsed Nd:YAG laser. The more superficial vessels are affected by the PDL because of the penetration characteristics at 595 nm, and because light at 1064 nm is better absorbed in deeper vessels. Additionally, the long-pulsed Nd:YAG laser can transform the hemoglobin in the target vessels into methemoglobin (MetHb), and MetHb absorbs 1064 nm extremely well. Some laser systems offer a handpiece tip that can deliver the laser energy in an oval pattern, and this makes the treatment of linear lesions such as telangiectasias more convenient. Vessels with powerful hemodynamics and thick vessels, such as those in the nose, can be particularly effectively treated with an oval tip using a long pulse duration (40 msec).

The KTP laser with long pulse duration is highly effective for treating superficial telangiectasia because it delivers a beam at 532 nm, and has been associated with less post-procedure purpura formation. As the 532 nm wavelength is highly absorbed by melanin, however, it poses a greater risk of epidermal damage or PIH in darker-skinned patients such as Asians, as already mentioned above. In addition, post-procedure erythema and swelling can persist for 6-12 hours or more, and the risk of crust and scar formation is higher than with the PDL. The long-pulsed alexandrite (755 nm) laser or the diode laser (800, 810, and 930 nm) is effective for the treatment of deep and thick telangiectatic vessels because the wavelengths of these systems are in the near-infrared and offer deeper penetration than the shorter visible wavelengths. Vessels with diameters of 0.4 mm or more are also known to respond to the long-pulsed alexandrite laser or the diode laser. The long-pulsed Nd:YAG laser is known to be effective for the treatment of thin vessels on the skin surface and also of thick vessels deep under the skin. Even a blue reticular vein that is not responsive to PDL treatment or a 532 nm laser can respond well to long-pulsed Nd:YAG laser treatment. Studies have reported that 97% of facial telangiectasia and periocular reticular veins treated with long-pulsed Nd:YAG laser led to a 75% or greater improvement. Long-pulsed Nd:YAG laser, however, is likely to cause a blister or scar when used to treat certain areas such as nose and perinasal areas, because of potential perivascular damage. In particular, when telangiectasia in the nasal area that does not respond well to the KTP or PDL lasers is treated with higher fluences of 1064 nm energy and shorter pulses, a depressed scar frequently occurs.

An IPL system with an appropriate cutoff filter is effective when the facial telangiectasia is distributed over a wide area, when there is poikiloderma of Civatte, or when the telangiectasia is accompanied by skin aging and pigmentation. In addition, IPL causes fewer adverse events such as purpura. Some IPL devices, however, may cause postage-stamp-like marks on the skin because the residual shorter wavelengths not filtered out by the cutoff filter can oxidize unoxidized melanin, or stimulate the epidermal melanocytes.In some cases, when an IPL is applied at a high energy level and a short wavelength cutoff filter for superficial cutaneous vessels in the presence of underlying melasma, the melasma may become exacerbated and darken. If there are areas of latent pigmentation in the skin, this can result in the unexpected appearance of freckles after IPL treatment. Thus, care must be taken when using an IPL to treat telangiectasia.

NOTE　**Pay particular attention to the following points**

- As the laser or IPL device that is used to treat a vascular lesion such as telangiectasia or flushing uses higher-level energy than that which is used to treat pigment diseases, care must be taken with the procedure.
- As Asians are more likely to develop adverse events such as PIH, blisters, and scars after the procedure than Caucasians, it is recommended that the treatment be performed conservatively on them.
- The appearance of melasma in the treated area post-procedure is common in Asians. Thus, the presence of any underlying melasma (latent pigmentation) must be checked before the treatment.
- When long-pulsed Nd:YAG laser is used to treat vessels in the nose area, a depressed scar is more likely to occur than in other areas. Thus, care must be taken.
- The standard treatment lasers for facial telangiectasia are the KTP, PDL and long-pulsed Nd:YAG lasers, with IPL systems as a non-laser light-based device. Particularly for Asians, the PDL causes less adverse events and is an effective treatment option. Table 02-1 lists lasers and parameters commonly used for the treatment of facial telangiectasias.

Tips for post-treatment care and follow-up

When telangiectasia has been treated with a laser or IPL, the application of an ice roller or gauze-wrapped ice should be carried out immediately after the treatment to cool down the treated site.This can reduce pain, swelling, and erythema, and increase patient comfort. The simple use of a cooling spray on the skin surface can be helpful, but when the treatment was

Table 02-1	Facial telangiectasia and suggested lasers systems with parameters					
Lesion	Laser	Spot size (mm)	Pulse width (ms)	Fluence (J/cm²)	Cryogen spray/delay (ms)	Clinical endpoint
Facial telangiectasia	V-beam (595 nm)	7	6, 10	7-12	medium, 30/20	vessels clear immmediately
		3x10	10	11-14	medium, 30/20	
Facial telangiectasia (vessels < 0.5 mm)	G-max (1064 nm)	1.5	20	340	10/20/10	vasoconstriction, vasospasm, and/ or darkening vessel contents
	Clarity (1064 nm)	2	12, 20	120-170	10/20/10	
Facial telangiectasia (vessels < 1.0 mm)	G-max (1064 nm)	3	30	130	40/30/0	vasoconstriction, vasospasm, and/ or darkening vessel contents
	Clarity (1064 nm)	3, 5	20-50	120-130	10/20/10	

V-Beam, Gmax, Syneron/Candela, USA; Clarity, Lutronic Corp, South Korea

performed with at high energy levels, soothing the treatment site for 15 minutes or more with a cooling mask or pack will be more helpful. Skin cooling reduces post-procedure pain, erythema, swelling, and secondary adverse events such as bruising, blistering, and burning. Application of near-infrared light emitting diode (LED) phototherapy post-treatment, such as the 830 nm Healite II (Lutronic Corp., South Korea), has been shown to reduce discomfort, erythema and edema more swiftly, and to enhance the final result.

Important

As Asians are more likely than Caucasians to develop post-procedure adverse events such as pigmentation, blistering, and scarring, adequate and appropriate skin cooling is required to reduce these events. Consider the adjunctive use of 830 nm LED phototherapy.

As post-procedure swelling or erythema may last for several days, it is recommended that the patient should sleep with his/her head elevated. A bruise sometimes occurs, and though it rarely occurs, a blister or a crust may be formed. In this case, it is recommended that the patient should visit a hospital for the appropriate dressing. Generally, as a blister caused by a PDL treatment is a very superficial burn, it often spontaneously resolves and leaves only mild pigmentation without a scar. Blisters caused by a long-pulsed Nd:YAG laser system, however, occasionally lead to scarring because of the depth of penetration of the 1064 nm wavelength, and the potential for deeper damage. Thus, in the case of long-pulsed Nd:YAG laser-mediated blisters, active and prompt post-treatment care is required, such as aggressive cooling, topical anti-burn ointment and so on.

Generally, about 1 week of follow-up monitoring is required to control the incidence of possible adverse events. Telangiectasia commonly improves after just one treatment session. In the case of recurrent telangiectasia, 3-5 treatment sessions at 1-month intervals are generally performed.

Concerning post-procedural home care, wearing makeup or washing the face is possible immediately after a procedure if there is no blister or crust, but irritating the treatment site severely with an exfoliating scrub, creams with an active exfoliating agent or rubbing the treated skin vigorously during washing should be avoided. Instruct patients to observe the following precautions for the optimum wound healing care: a good approach is to issue these to the patient on a post-care card which they can attach to their refrigerator door or other often-looked-at location.

- Do not rub, scratch, or pick at the treated area if bruising/red discoloration (purpura) is present.
- Please call the office immediately if the area becomes tender, reddened or shows signs of infection.
- Avoid swimming, contact sports, saunas and hot tubs until the redness or irritation has completely disappeared.

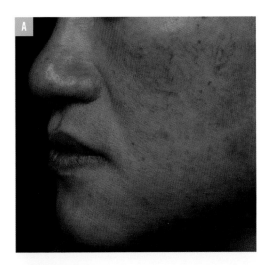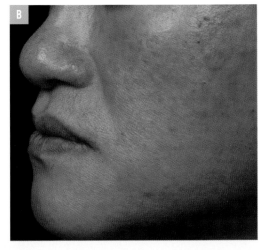

Figure 02-1 Facial telangiectasia: Clinical photography showing telagiectasia before and 1 month after a PDL treatment.

- Avoid rubbing or pressure (caused by clothing) on the treated areas. Wear loose-fitting clothing if your treated area is on a non-exposed area of the body.
- Avoid exposure to the sun. If sun exposure is expected, apply an SPF 50 or higher UVA/B sunscreen to prevent pigmentation changes until the lesion has healed.

REFERENCES

1. C Travelute Ammirati, et al. Laser treatment of facial vascular lesions. Facial Plast Surg 2001;17:193-201.
2. D Railan, et al. Laser treatment of vascular lesions. Clin Dermatol 2006;24:8-15.
3. EV Ross, et al. Intense pulsed light and laser treatment of facial telangiectasias and dyspigmentation: some theroretical and practical comparisons. Dermatol Surg 2005;31:1188-1198.
4. HH Hare McCoppin, et al. Laser treatment of facial telangiectases: an update. Dermatol Surg 2010;36:1221-1230.
5. V Madan, et al. Using the ultra-long pulse width pulsed dye laser and elliptical spot to treat resistant nasal telangiectasia. Lasers Med Sci 2010;25:151-154.

Miscellaneous others / Special issues

C/O/N/T/E/N/T/S

Hyperhidrosis & osmidrosis

▶ Il Hwan Kim, MD, PhD

Axillary hyperhidrosis and osmidrosis

Axillary hyperhidrosis

Axillary hyperhidrosis refers in general to primary (intrinsic) excessive sweating limited to the armpit, without particular reasons or comorbidity. It occurs when the hypothalamus, cerebral cortex, and nervous system (sudomotor: acetylcholine acts in the cholinergic fibers of the sympathetic nervous system) that control perspiration act excessively in response to emotions or stress-related stimulation, leading to increased secretion of the eccrine sweat gland that is morphologically and functionally normal. Though it is rare, it may occur secondary to obesity, menopause, taking antidepressants, neural disorder, endocrine disorder (hypoglycemia and hyperthyroidism), spinal cord injury, chemical weapons (acetylcholinesterase inhibitors), and other causes. Axillary hyperhidrosis is the second most common form of hyperhidrosis, next to hand and foot hyperhidrosis. It can occur alone or together with hand and foot hyperhidrosis. A U.S. study reported that the prevalence rate of primary hyperhidrosis was 2.0%, more than half (1.4%) of which was accounted for by axillary hyperhidrosis and the remaining 1/6 (0.5%) of which affected daily life.

Axillary osmidrosis

Body odor originates from sweat. It develops mostly in hairy areas where there are profuse sweat glands. Osmidrosis broadly refers to the unpleasant odor that emanates in relation to the sweat glands, and is defined as any form of abnormally severe body odor. As such, axillary osmidrosis includes hyperhidrosis, osmidrosis, and extrinsic osmidrosis. From a clinical treatment viewpoint, it is useful to classify axillary osmidrosis according to the type of sweat gland—i.e., into apocrine bromidrosis that is related to the apocrine sweat glands, and to eccrine bromidrosis that is related to the eccrine sweat glands. Eccrine (non-apocrine) bromidrosis can be further classified into keratolysis-related bromidrosis such as foot odor caused by bacteria, and metabolic-amino-acid-related bromidrosis caused by a metabolic abnormality. Of the body odors, those that emanate from the armpit, pubic area, scalp, perianal area, and sole of the foot are causes for concern, and the body odor that hinders social activity most seriously is broadly axillary osmidrosis.

Tips for the diagnosis

▌ Axillary hyperhidrosis

1. Axillary hyperhidrosis can be diagnosed based on clear clinical features such as increased perspiration (a subjective symptom), and objective findings. It can be conclusively diagnosed based on the patient's medical history, familial history, and physical examination findings. A Minor test (Figure 01-1) using an iodine-starch solution can reveal the perspiration area and activity. In addition, the perspiration and body heat can be measured both qualitatively and quantitatively to come up with an accurate diagnosis.

2. The extent of the impact on the patient's social life and quality of life should be assessed; and if the impact on the patient's daily life is significant (e.g., loss of confidence), aggressive treatment is required.

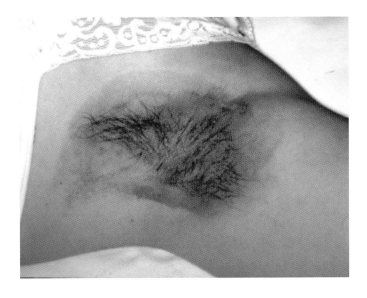

Figure 01-1   Minor test for left axillary hyperhidrosis

Diagnosis of axillary osmidrosis

The patient should meet several criteria to be diagnosed as having apocrine axillary osmidrosis. First, a familial history of autosomal dominant inheritance should be present. Second, a characteristic odor attributable to secretion from the apocrine sweat glands should emanate from the armpit (this should be differentiated from the odor attributable to the eccrine sweat glands). Third, the onset of axillary osmidrosis takes place during or after adolescence. As patients with axillary osmidrosis may also have odor and most of them also have wet ear-wax, their family history is important. Axillary osmidrosis is known to be rarest among Far East Asians. Thus, patients with severe symptoms may have more serious social and cultural problems. The mechanism of occurrence of armpit odor can be explained by the bacterial level. That is, even in normal people, various bacteria such as micrococcaceae, diptheroid, and propionibacteria coexist in the armpits. Studies have shown, however, that the distribution of these bacteria varies by the type of body odor, and it is known that in the case of non-apocrine body odor, micrococci are most profuse, whereas in the case of apocrine body odor (i.e., axillary osmidrosis), aerobic diptheroids abound most. These bacteria degenerate secretions from the sweat glands, and the odor-emitting acid that arises from the degeneration varies by bacteria (axillary osmidrosis: short-chain fatty acid (E)-3-methyl-2-hexanoic acid (E-3M2H) and eccrine osmidrosis: isovaleric acid). Few studies have investigated the method of objective assessment of underarm odor.

Methods of analysis of apocrine body odor

Gas chromatography is the most accurate method of analyzing apocrine body odor, but it is not applicable in clinical practice.

To come up with a diagnosis based on the odor, a test using olfaction, a sensory receptor, and memory related to the olfactory center is the most reliable method but is subjective and has the disadvantage of producing variable results depending on the examiner. Thus, to differentiate eccrine bromidrosis from apocrine bromidrosis, repeated training on olfaction is needed. No device that can objectively quantify the odor and is more sensitive than the human nose has been developed yet.

Therefore, currently the most widely used diagnostic method is to directly smell the odor from the clothes or in the underarms (the method can detect a 1/1 billion concentration). Since many cases of axillary osmidrosis among South Korean patients involve eccrine bromidrosis, differential diagnosis is important from the therapeutic viewpoint for both the clinician and the patient.

> • Among Far East Asians, osmidrosis is rare, but is a more sensitive concern.
> • Among Far East Asians, osmidrosis seriously affects the patient's quality of life, and patients want a radical operation rather than temporary drug therapy.

Tips for treatment

The stepwise approach based on symptoms should be used for axillary osmidrosis

If the patient has symptoms that are attributable to emotional or psychological causes, the administration of a systemic anticholinergic drug should be considered under consultation with specialists. For other cases, the following stepwise treatments should be performed.

Step 1: If there is no emotional and psychological cause, a topical antiperspirant (ingredients: aluminum chloride hexahydrate, Drysol, Xerac AC) can be used at concentrations of 10-15% for the underarms and 30% for the hands and feet.

Step 2: If not controlled well with step 1 treatment, the use of the following two options can be considered.

   A. Iontophoresis: It is difficult to apply this method in the case of axillary osmidrosis, and this method has the disadvantage of recurrence after discontinuation of treatment. Due to this, this method is rarely used in clinical practice.

   B. Botulinum Toxin Type A injection: This method has been approved by the regulatory authroities for the treatment of severe primary axillary osmidrosis that is resistant to topical treatment and hinders daily life.

▌ Topical application and botulinum toxin injection

For primary axillary osmidrosis, a topical treatment such as topical application of aluminum chloride ($AlCl_3$), and iontophoresis can be used as forms of non-invasive treatment. The treatment effect of these methods is short-term and temporary, however. The administration of a systemic anticholinergic drug is seldom chosen as a primary form of treatment because of its inducement of adverse events. Additionally, invasive treatment methods such as axillary sweat gland removal, liposuction, and sympathetic blocking are also seldom selected as primary forms of treatment. Recently, however, numerous studies have reported a long-term good treatment outcome for primary axillary hyperhidrosis treated with the use of botulinum toxin, which is increasing because of its high success rate and the convenience of performing the procedure. Botulinum toxin is a neurotoxin produced from Clostridium botulinum, an anaerobic bacterium. The nerves distributed around the sweat glands are mostly sympathetic postganglionic fibers. Acetylcholine, a neurotransmitter that is secreted from these neuroterminals, promotes perspiration. Botulinum toxin inhibits perspiration by interrupting the secretion of acetylcholine from the neuroterminals. To treat axillary eccrine osmidrosis, an antiperspirant is most widely used, though it has limitations as far as inhibiting the odor. An antiperspirant is helpful for mild cases that involve slight odor and hyperhidrosis. Aluminum chloride is the most effective antiperspirant and can be used after it is diluted to a 20% concentration, or else a commercial antiperspirant (Drysol, Xerac AC) is available. Eccrine osmidrosis related to keratolytic bacteria can be easily resolved and controlled with the addition of a topical form of treatment such as an antibacterial soap, and with the addition of antibiotics to the antiperspirant. Because it is known that, in many patients with apocrine osmidrosis, the apocrine sweat glands are responsible for the increased perspiration, topical application of an antiperspirant is expected to help inhibit the odor, although axillary osmidrosis is unrelated to perspiration. Moreover, the effect of a topical antiperspirant is transient. Recently, a study reported that topical injection therapy using botulinum toxin A was performed. In this study, the applicability of botulinum toxin A was examined, and it was found that the patient's satisfaction with his quality of life was quite high, though the effect was transient. Thus, it is believed that botulinim toxin A will be a standard treatment in the future. In addition, botulinum toxin A was reported to be effective for axillary osmidrosis, though temporarily, and this effect is considered related to the inhibition of the perspiration mechanism, as in hyperhidrosis.

▌ Far east Asians prefer a radical operation to non-surgical treatment of axillary osmidrosis because the effect of non-surgical treatment is transient and poor.

▌ The principle of surgical treatment of axillary hyperhidrosis and osmidrosis is shown in the following figure.

The sweat glands are distributed in the dermis and the subcutaneous adipose layer. As such, to remove the sweat glands completely, the tissues from the upper region of the subcutaneous adipose layer to the regions just below the pilosebaceous unit should be removed by undermining the tissue at the subcutaneous level (Figure 01-2 & 01-3). Removal of part of the deep dermis around the adipose layer cannot remove the sweat glands completely. In contrast, excessive removal of the tissue, including the sebaceous glands, in the upper dermis may cause full-thickness skin necrosis by damaging the dermal vascular plexus (Figure 01-3, upper box area).

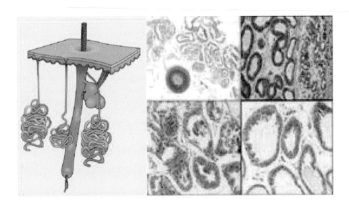

Figure 01-2 Schematic view of the axillary sweat glands (left: eccrine and right: apocrine) and histological findings (top: eccrine gland and bottom: apocrine gland).

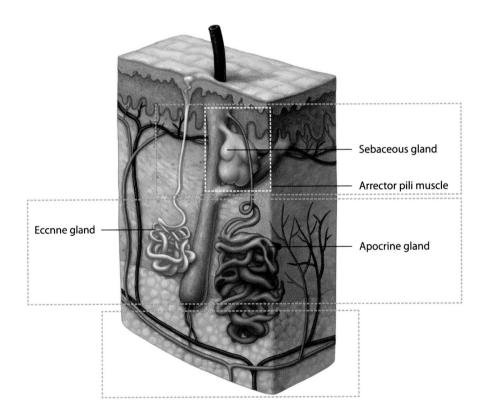

Sebaceous gland

Arrector pili muscle

Eccnne gland

Apocrine gland

Figure 01-3 **Schematic view of the subdermal appendages.** To remove the sweat glands completely, the tissues from the upper adipose layer to the regions just below the pilosebaceous glands should be removed (middle box area).

Surgical treatment

The most effective and permanent treatment for axillary hyperhidrosis and osmidrosis is surgery. Bisbal et al. classified the surgical treatment methods into three types; and since then, various methods have been introduced. Wide excision of the axillary tissue was used in the past but is rarely used nowadays because it requires a long recovery time and has a high risk of complications after the procedure. Possible complications of a wide excision include infection/phlegmon/fasciitis, ecchymosis, hematoma, damage to neighboring nerves (paresthesia and sensoparalysis), damage to neighboring vessels, secondary permanent malformation, cosmetic malformation, serious scarring with contracture, muscular damage or irritation, fat formation, fat embolism, periostitis, osteomyelitis, and seroma. Skoog and Inaba et al. reported methods that remove only the subcutaneous adipose layer, are highly effective for skin preservation and cosmetic restoration, and cause less complications. Among these methods, the subcutis tissue shaver, which was introduced by Inaba et al., is most effective but takes a long operating time (a double tie-over dressing is required), requires a long time for learning the surgical technique, and still has a risk of complication (hematoma, skin necrosis, and scarring). Thoracoscopy-guided sympathectomy was reported for axillary hyperhidrosis, but its current use is limited because of surgery-related complications (pneumothorax, Horner syndrome, etc.) and the high incidence of compensatory hyperhidrosis.

Authors' procedure: Minimally invasive surgery and subdermal laser coagulation

A. Subcutaneous tissue removal using a device after minimal incision. This method has overcome the disadvantages of Inaba's surgical technique. Its surgical procedure is as follows (Figure 01-4).

a. With the patient's arm 100-120° open to expose the underarm, the underarm skin was disinfected. Then a demarcation line was made about 0.5-1 cm outward from the hair areas. A skin test for hypersensitivity to lidocaine was performed, and tumescent anesthesia was administered using a 26-gauge needle on the skin area that was about 1.5 times thicker than the lesion. A tumescent local anesthetic was mixed with 20 cc of 2% lidocaine, 80 ml of 0.9% physiological saline, and 0.1 ml of epinephrine. According to the patient's weight, 20-30 ml of the mixed anesthetic was injected into the one side of the underarm. After local anesthesia was administered using a 0.5% lidocaine solution (1:20 epinephrine), a 1.5 cm incision parallel to the wrinkle line was made on the area 1/3 outwards from the underarm. In the upper adipose layer, tissue was detached using Metzenbaum scissors, and hemostasis was performed. It is important to use a skin hook instead of forceps when handling the skin flap to prevent trauma or necrosis due to sub-

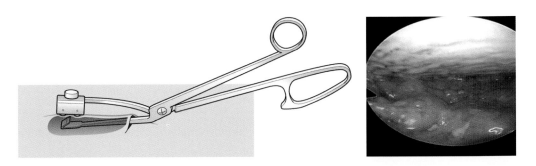

Figure 01-4 **Subcutaneous tissue shaving after minimal incision.** (left: schematic view of intra-op, right: post-op endoscopic finding) (supplement from Lutronic Corp.)

dermal blood flow impairment on account of the skin flap.

b. The adipose layer and the lower dermis in the hypodermis around the incision line were removed using Metzenbaum scissors until the pilosebaceous unit became visible (manual removal, Figure 01-4), and the medial part (toward the trunk from the incision line) was shaved using a modified-Inaba device (Figure 01-4) (subdermal tissue shaving with a modified Inaba device). As excessive excision may cause skin necrosis by inducing subdermal vascular damage, the device was used with 2-3 passes while taking care not to change the skin color.

c. After the surgical site was washed with normal physiological saline, a drainage tube was placed when drainage of blood was required. When there was only slight bleeding, 3-6 incisions (2 mm each) were made or simply 8-10 skin flaps and subcutaneous adipose layers were sutured using No. 4 nylon (quilting suture), and fixed using a gauze and compression bandage. Most of the patients were discharged right after the surgery and received treatment for their wound at the post-operative days 2, 4, 6, and 10. As an absorbable suture was used, it was not removed in most of the patients but was partly removed in some patients depending on their condition at day 10. As steri-strip tape and a film dressing were used, the patients could take showers.

B. Laser: Subdermal laser coagulation using a long-pulse 1444 nm Nd: YAG laser

The rationale for using a 1444 nm Nd:YAG laser was as follows. (1) 20% of the sweat gland tissue consists of water. (2) The 1444 nm wavelength (absorbance in water and fat is ×100 and ×15, respectively, compared with 1064 nm) (Figure 01-5) is absorbed more in water and fatty tissue than in the neighboring tissues. (3) A minimally invasive procedure is possible because the laser is delivered via a fiber (Figure 01-6, 01-7). This procedure can be performed under local anesthesia without the need for hospitalization. Point-by-point subdermal

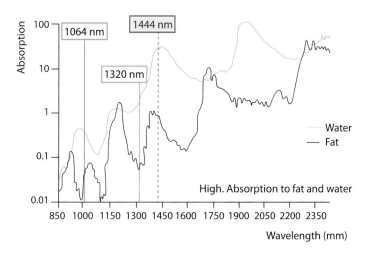

Absorption coefficient curves according to the laser wavelength

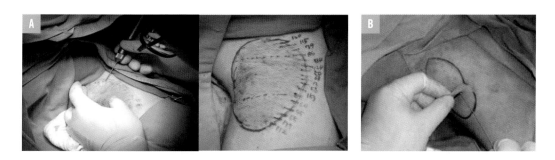

Figure 01-6 **Subcutaneous interstitial laser application to the axilla.** Point by point subdermal coagulation was performed (**A**). The laser light is conveyed through a 1 mm diameter microcannula or with the bare fiber. Position and depths of the cannula tip were controlled by transcutaneous guidance with a red aiming beam from a laser diode (**B**).

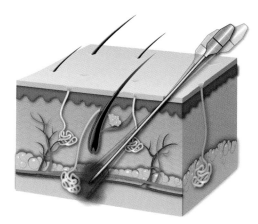

Figure 01-7 Schematic view of procedure with interstitial laser application. (supplement from Lutronic Corp.)

interstitial coagulation was performed by inserting the laser fiber through an entry point created with an 18 G needle. The detailed procedure protocol is as follows.

Procedure:
- The Minor starch-iodine test was done (Preop, and at 180 days postop).
- Infiltration anesthesia was performed in both operative fields using each 20-30 ml of 0.5% lidocaine mixed with 1:100,000 epinephrine.
- The laser irradiation area was marked in both axillae.
- Subdermal layers were destroyed with the fiber-delivered laser energy.
  (pulse energy 175 mJ / pulse rate 40 Hz/power 7 W/ total energy 1,000-2,500 J)
- The total amount of energy delivered was based on the elevation of surface temperature and the degree of fat dissolution which the operator could sense with their hands
- No liposuction was done after laser irradiation
- No compression dressing was applied.

A preliminary clinical study was performed to objectively compare the difference between minimally invasive surgery and the aforementioned laser procedure. The laser procedure was more advantageous because it caused less pain and no scarring, and involved shorter activity restriction. A long-term prospective follow-up study was performed on 18 patients with axillary hyperhidrosis and osmidrosis to investigate the long-term clinical effect. The resulting of effect (Figure 01-8) and complications are shown in the following Table 01-1 and 01-2.

> Features of Asians: Many patients are young, either adolescent or post-adolescent. For these patients, non-surgical laser treatment can be indicated.

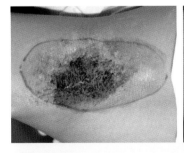 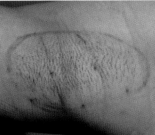 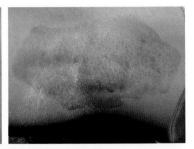

Figure 01-8 Pictures of the pre-, intra-, and post-procedure underarm showing the preop positive and postop negative results of the Minor test.

Table 01-1	Effectiveness of the laser treatment of axillary osmidrosis
Total number of patients	18 (11 females, 7 males)
Total number of operated axillae	36
Follow up months (mean)	11.9 months (10-13)
Mean age	33.2 years (18-52)
Malodour elimination	
Good	20/36 axillae (56%)
Fair	12/36 axillae (33%)
Poor	4/36 axillae (11%)
Patient satisfaction	
Totally satisfied	14/18 patients (78%)
Partially satisfied	3/18 patients (17%)
Dissatisfied	1/18 patients (5%)
Axillary sweating reduction	
Significant	26/36 axillae (72%)
Improved	8/36 axillae (22%)
No change	2/36 axillae (6%)

Table 01-2	Complications of the laser treatment of axillary osmidrosis
Intraoperation complicarions	
Brachial nerve injury	0/36 axillae (0%)
Early complications	
Ecchymosis	20/36 axillae (55.6%)
Hematoma	0/36 axillae (0%)
Seroma	0/36 axillae (0%)
Pressure blister at shoulder	0/36 axillae (0%)
Contact dermatitis (bandage)	0/36 axillae (0%)
Superficial epidermal mecrosis	4/36 axillae (11%)
Small granuloma	0/36 axillae (0%)
Wound infection	0/36 axillae (0%)
Wound dehiscence	0/36 axillae (0%)
Late complications	
Comedones/milia	0/36 axillae (0%)
Sebaceous cyst (or with abscess)	0/36 axillae (0%)
Hypertrophic scar	2/36 axillae (6%)
Temporary skin pigmentation	6/36 axillae (17%)

Tips for post-treatment care and follow-up

At post-procedure day 3, the treatment site and the status of the sutured wound where the laser fiber was inserted were checked. No adverse events that required additional treatment were found in any of the patients. In some primary patients, local skin necrosis occurred after the laser tip was directed to the epidermis by mistake. After the procedure was modified to direct the laser fiber parallel to the epidermis, however, skin necrosis no longer occurred. The wound in the insertion site healed within several days after the patient's self-application of antibiotics. The patients were asked to apply antibiotics for 7 days after the procedure; and on day 7, they visited the hospital and had the suture removed. Then the patients were allowed to take a shower and perform all other activities normally.

REFERENCES

1. Eisenach JH, Atkinson JLD, Fealey RD. Hyperhidrosis: Evolving Therapies for a Well-Established Phenomenon. Mayo Clin Proc May 2005;80:657-666.
2. IH Kim, SL Seo, CH Oh. Minimally Invasive Surgery for Axillary Osmidrosis: Combined Operation with CO2 Laser and Subcutaneous Tissue Remover. Dermatol Surg 1999;25:875-879.
3. KC Hwang and IH Kim. Study of the Skin Barrier Function and the Change in the Quality of Life after Treatment of Primary Axillary Hyperhidrosis using Botulinum Toxin A. Korean J Dermatol 2004;42:406-412.
4. KG Lee, SA Kim, SM Yi, JH Kim, IH Kim. Subdermal Coagulation Treatment of Axillary Bromhidrosis by 1444nm Nd:YAG Laser: A Comparison with Surgical Treatment. Ann Dermatol 2014;26:99-102.
5. Naver H, Swartling C, Aquilonius SM. Palmar and axillary hyperhidrosis treated with botulinum toxin: one-year clinical follow-up. Eur J Neurol 2000;7:55-62.
6. Rusciani L, Severino E, Rusciani A. Type A botulinum toxin: a new reatment for axillary and palmar hyperhidrosis. J Drugs Dermatol 2002;1:147-151.
7. SK Jung, HW Jang, HJ Kim, SG Lee, KG Lee, SY Kim, SM Yi, JH Kim, IH Kim. A Prospective, Long-term Follow up Study of 1444nm Nd:YAG Laser: A New Modality for the Treatment of Axillary Bromhidrosis. Ann Dermatol 2014;26:184-188.
8. Stolman LP. Treatment of hyperhidrosis. Dermatol Clin 1998;16:863.
9. Tark KC, Song SY. Superior lipolytic effect of the 1,444 nm Nd:YAG laser:comparison with the 1,064 nm Nd:YAG laser. Lasers Surg Med 2009;41:721-727.

02

Lipomas

▶ Kee Yang Chung, MD, PhD

Introduction

Lipomas are benign fatty tumors composed of mature fat cells. They are the most common benign mesenchymal tumors of soft tissue. The incidence of lipomas is approximately 2.1/1000 individuals, and they appear as single lesions in 95% of all cases.

Tips for diagnosis

The most common presentation is a painless, slowly enlarging mass involving the subcutaneous tissue of the trunk, neck or proximal extremities. Lipomas can range in size from less than 1 cm to over 25 cm in diameter. Ultrasonography may help to identify the exact depth of the lipoma before treatment. They are frequently removed due to cosmetic concerns, but may also be removed to improve pain or paresthesia associated with compression of surrounding structures.

Tips for treatment

Surgical excision remains the treatment of choice for small lipomas. However, in patients with large or multiple lipomas, excision may result in a large or numerous scars. More cosmetically acceptable approaches have been successful in these situations, including modified incisional approaches, liposuction, intralesional laser therapy with or without liposuction, and injection with deoxycholate to partially or completely dissolve the lipoma.

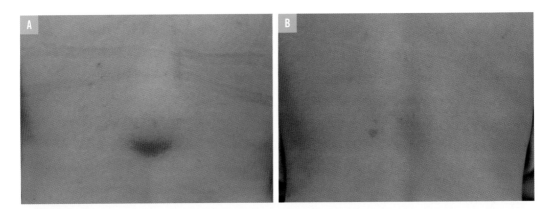

Recently, subcutaneous intralesional application of a micropulsed 1,444 nm Nd:YAG laser has been suggested as an option for the treatment of lipomas (Figure 02-1). Laser lipolysis of adipose tissue works via the concept of selective photohyperthermia. The optical fiber is inserted into the target area either via a dedicated cannula or as bare fiber via a puncture with a hypodermic needle. Laser energy delivered through the optical fiber is converted into heat and absorbed by the surrounding adipocytes. Histologic studies have demonstrated that the heat melts adipocytes via creation of pores in the cell membrane. The laser is passed in a fan-like motion throughout the targeted adipose tissue in the same pattern as traditional liposuction, leading to the creation of tunnels lined by thermally damaged adipocytes

The procedure is initiated after the tumor is anesthetized using 1% lidocaine with 1:100,000 epinephrine and 10 mEq/L of sodium bicarbonate The anesthetic solution is infiltrated into the tumor, and not the surrounding tissue, just enough to make the tumor stand out for easier removal. Excessive use of the anesthetic solution will result in ineffective delivery of laser energy to the adipocytes Next, a 600 μm optical fiber connected to a 1,444 nm micropulsed Nd:YAG laser system (AccuSculpt®, Lutronic Corporation, Goyang, Korea) is inserted directly into the lipoma via a 1-mm-diameter stainless steel microcannula of variable length. Parameters are as follows: pulse rate 30 Hz, pulse energy 200 mJ, pulse width 100 μs and power of 6 W. The total accumulated energy is determined by the lipoma size. After the laser treatment, dissolved lipid and fat cell debris are aspirated with a suction cannula.

Tips for post-treatment care and follow-up

Adverse effects are generally mild, and include ecchymosis and edema. However, infection and bleeding may occur. Also, multiple treatment sessions may be required for complete removal of the tumor.

From a comparison of the various treatment techniques available, surgery is the gold standard, but has the disadvantages of leaving large scars and causing adverse effects. Liposuction is less invasive, but its effect is limited in fibromatous lipomas as well as very small tumors. Recurrence rates are higher as remnants of the capsule may be left in situ. However, since the capsule can be destroyed at the same time with the 1,444 nm Nd:YAG laser, it can overcome the limitations of classical tumescent liposuction. In addition, because of excellent cosmetic results, the need for multiple treatments in some patients does not seem to be a major disadvantage. The recovery time is quicker with subdermal laser lipolysis, although the cost may be higher as compared to classical surgery or liposuction.

REFERENCES

1. A Goldman, et al. Lipoma treatment with a subdermal Nd:YAG laser technique. Int J Dermatol 2009;48:1228-1232.
2. SH Lee, et al. Treatment of Lipomas Using a Subdermal 1,444 nm Micropulsed Neodymium-YAG laser. Dermatol Surg 2011 (Epub).
3. WG Stebbins, et al. Novel method of minimally invasive removal of large lipoma after laser lipolysis with 980 nm diode laser. Dermatol Ther 2011;24:125-130.

Neurofibromas

▶ Il Hwan Kim, MD, PhD

Definition

Neurofibromatosis

The common dermatological finding of neurofibromatosis is a type of neurofibroma that occurs in the skin and the subcutaneous region. Type 1 neurofibromatosis (NF-1) is an autosomal dominant genetic disease (chromosome 17 long-arm gene mutation 17q11.2), and is diagnosed according to the following criteria (Table 03-1). Multiple slowly growing skin neurofibromas (500-1000) that originate from peripheral nerves characteristically occur throughout the patient's lifetime. In patients with NF-1, multiple neurofibromas considerably affect their quality of life from a cosmetic point of view.

Tips for the diagnosis

Type 1 neurofibromatosis is diagnosed based on the patient's characteristic clinical and familial history and histological findings (Table 03-1). Café au lait spots (6 or more), armpit freckles (both sides), scoliosis, and dozens of nodular neurofibromas with various sizes are found all over the body. An accurate diagnosis can be made from a histological examination of such nodules. In the histological findings (Figure 03-1), a flabby structure without encapsulation is observed, and a tumor that consists of spindle cells and thin wavy collagenous strands is observed mostly in the dermis and to have infiltrated the subcutaneous fat layer. Multinuclear giant cells are found or a grenz zone is formed between the lesion and the skin. The substrate is weakly stained and consists of winding collagen bundles and fibers.

Table 03-1	**Diagnostic criteria for NF-1**
≥ 6 café-au-lait macules (>5 mm in prepubertal, >15 mm in postpubertal age)	
≥ Neurofibromas of any type or 1 plexiform neurofibroma	
Freckling in the axillary or inguinal regions	
Optic glioma	
≥ iris Lisch nodules	
Distinctive osseous lesion (e.g., spenoid dysplasia or thinning of long bone cortex with or without pseudoarthrosis)	
1st degree relative (parent, sibling, offspring) with NF-1 by the above criteria	

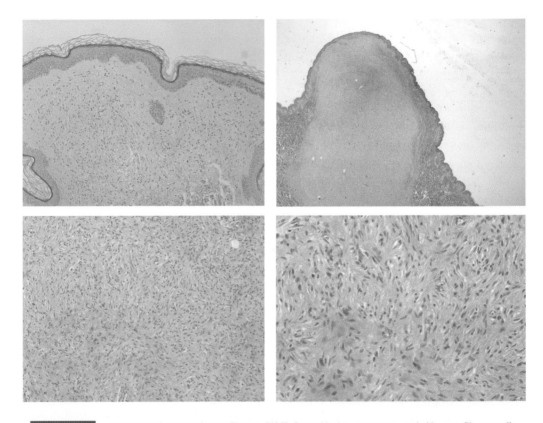

Figure 03-1 **Histological findings of neurofibroma (H&E).** Dermal lesion, grenz zone, and skin neurofibroma cells.

Tips for the treatment

Multiple skin neurofibromas are a major source of morbidity and cosmetic and psychological concern in NF-1 because of the sheer number, visibility, and size of the tumor. Surgical excision of the neurofibroma is required when neurological symptoms occur, malignancy is suspected, or cosmetic concern is involved. Patients generally want to have as many skin neurofibromas as possible excised, but because of the difficulty in repeating the excision due to anesthesia-related pain, the long healing time, and surgical scarring, there is no widely accepted standard surgical treatment. Generally, a large neurofibroma is excised under general anesthesia, but the number of neurofibromas that can be removed per surgery is limited due to the limited operating time. In most cases, numerous small and flat nodular lesions occur in the early stage, and non-surgical treatment methods have been used. Excision using electrocautery was the first non-surgical treatment method used for neurofibroma. This excision procedure could remove numerous lesions in one or more sessions, but had the disadvantages of a long healing time, post-surgical scarring, and discomfort. Afterwards, the CO_2 laser was developed and used to treat skin neurofibroma. It was inefficient, however, because it took a longer time to treat a neurofibroma than electrocautery. A study in 2008 reported the superficial laser coagulation technique using the Nd:YAG laser. In that study, the authors reported that the treatment of a flat superficial lesion using the Nd-YAG laser had a better cosmetic outcome than previous treatment methods. The authors recommended, however, that the CO_2 laser be used only for large lesions in exposed areas, as interstitial laser photocoagulation commonly resulted in hypertrophic and atrophic scars. A recent study reported a new surgical procedure that can selectively remove only neurofibromas by distinguishing normal tissue from neurofibromas using confocal laser microscopy. This new procedure is too complex to apply to numerous small skin neurofibromas, however, and is inefficient. As such, this author applied the 1444 nm Neodymium:Yttrium Aluminum Garnet (Nd:YAG) laser (Accusculpt™, Lutronic, Goyang, South Korea), a recently developed form of lipolytic laser, to various types of skin diseases, and called this approach selective photothermal coagulation (SPTC), which combines the principle that the wavelength of this laser is characteristically absorbed more by fat and water with the principle that the beam (2-8 mm) from the internal fiber or the external headpiece could selectively coagulate targets by minimizing damage to neighboring tissues. This author observed that SPTC effectively treated water-rich tissues or vascular lesions both clinically and histologically, and reported the outcome.

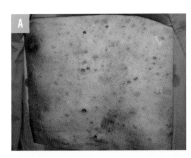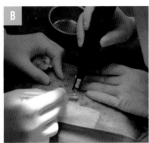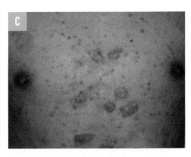

Figure 03-2   **The process of laser treatment. A.** Shave excision. **B.** Selective photothermocoagulation with an external handpiece (2.0 W, 3 mm spot, multiple pass). **C.** After dressing with silver (Acticoat) and hydrocolloid (Duoderm).

Small, flat neurofibromas were treated using the non-surgical photo-coagulation method based on SPTC. For numerous large and protruding neurofibromas, the base of the tumor was first shave-excised, and then the residual subcutaneous neurofibroma was photocoagulated using STPC, almost without damaging the neighboring tissues (Figure 03-2).

This method more simply removed the skin neurofibroma than did the existing surgical methods, and caused less pain. Besides, it was highly efficient because it could remove numerous lesions within a short time while watching the base of the lesions and checking the end-point of the lesions that were being coagulated. When a whole tumor is coagulated externally, it is difficult to see if the base of the lesion was completely removed. As such, this new procedure more efficiently removed the neurofibroma and resulted in a higher degree of patient satisfaction and a better cosmetic outcome than simple surface photocoagulation,

Table 03-2   **Comparison with conventional method - Pros and Cons**

	1444 nm Nd-YAG laser SPTC by internal fiber or external handpiece	Surgical excision	CO$_2$ ablative laser
Pros	Convenient repeated procedure Patient satisfaction with less pain, higher quality of life No need for suture → easier wound care Less scarring (cosmetically superior) More treatable lesions at one time Able to remove small, flat lesions (<5 mm) Less perilesional damage	Complete excision	More lesions can be treated in the one session
Cons	Less efficient for large lesions Operator-dependent Difficult to confirm complete removal → Need follow-up	Limited number of excision at one time Time-consuming Need suture and stitch-out Postoperative pain Scarring	Hypertrophic scarring Perilesional heat damage

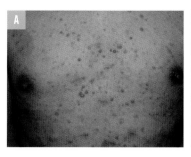
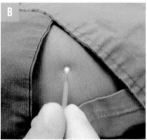
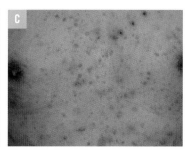

Figure 03-3   **Treatment results with internal fiber. A.** Pre-treatment. **B.** Aiming beam can show the position of the tip in the skin. **C.** Post-treatment.

a sort of blind technique that uses CO_2 or radio frequency. Thus, the use of SPTC to remove multiple skin neurofibroma made it possible to remove flat lesions non-surgically using surface photocoagulation while watching the lesion, and to coagulate large lesions safely and effectively while watching the subcutaneous tumor areas that were not removed by shave-excision without the need for the patient to be hospitalized. In conclusion, the STPC technique using the 1444 nm Nd:YAG laser is considered the best minimally invasive procedure among the existing forms of treatment, as it is possible to watch the process of photocoagulation and selectively treat targets, thus allowing rapid wound healing while causing little thermal damage to neighboring tissues.

Tip for post-treatment care and follow-up

After the procedure, the patients were asked to apply an antibiotic ointment 2-3 times a day for 5-7 days. Following that, moisturizing treatment using a moisturizer was recommended until the crust fell off. As of now, 1 day after the procedure, the treated sites were observed to have healed without recurrence in most cases. Some incompletely treated sites were also cured via re-treatment under local anesthesia.

REFERENCES

1. Kim HJ, Lee KG, Yi SM, Kim JH, Kim IH. Successful Treatment of Multiple Cutaneous Neurofibromas Using a Combination of Shave Excision and Laser Photothermocoagulation with a 1,444-nm Neodymium-Doped Yttrium Aluminum Garnet Laser. Dermatol Surg 2012;38:960-963.
2. Elwakil TF, Samy NA, Elbasiouny MS. Non-excision treatment of multiple cutaneous neurofibromas by laser photocoagulation. Lasers Med Sci 2008;23:301-306.
3. K. P. Boyd, B. R. Korf, A. Theos. Neurofibromatosis type 1. J m Acad Dermatol 2009;61:1-14.

4. KG Lee, SG Lee, SM Yi, JH Kim, JE Choi, Il-Hwan Kim. Proposing Concept Of Selective Photothermocoagulation (SPTC) and Various Dermatologic Indications By Using 1444nm Nd:YAG LASER. Grapevine, Texas, 31th ASLMS annual conference March. 30~April 2, 2011 (Oral Presentation).

5. Koller S, Horn M, Weger W, Massone C, Smolle J, Gerger. A. Confocal laser scanning microscopy-guided surgery for neurofibroma. Clin Exp Dermatol 2009;34:e670-672.

6. Levine SM, Levine E, Taub PJ, Weinberg H. Electrosurgical excision technique for the treatment of multiple cutaneous lesions in neurofibromatosis type I. J Plast Reconstr Aesthet Surg 2008;61:958-962.

7. Moreno JC, Mathoret C, Lantieri L, Zeller J, Revuz J, Wolkenstein P. Carbon dioxide laser for removal of multiple cutaneous neurofibromas. Br J Dermatol 2001;144:1096-1098.

8. Ostertag JU, Theunissen CC, Neumann HA. Hypertrophic scars after therapy with CO2 laser for treatment of multiple cutaneous neurofibromas. Dermatol Surg 2002;28:296-298.

9. R. R. Anderson, W. Farinelli, H. Laubach, et al. Selective photothermolysis of lipid-rich tissues: a free electron laser study. Lasers Surg Med 2006;38:913-919.

10. Roberts AH, Crockett DJ. An operation for the treatment of cutaneous neurofibromatosis. Br J Plast Surg 1985;38:292-293.

11. Roenigk RK, Ratz JL. CO2 laser treatment of cutaneous neurofibromas. J Dermatol Surg Oncol 1987;13:187-190.

12. T. F. Elwakil, N. A. Samy, M. S. Elbasiouny. Non-excision reatment of multiple cutaneous neurofibromas by laser photocoagulation. Lasers Med Sci 2008;23:301-306.

Syringomas

▶ Won Serk Kim, MD, PhD

Introduction

The syringoma is a neoplasm of the skin appendages occurring frequently in women after adolescence. Although its origin is still controversial, it is now considered an adenoma originating from an eccrine sweat gland in the epidermis. The lesion is generally a 1- to 3-mm-wide skin-colored papule occurring mostly at and around the lower eyelid in a symmetrical fashion. Some cases of its occurrence on the chin, neck, chest and abdomen have been reported. Syringomas limited to the genital area have also been reported. Syringomas in the periorbital area are generally asymptomatic, although they may occasionally be itchy. The lesion generally progresses gradually, although it is rarely disseminated. The pathogenesis of syringomas remains uncertain, and the lesion becomes larger in pregnancy and before the premenstrual period. Given that the lesion becomes elevated after the administration of estrogen, and that the incidence is high in women after adolescence, it is believed that the hormones may have an influence on the development of syringomas.

Tips for diagnosis

Syringomas come in the form of small skin-colored papules and occur in multiple numbers in limited areas. Syringomas can be classified into the localized type, where a single lesion or multiple lesions occur in a single anatomical areaand the generalized type, where multiple lesions are disseminated over a wide range of anatomical areas. In most cases, diagnosis of a syringoma is based on the clinical findings, and when a differential diagnosis from collid milium, flat wart, and angiofibroma is difficult, histological examination is performed. Histopathological findings include multiple small tubes surrounded by fibrous matrices, and some tubes characteristically appear tadpole-like. Other histopathological findings include acanthosis, hyper-pigmentation of the epidermal basal layer, vacuolar degeneration of the luminal cells, keratin-filled cysts, luminal calcification, and the presence or proliferation of fibrous matrices.

Tips for treatment

As most syringomas occur on the faces of female patients, aesthetic consideration must be borne in mind when treating them. Surgical removal or topical application of atropine or tretinoin can be used. It has been reported that cryosurgery, electrodesiccation, and cauterization using various chemical ablation and laser techniques could achieve various treatment responses. Despite the advantage of being capable of completely removing syringoma, surgical removal is limited in its application to only very small lesions as it may cause such postoperative complications as scarring or ectropion. Cryosurgery has the disadvantages of poor accuracy and of causing scar and pigmentary changes. Although it can be more selectively used for the treatment of syringoma than surgery or cryosurgery, electrodesiccation involves procedural difficulties as it causes thermal damage to the neighboring normal tissues. With the development of various laser procedures, however, the conventional treatments are now rarely performed. The argon, superpulsed, and ultra-pulse CO_2 laser as well as the erbium:YAG laser have been used for the removal of syringomas. For the ideal treatment, it is important to minimize the damage to the normal tissues. As syringomas, however, characteristically involve multiple proliferation of the eccrine sweat glands in the deep dermis, the selective destruction of syringomas is difficult.

No laser can selectively destroy a syringoma without destroying some normal tissues. A procedure where the surface was shaved off using laser with TCA application, however, and a procedure where Q-switched Nd-YAG laser was applied after creating a temporary tattoo, were reported to have achieved aesthetically superior outcomes. Syringomas consisting of small scattered papules can be easily removed by applying the conventional laser deep in the skin, whereas syringomas in the form of fused plaques frequently have problems, such as scar formation, pigmentation, or prolonged healing time. This author has effectively cured syringomas using the CO_2 laser in the superpulse mode, and by performing multiple drilling or creating multiple deep, narrow and high-density ablation (Figure 04-1). The advantage of this procedure is that a neoplasm located in the deep skin can be removed, and rapid healing of the treatment site can be achieved via the normal tissues between the ablations. Thus, the damage to the normal tissues can be minimized, and neoplasms in aggregated forms can be effectively removed. Besides, the treatment method is easy. The procedure has the disadvan-

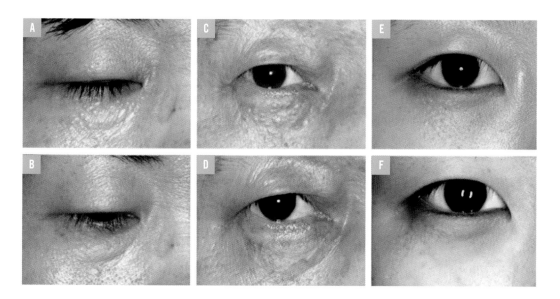

Figure 04-1   Clinical results: (**A and B**) Before treatment and 7 months after three laser sessions, respectively. (**C** and **D**) Before treatment and 2 months after two laser sessions, respectively. (**E** and **F**) Before treatment and 5 months after one laser session, respectively.

tages, however, of a limited treatment area and the requirement of multiple treatments for a complete cure. Before laser, local anesthesia is performed, and then the syringoma area is irradiated with laser in the superpulse mode for 0.15 sec, at 4.0 W, in the single-pulse mode. Depending on the case, the treatment can be completed in one session. For multiple lesions, however, more sessions are required.

Tips for post-treatment care and follow-up

After the treatment, the application of a topical antibiotic ointment and a low-potency steroid ointment can achieve rapid healing of the treated site.

REFERENCES

1. Belardi MG, Maglione MA, Vighi S, di Paola GR. Syringoma of the vulva: a case report. J Reprod Med 1994;39:957–959.
2. Castro DJ, Tartell PB, Soudant J, Saxton RE. The surgical management of facial syringomas using the superpulsed CO2 laser. J Clin Laser Med Surg 1993;11:33–37.
3. Gomez MI, Perez B, Azana JM, Nunez M, Ledo A. Eruptive syringoma: treatment with topical tretinoin. Dermatology

1994;189:105–106.

4. Goyal S, Martins CR. Multiple syringomas on the abdomen, thighs, and groin. Cutis 2000;66:259–262.

5. Kang WH, Kim NS, Kim YB, Shim WC. A new treatment for syringoma: combination of carbon dioxide laser and trichloroacetic acid. Dermatol Surg 1998;24:1370–1374.

6. Karam P, Benedetto AV. Intralesional electrodesiccation of syringoma. Dermatol Surg 1997;23:921–924.

7. Karam P, Benedetto AV. Syringomas: new approach to an old technique. Int J Dermatol 1996;35:219–220.

8. Moreno-Gonzalez J, Rios-Arizpe S. A modified technique for excision of syringomas. J Dermatol Surg Oncol 1989;15:796–798.

9. Nerad JA, Anderson RL. CO2 laser treatment of eyelid syringomas. Ophthal Plast Reconstr Surg 1988;4:91–94.

10. Sajben FP, Ross EV. The use of the 1.0mm handpiece in high energy, pulsed CO2 laser destruction of facial adnexal tumors. Dermatol Surg 1999;25:41–44.

11. Sanchez TS, Dauden E, Casas AP, Garcia-Diez A. Eruptive pruritic syringomas: treatment with topical atropine. J Am Acad Dermatol 2001;44:148–149.

12. Soler-Carrillo J, Estrach T, Mascaro JM. Eruptive syringoma: 27 new cases and review of the literature. J Eur Acad Dermatol Venereol 2001;15:242–246.

13. Stevenson TR, Swanson NA. Syringoma: removal by electrodesiccation and curettage. Ann Plast Surg 1985;15:151–154.

14. Wang JI, Roenigk HH Jr. Treatment of multiple facial syringomas with the carbon dioxide (CO2) laser. Dermatol Surg 1999;25:136–139.